T0327442

USING STATISTICS IN THE SOCIAL AND HEALTH SCIENCES WITH SPSS® AND EXCEL®

USING STATISTICS IN THE SOCIAL AND HEALTH SCIENCES WITH SPSS® AND EXCEL®

MARTIN LEE ABBOTT

WILEY

Published by John Wiley & Sons, Inc., Hoboken, New Jersey
Published simultaneously in Canada

For general information on our other products and services or for technical support, please contact our Customer Care Department within the United States at (800) 762-2974, outside the United States at (317) 572-3993 or fax (317) 572-4002.

Wiley also publishes its books in a variety of electronic formats. Some content that appears in print may not be available in electronic formats. For more information about Wiley products, visit our web site at www.wiley.com.

Library of Congress Cataloging-in-Publication Data:

Names: Abbott, Martin, 1949-
Title: Using statistics in the social and health sciences with SPSS® and Excel®
    / Martin Lee Abbott.
Description: Hoboken, New Jersey : John Wiley & Sons, Inc., [2017] | In the
    title, both SPSS and Excel are accompanied by the trademark symbol. |
    Includes bibliographical references and index.
Identifiers: LCCN 2016009168| ISBN 9781119121046 (cloth) | ISBN 9781119121060
    (epub) | ISBN 9781119121053 (epdf)
Subjects: LCSH: Mathematical statistics–Data processing. | Multivariate
    analysis–Data processing. | Social sciences–Statistical methods. |
    Medical sciences–Statistical methods. | Microsoft Excel (Computer file) |
    SPSS (Computer file)
Classification: LCC QA276.45.M53 A23 2017 | DDC 005.5/5–dc23 LC record available at
    https://lccn.loc.gov/2016009168

Set in 10/12pt, TimesLTStd by SPi Global, Chennai, India.

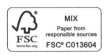

To my longsuffering, wonderful wife Kathy;
-and-
To those seeking to understand the nature of social systems so that, like Florence Nightingale, they might better understand God's character.

CONTENTS

Preface   **xv**

Acknowledgments   **xix**

1 INTRODUCTION   **1**

Big Data Analysis, 1
Visual Data Analysis, 2
Importance of Statistics for the Social and Health Sciences and Medicine, 3
Historical Notes: Early Use of Statistics, 4
Approach of the Book, 6
Cases from Current Research, 7
Research Design, 9
Focus on Interpretation, 9

2 DESCRIPTIVE STATISTICS: CENTRAL TENDENCY   **13**

What is the Whole Truth? Research Applications (Spuriousness), 13
Descriptive and Inferential Statistics, 16
The Nature of Data: Scales of Measurement, 16
Descriptive Statistics: Central Tendency, 23
Using SPSS$^{®}$ and Excel to Understand Central Tendency, 28
Distributions, 35
Describing the Normal Distribution: Numerical Methods, 37
Descriptive Statistics: Using Graphical Methods, 41
Terms and Concepts, 47

Data Lab and Examples (with Solutions), 49
Data Lab: Solutions, 51

3 DESCRIPTIVE STATISTICS: VARIABILITY   55

Range, 55
Percentile, 56
Scores Based on Percentiles, 57
Using SPSS® and Excel to Identify Percentiles, 57
Standard Deviation and Variance, 60
Calculating the Variance and Standard Deviation, 61
Population SD and Inferential SD, 66
Obtaining SD from Excel and SPSS®, 67
Terms and Concepts, 70
Data Lab and Examples (with Solutions), 71
Data Lab: Solutions, 73

4 THE NORMAL DISTRIBUTION   77

The Nature of the Normal Curve, 77
The Standard Normal Score: *Z Score*, 79
The *Z* Score Table of Values, 80
Navigating the *Z* Score Distribution, 81
Calculating Percentiles, 83
Creating Rules for Locating *Z* Scores, 84
Calculating *Z* Scores, 87
Working with Raw Score Distributions, 90
Using SPSS® to Create *Z* Scores and Percentiles, 90
Using Excel to Create *Z* Scores, 94
Using Excel and SPSS® for Distribution Descriptions, 97
Terms and Concepts, 99
Data Lab and Examples (with Solutions), 99
Data Lab: Solutions, 101

5 PROBABILITY AND THE Z DISTRIBUTION   105

The Nature of Probability, 106
Elements of Probability, 106
Combinations and Permutations, 109
Conditional Probability: Using Bayes' Theorem, 111
Z Score Distribution and Probability, 112
Using SPSS® and Excel to Transform Scores, 117
Using the Attributes of the Normal Curve to Calculate Probability, 119
"Exact" Probability, 123
From Sample Values to Sample Distributions, 126
Terms and Concepts, 127

Data Lab and Examples (with Solutions), 128
Data Lab: Solutions, 129

6 RESEARCH DESIGN AND INFERENTIAL STATISTICS   **133**

Research Design, 133
Experiment, 136
Non-Experimental or Post Facto Research Designs, 140
Inferential Statistics, 143
Z Test, 154
The Hypothesis Test, 154
Statistical Significance, 156
Practical Significance: Effect Size, 156
Z Test Elements, 156
Using SPSS$^{®}$ and Excel for the Z Test, 157
Terms and Concepts, 158
Data Lab and Examples (with Solutions), 161
Data Lab: Solutions, 162

7 THE *T* TEST FOR SINGLE SAMPLES   **165**

Introduction, 166
Z Versus *T*: Making Accommodations, 166
Research Design, 167
Parameter Estimation, 169
The *T* Test, 173
The *T* Test: A Research Example, 176
Interpreting the Results of the *T* Test for a Single Mean, 180
The *T* Distribution, 181
The Hypothesis Test for the Single Sample *T* Test, 182
Type I and Type II Errors, 183
Effect Size, 187
Effect Size for the Single Sample *T* Test, 187
Power, Effect Size, and Beta, 188
One- and Two-Tailed Tests, 189
Point and Interval Estimates, 192
Using SPSS$^{®}$ and Excel with the Single Sample *T* Test, 196
Terms and Concepts, 201
Data Lab and Examples (with Solutions), 201
Data Lab: Solutions, 203

8 INDEPENDENT SAMPLE *T* TEST   **207**

A Lot of "Ts", 207
Research Design, 208
Experimental Designs and the Independent *T* Test, 208
Dependent Sample Designs, 209

Between and Within Research Designs, 210
Using Different *T* Tests, 211
Independent *T* Test: The Procedure, 213
Creating the Sampling Distribution of Differences, 215
The Nature of the Sampling Distribution of Differences, 216
Calculating the Estimated Standard Error of Difference with Equal Sample
    Size, 218
Using Unequal Sample Sizes, 219
The Independent *T* Ratio, 221
Independent *T* Test Example, 222
Hypothesis Test Elements for the Example, 222
Before–After Convention with the Independent *T* Test, 226
Confidence Intervals for the Independent *T* Test, 227
Effect Size, 228
The Assumptions for the Independent *T* Test, 230
SPSS$^{®}$ Explore for Checking the Normal Distribution Assumption,
    231
Excel Procedures for Checking the Equal Variance Assumption, 233
SPSS$^{®}$ Procedure for Checking the Equal Variance Assumption, 237
Using SPSS$^{®}$ and Excel with the Independent *T* Test, 239
SPSS$^{®}$ Procedures for the Independent *T* Test, 239
Excel Procedures for the Independent *T* Test, 243
Effect Size for the Independent *T* Test Example, 245
Parting Comments, 245
Nonparametric Statistics: The Mann–Whitney *U* Test, 246
Terms and Concepts, 249
Data Lab and Examples (with Solutions), 249
Data Lab: Solutions, 251
Graphics in the Data Summary, 254

9 ANALYSIS OF VARIANCE   **255**

A Hypothetical Example of ANOVA, 255
The Nature of ANOVA, 257
The Components of Variance, 258
The Process of ANOVA, 259
Calculating ANOVA, 260
Effect Size, 268
Post Hoc Analyses, 269
Assumptions of ANOVA, 274
Additional Considerations with ANOVA, 275
The Hypothesis Test: Interpreting ANOVA Results, 276
Are the Assumptions Met?, 276
Using SPSS$^{®}$ and Excel with One-Way ANOVA, 282

The Need for Diagnostics, 289
Non-Parametric ANOVA Tests: The Kruskal–Wallis Test, 289
Terms and Concepts, 292
Data Lab and Examples (with Solutions), 293
Data Lab: Solutions, 294

10 FACTORIAL ANOVA   297

Extensions of ANOVA, 297
ANCOVA, 298
MANOVA, 299
MANCOVA, 299
Factorial ANOVA, 299
Interaction Effects, 299
Simple Effects, 301
2XANOVA: An Example, 302
Calculating Factorial ANOVA, 303
The Hypotheses Test: Interpreting Factorial ANOVA Results, 306
Effect Size for 2XANOVA: Partial η^2, 308
Discussing the Results, 309
Using SPSS$^{®}$ to Analyze 2XANOVA, 311
Summary Chart for 2XANOVA Procedures, 319
Terms and Concepts, 319
Data Lab and Examples (with Solutions), 320
Data Lab: Solutions, 320

11 CORRELATION   329

The Nature of Correlation, 330
The Correlation Design, 331
Pearson's Correlation Coefficient, 332
Plotting the Correlation: The Scattergram, 334
Using SPSS$^{®}$ to Create Scattergrams, 337
Using Excel to Create Scattergrams, 339
Calculating Pearson's r, 341
The Z Score Method, 342
The Computation Method, 344
The Hypothesis Test for Pearson's r, 345
Effect Size: the Coefficient of Determination, 347
Diagnostics: Correlation Problems, 349
Correlation Using SPSS$^{®}$ and Excel, 352
Nonparametric Statistics: Spearman's Rank Order Correlation (r_s), 358
Terms and Concepts, 363
Data Lab and Examples (with Solutions), 364
Data Lab: Solutions, 365

12 BIVARIATE REGRESSION 371

The Nature of Regression, 372
The Regression Line, 374
Calculating Regression, 376
Effect Size of Regression, 379
The Z Score Formula for Regression, 380
Testing the Regression Hypotheses, 382
The Standard Error of Estimate, 383
Confidence Interval, 385
Explaining Variance Through Regression, 386
A Numerical Example of Partitioning the Variation, 389
Using Excel and SPSS® with Bivariate Regression, 390
The SPSS® Regression Output, 390
The Excel Regression Output, 396
Complete Example of Bivariate Linear Regression, 398
Assumptions of Bivariate Regression, 398
The Omnibus Test Results, 404
Effect Size, 404
The Model Summary, 405
The Regression Equation and Individual Predictor Test of Significance, 405
Advanced Regression Procedures, 406
Detecting Problems in Bivariate Linear Regression, 408
Terms and Concepts, 409
Data Lab and Examples (with Solutions), 410
Data Lab: Solutions, 411

13 INTRODUCTION TO MULTIPLE LINEAR REGRESSION 417

The Elements of Multiple Linear Regression, 417
Same Process as Bivariate Regression, 418
Some Differences between Bivariate Linear Regression and Multiple Linear
    Regression, 419
Stuff not Covered, 420
Assumptions of Multiple Linear Regression, 421
Analyzing Residuals to Check MLR Assumptions, 422
Diagnostics for MLR: Cleaning and Checking Data, 423
Extreme Scores, 424
Distance Statistics, 428
Influence Statistics, 429
MLR Extended Example Data, 430
Assumptions Met?, 431
Analyzing Residuals: Are Assumptions Met?, 433
Interpreting the SPSS® Findings for MLR, 436
Entering Predictors Together as a Block, 437
Entering Predictors Separately, 442

Additional Entry Methods for MLR Analyses, 447
Example Study Conclusion, 448
Terms and Concepts, 448
Data Lab and Example (with Solution), 450
Data Lab: Solution, 450

14 CHI-SQUARE AND CONTINGENCY TABLE ANALYSIS   455

Contingency Tables, 455
The Chi-square Procedure and Research Design, 456
Chi-square Design One: Goodness of Fit, 457
A Hypothetical Example: Goodness of Fit, 458
Effect Size: Goodness of Fit, 462
Chi-square Design Two: The Test of Independence, 463
A Hypothetical Example: Test of Independence, 464
Special 2×2 Chi-square, 468
Effect Size in 2×2 Tables: PHI, 470
Cramer's V: Effect Size for the Chi-square Test of Independence, 471
Repeated Measures Chi-square: Mcnemar Test, 472
Using SPSS® and Excel with Chi-square, 474
Using SPSS® for the Chi-square Test of Independence, 475
Using Excel for Chi-square Analyses, 481
Terms and Concepts, 483
Data Lab and Examples (with Solutions), 483
Data Lab: Solutions, 484

15 REPEATED MEASURES PROCEDURES: T_{dep} AND ANOVA$_{WS}$ 489

Independent and Dependent Samples in Research Designs, 490
Using Different T Tests, 491
The Dependent T Test Calculation: The "Long" Formula, 491
Example: The Long Formula, 492
The Dependent T Test Calculation: The "Difference" Formula, 494
T_{dep} and Power, 496
Conducting The T_{dep} Analysis Using SPSS®, 496
Conducting The T_{dep} Analysis Using Excel, 498
Within-Subject ANOVA (ANOVA$_{WS}$), 498
Experimental Designs, 499
Post Facto Designs, 500
Within-Subject Example, 501
Using SPSS® for Within-Subject Data, 501
The SPSS® Procedure, 502
The SPSS® Output, 504
Nonparametric Statistics, 508
Terms and Concepts, 508

APPENDICES

Appendix A   SPSS® BASICS   **509**
Using SPSS®, 509
General Features, 510
Management Functions, 513
Additional Management Functions, 517

Appendix B   EXCEL BASICS   **531**
Data Management, 531
The Excel Menus, 533
Using Statistical Functions, 541
Data Analysis Procedures, 543
Missing Values and "0" Values in Excel Analyses, 544
Using Excel with "Real Data", 544

Appendix C   STATISTICAL TABLES   **545**
Table C.1: Z-Score Table (Values Shown are Percentages – %), 545
Table C.2: Exclusion Values for the T-Distribution, 547
Table C.3: Critical (Exclusion) Values for the Distribution of F, 548
Table C.4: Tukey's Range Test (Upper 5% Points), 551
Table C.5: Critical (Exclusion) Values for Pearson's Correlation
        Coefficient, r, 552
Table C.6: Critical Values of the χ^2 (Chi-Square) Distribution, 553

REFERENCES   **555**
Index   **557**

PREFACE

The study of statistics is gaining recognition in a great many fields. In particular, researchers in the social and health sciences note its importance for problem solving and its practical importance in their areas. Statistics has always been important, for example, among those hoping to enter careers in medicine but more so now due to the increasing emphasis on "Scientific Inquiry & Reasoning Skills" as preparation for the Medical College Admission Test (MCAT). Sociology, always relying on statistics and research for its core emphases, is now included in the MCAT as well.

This book focuses squarely on the procedures important to an essential understanding of statistics and how it is used in the real world for problem solving. Moreover, my discussion in the book repeatedly ties statistical methodology with research design (see the "companion" volume my colleague and I wrote to emphasize research and design skills in social science; Abbott and McKinney, 2013).

I emphasize applied statistical analyses and as such will use examples throughout the book drawn from my own research as well as from national databases like GSS and Behavioral Risk Factor Surveillance System (BRFSS). Using data from these sources allow students the opportunity to see how statistical procedures apply to research in their fields as well as to examine "real data." A central feature of the book is my discussion and use of SPSS® and Microsoft Excel® to analyze data for problem solving.

Throughout my teaching and research career, I have developed an approach to helping students understand difficult statistical concepts in a new way. I find that the great majority of students are visual learners, so I developed diagrams and figures over the years that help create a conceptual picture of the statistical procedures that are often problematic to students (like sampling distributions!).

Another reason for writing this book was to give students a way to understand statistical computing without having to rely on comprehensive and expensive statistical software programs. Since most students have access to Microsoft Excel, I developed a step-by-step approach to using the powerful statistical procedures in Excel to analyze data and conduct research in each of the statistical topics I cover in the book.[1]

I also wanted to make those comprehensive statistical programs more approachable to statistics students, so I have also included a "hands-on" guide to SPSS in parallel with the Excel examples. In some cases, SPSS has the only means to perform some statistical procedures, but in most cases, both Excel and SPSS can be used.

Here are some of the features of the book:

1. Emphasis on the interpretation of findings.

2. Use of clear examples from my existing and former research projects and large databases to illustrate statistical procedures. "Real-world" data can be cumbersome, so I introduce straightforward procedures and examples in order to help students focus more on interpretation of findings.

3. Inclusion of a data lab section in each chapter that provides relevant, clear examples.

4. Introduction to advanced statistical procedures in chapter sections (e.g., regression diagnostics) and separate chapters (e.g., multiple linear regression) for greater relevance to real-world research needs.

5. Strengthening of the connection between statistical application and research designs.

6. Inclusion of detailed sections in each chapter explaining applications from Excel and SPSS.

I use SPSS[2] (versions 22 and 23) screenshots of menus and tables by permission from the IBM® Company. IBM, the IBM logo, ibm.com, and SPSS are trademarks or registered trademarks of **International Business Machines Corporation**, registered in many jurisdictions worldwide. Other product and service names might be trademarks of IBM or other companies. A current list of IBM trademarks is available on the Web at "IBM Copyright and trademark information" at www.ibm.com/legal/

---

[1]One limitation to teaching statistics procedures with Excel is that the data analysis features are different depending on whether the user is a "Mac" user or a "PC" user. I am using the PC version, which features a "Data Analysis" suite of statistical tools. This feature may no longer be included in the Mac version of Excel.

[2]SPSS screen reprints throughout the book are used courtesy of International Business Machines Corporation, ©International Business Machines Corporation. SPSS was acquired by IBM in October 2009.

copytrade.shtml. Microsoft Excel references and screenshots in this book are used with permission from Microsoft. I use Microsoft Excel® 2013 in this book.[3]

I use GSS (2014) data and codebook for examples in this book.[4] The BRFSS Survey Questionnaire and Data are used with permission from the CDC.[5]

[3]Excel references and screenshots in this book are used with permission from Microsoft®.

[4]Smith, Tom W., Peter Marsden, Michael Hout, and Jibum Kim. General Social Surveys, 1972–2012 [machine-readable data file]/Principal Investigator, Tom W. Smith; Coprincipal Investigator, Peter V. Marsden; Coprincipal Investigator, Michael Hout; Sponsored by National Science Foundation. NORC ed. Chicago: National Opinion Research Center [producer]; Storrs, CT: The Roper Center for Public Opinion Research, University of Connecticut [distributor], 2013. 1 data file (57,061 logical records) + 1 codebook (3432 pp.). (National Data Program for the Social Sciences, No. 21).

[5]Centers for Disease Control and Prevention (CDC). *Behavioral Risk Factor Surveillance System Survey Questionnaire*. Atlanta, Georgia: U.S. Department of Health and Human Services, Centers for Disease Control and Prevention, 2013 and Centers for Disease Control and Prevention (CDC). *Behavioral Risk Factor Surveillance System Survey Data*. Atlanta, Georgia: U.S. Department of Health and Human Services, Centers for Disease Control and Prevention, 2013.

ACKNOWLEDGMENTS

I wish to thank my daughter Kristin Hovaguimian for her outstanding work on the Index to this book (and all the others!) – not an easy task with a book of this nature.

I thank my wife Kathleen Abbott for her dedication and amazing contributions to the editing process.

I thank my son Matthew Abbott for the inspiration he has always provided in matters statistical and philosophical.

Thank you Jon Gurstelle and the team at Wiley for your continuing support of this project.

1

INTRODUCTION

The world suddenly has become awash in data! A great many popular books have been written recently that extol "big data" and the information derived for decision makers. These data are considered "big" because a certain "catalog" of data may be so large that traditional ways of managing and analyzing such information cannot easily accommodate it. The data originate from you and me whenever we use certain social media, or make purchases online, or have information derived from us through radio frequency identification (RFID) readers attached to clothing and cars, even implanted in animals, and so on. The result is a massive avalanche of information that exists for businesses leaders, decision makers, and researchers to use for predicting related behaviors and attitudes.

BIG DATA ANALYSIS

Decision makers are trying to figure out how to manage and use the information available. Typical computer software used for statistical decision making is currently limited to a number of cases far below that which is available for consideration of big data. A traditional approach to address this issue is known as "data mining" in which a number of techniques, including statistics, are used to discover patterns in a large set of data.

Researchers may be overjoyed with the availability of such rich data, but it provides both opportunities and challenges. On the opportunity side, never before have

Using Statistics in the Social and Health Sciences with SPSS® and Excel®, First Edition.
Martin Lee Abbott.
© 2017 John Wiley & Sons, Inc. Published 2017 by John Wiley & Sons, Inc.

such large amounts of information been available to assist researchers and policy makers understand widespread public thinking and behavior. On the challenge side however are several difficult questions:

- How are such data to be examined?
- Do current social science methods and processes provide guidance to examining data sets that surpass historical data-gathering capacity?
- Are big data representative?
- Do data sets so large obviate the need for probability-based research analyses?
- Do decision makers understand how to use social science methodology to assist in their analyses of emerging data?
- Will the decisions emerging from big data be used ethically, within the context to social science research guidelines?
- Will effect size considerations overshadow questions of significance testing?

Social scientists can rely on existing statistical methods to manage and analyze big data, but the *way in which the analyses are used for decision making will change*. One trend is that prediction may be hailed as a more prominent method for understanding the data than traditional hypothesis testing. We will have more to say about this distinction later in the book, but it is important at this point to see that researchers will need to adapt statistical approaches for analyzing big data.

VISUAL DATA ANALYSIS

Another emerging trend for understanding and managing the swell of data is the use of visuals. Of course, visual descriptions of data have been used for centuries. It is commonly acknowledged that the first "pie chart" was published by Playfair (1801). Playfair's example in Figure 1.1 compares the dynamics of nations over time.

Figure 1.1 compared nations using size, color, and orientation over time. Using this method for comparing information has been useful for viewing the patterns in data not readily observable from numerical analysis.

As with numerical methods, however, there are opportunities and challenges in the use of visual analyses:

- Can visual means be used to convey complex meaning?
- Are there "rules" that will help to insure a standard way of creating, analyzing, and interpreting such visual information?
- Will visual analyses become divorced from numerical analysis so that observers have no way of objectively confirming the meaning of the images?

Several visual data software analysis programs have appeared over the last several years. Simply running an online search will yield several possibilities including many that offer free (initial) programs for cataloging and presenting data from the user. I offer one very important caveat (see the final bullet point earlier), which is that it is

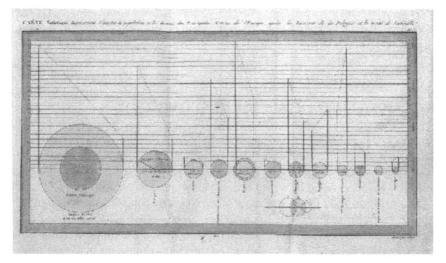

Figure 1.1   William Playfair's pie chart. *Source*: https://commons.wikimedia.org/wiki/File :Playfair_piecharts.jpg. Public domain.

important to perform visual data analysis in concert with numerical analysis. As we will see later in the book, it is easy to intentionally or unintentionally mislead readers using visual presentations when these are divorced from numerical statistical means that discuss the "significance" and "meaningfulness" of the visual data.

IMPORTANCE OF STATISTICS FOR THE SOCIAL AND HEALTH SCIENCES AND MEDICINE

The presence of so much rich information presents meaningful opportunities for understanding many of the processes that affect the social world. While much of the time big data analyses are used for understanding business dynamics and eco-nomic trends, it is also important to focus on those data patterns that can affect the social sphere beyond these indicators: social and psychological behavior and atti-tudes, changes in understanding health and medicine, and educational progress. These social indicators have been the subject of a great deal of analyses over the decades and now may make significant advances depending on how big data are analyzed and managed. On a related note, the social sciences (especially sociology and psychol-ogy) are now areas included in the new Medical College Admission Test (MCAT), which also includes greater emphasis upon "Scientific Inquiry & Reasoning Skills." The material we will learn from this book will help to support study in these areas for aspiring health and medical professionals.

In this book, I intend to focus on how to use and analyze data of all sizes and shapes. While we will be limited in our ability to dive into the world of big data fully, we can study the basics of how to recognize, generate, interpret, and critique analyses of data for decision making. One of the first lessons is that *data can be understood both numerically and visually*. When we describe information, we are attempting to see and convey underlying meaning in the numbers and visual expressions. If I have a collection of data, I cannot recognize its meaning by simply looking at it. However, if I apply certain numerical and visual methods to <u>organize</u> the data, I can see what patterns lay below the surface.

HISTORICAL NOTES: EARLY USE OF STATISTICS

Statistics as a field has had a long and colorful history. Students will recognize some prominent names as the field developed its mathematical identity: Pearson, Fisher, Bayes, Laplace, and others. But it is important to note that some of the earliest statistical studies were based in solving social and political problems.

One of the earliest of such studies was developed by John Graunt who compiled information from Bills of Mortality to detect, among other things, the impact and origins of deaths by plague. Parish records documented christenings, weddings, and burials at the time, so Graunt's study tracked the number of deaths in the parishes as

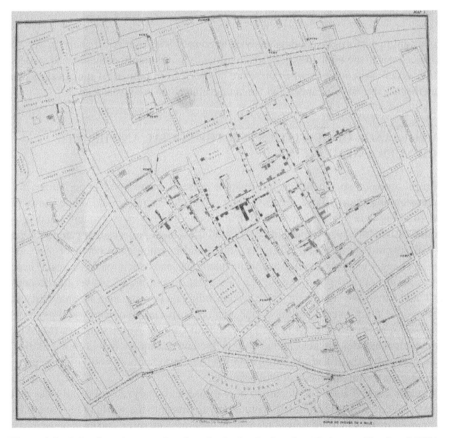

Figure 1.2 John Snow's map showing deaths in the London cholera epidemic of 1854. *Source*: https://commons.wikimedia.org/wiki/File:Snow-cholera-map-1.jpg. Public domain.

a way to understand the dynamics of the plague. His broader goal was to predict the population of London using extant data from the parish records.

Another early use of statistics was Dr John Snow's map showing deaths in the houses of London's Soho District during the 1854 cholera epidemic, as popularized by Johnson's book, *The Ghost Map* (2006). In order to investigate the reasons for the spread of cholera other than odor ("miasma theory"), Snow created a map showing each death as a black line outside each household, along with features of the neighborhood including the water sources located throughout the district. The map created a visual picture of the concentration of deaths across the district and led to hypotheses about cholera spreading by waterborne contamination rather than smell. (If you were to walk across the same London district today, you will see that the great social theorist Karl Marx lived just a few streets away from the center of the cholera deaths.)

Figure 1.2 shows Snow's map. You can see that near the center of the map is the "Broad Street Pump" which Snow determined to be the source for the spread of cholera. (At the time, Karl Marx lived on Dean Street, just to the east of the Broad Street Pump.) Notice that the houses nearest this pump recorded the highest numbers of deaths.

Figure 1.2 example not only shows how descriptive statistics underscored the use of visual means of representing data, but it also helped to clarify possible reasons for an epidemic. Graunt's tables based on the Bills of Mortality were rudimentary visuals, but Snow's map was a more effective means of portraying complex data by visual means. A still later statistician made even greater advancements in using visual information to communicate trends in data.

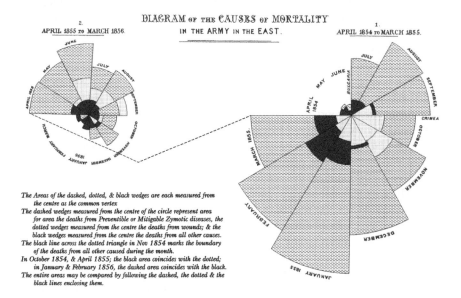

Figure 1.3 Florence Nightingale's polar chart comparing battlefield and nonbattlefield deaths. *Source*: https://en.wikipedia.org/wiki/Pie_chart#/media/File:Nightingale-mortality.jpg. Public domain.

Note: The original color version of this figure can be found in the online version of this book.

Nightingale (1858) is most often remembered as the founder of modern nursing. She is often represented in paintings as "the lady with the lamp," since she was known to walk among the bedsides checking on the sick and wounded of the war. But Nightingale was also an astute statistician who used statistics to capture the dramatic need in hospitals during the Crimean War. She is credited as being one of the first to use a "pie chart" (more accurately, a "polar chart"). Figure 1.3 shows comparisons in her original polar chart of differences between soldiers who died of battlefield wounds ("dotted" wedges near the center) and those who died from other causes ("dashed" wedges measured from the center of the graph) over time. The original color version of Figure 1.3 can be found in the online version of this book. The relationship between these groups fueled Nightingale's efforts to obtain further funding for sanitary hospital conditions since those who died of infections were greater in number than those dying of battlefield wounds.

APPROACH OF THE BOOK

Many students and researchers are intimidated by statistical procedures, which may be due to fear of math, problematic math teachers in earlier education, or the lack of exposure to a "discovery" method for understanding difficult procedures. This book is an introduction to understanding statistics in a way that allows students to discover patterns in data and developing skill at making interpretations from data analyses. I describe how to use statistical programs (SPSS and Excel) to make the study more understandable and to teach students how to approach problem solving. Ordinarily, a first course in statistics leads students through the worlds of descriptive and inferential statistics by highlighting the formulas and sequential procedures that lead to statistical decision making. We will do all this in this book, but I place a good deal more attention on conceptual understanding. Thus, rather than memorizing a specific formula and using it in a specific way to solve a problem, I want to make sure the student first understands the nature of the problem, why a specific formula is needed, and how it will result in the appropriate information for decision making.

By using statistical software, we can place more attention on understanding how to *interpret findings*. Statistics courses taught in mathematics departments, and in some social science departments, often place primary emphases on the formulas/processes themselves. In the extreme, this can limit the usefulness of the analyses to the practitioner. My approach encourages students to focus more on how to understand and make applications of the results of statistical analyses. SPSS and other statistical programs are much more efficient at performing the analyses; the key issue in my approach is how to interpret the results in the context of the research question.

Beginning with my first undergraduate course teaching statistics with conventional textbooks, I have spent countless hours demonstrating how to conduct statistical tests manually and teaching students to do likewise. This is not always a bad strategy; performing the analysis manually can lead the student to understand how formulas treat data and yield valuable information. However, it is often the case that the student gravitates to memorizing the formula or the steps in an analysis. Again, there is nothing wrong with this approach as long as the student does not stop there. *The outcome of the analysis is more important than memorizing the steps to the outcome.* Examining the appropriate output derived from statistical software shifts the attention from the nuances of a formula to the wealth of information obtained by using it.

It is important to understand that I do indeed teach the student the nuances of formulas, understanding why, when, how, and under what conditions they are used. But in my experience, forcing the student to scrutinize statistical output files accomplishes this and teaches them the appropriate use and limitations of the information derived.

Students in my classes are always surprised (ecstatic) to realize they can use their textbooks and notes on my exams. But they quickly find that, unless they really understand the principles and how they are applied and interpreted, an open book is not going to help them. Over time, they come to realize that the analyses and the outcomes of statistical procedures are simply the ingredients for what comes next: building solutions to research problems. Therefore, their role is more detective and constructor than number juggler.

This approach mirrors the recent national and international debate about math pedagogy. In our recent book, *Winning the Math Wars* (2010), my colleagues and I addressed these issues in great detail, suggesting that, while traditional ways of teaching math are useful and important, the emphases of reform approaches are not to be dismissed. Understanding and memorizing detail are crucial, but problem solving requires a different approach to learning.

CASES FROM CURRENT RESEARCH

I focus on using real-world data in this book. There are several reasons for doing so, primarily because students need to be grounded in approaches for using data from the real world with all their problems and "grittiness." When people respond to surveys or interviews, they inevitably fill out information in ways not asked by interviewers (e.g., respondents may choose two possible answers when one is required, etc.). Moreover, transferring data to electronic form may result in miscoded responses or categorization problems. Researchers always confront these issues, and I believe it is important for students to leave the classroom aware of the range of possible problems with real-world data and prepared for dealing with them. Of course, much of the data we will examine will already have been put in standard forms, but other research issues will arise (e.g., how do I recategorize data, assign missing cases, compute new variables, etc.?).

Another reason I use real-world data is to familiarize students with contemporary research questions in the social and health science fields. Classroom data often are contrived to make a certain point or show a specific procedure, which are both helpful. But I believe it is important to draw the focus away from the procedure per se and understand how the procedure will help the researcher resolve a research question. The research questions are important. Policy reflects the available information on a research topic, to some extent, so it is important for students to be able to generate that information as well as to understand it. This is an "active" rather than "passive" learning approach to understanding statistics.

Data Labs are a very important part of this course since they allow students to take charge of their learning. This is the heart of discovery learning. Understanding a statistical procedure in the confines of a classroom is necessary and helpful. However, learning that lasts is best accomplished by students directly engaging the processes with actual data and observing what patterns emerge in the findings that can be applied to real research problems.

Some practice problems may use data created for classroom use, but real-world data from actual research databases will enable a deepening of understanding. In addition to national databases, I use results from my own research for classroom learning. In every case, researchers know that they will discover knotty problems and unusual, sometimes idiosyncratic, information in their data. If students are not exposed to this real-world aspect of research, it will be confusing when they engage in actual research beyond the confines of the classroom.

In this course, we will have several occasions to complete Data Labs that pose research problems with actual data. Students take what they learn from the book material and conduct a statistical investigation using SPSS and Excel. Then, they have the opportunity to examine the results, write research summaries, and compare findings with the solutions presented at the end of the book.

The project labs also introduce students to two software approaches for solving statistical problems. These are quite different in many regards, as we will see in the chapters that follow. SPSS provides additional advanced procedures educational researchers utilize for more complex and extensive research questions. Excel is widely accessible and provides a wealth of information to researchers about many statistical processes they encounter in actual research. The Data Labs provide solutions in both formats so the student can learn the capabilities and approaches of each.

This book makes use of publically available research data. The General Social Survey or GSS[1] is a nationally representative survey designed to be part of a program of social research to monitor changes in Americans' social characteristics and attitudes. Funded through the National Science Foundation and administered by the National Opinion Research Center (NORC), the GSS has been administered annually or biannually since 1972. As a general survey, the GSS asks a variety of questions on a series of topics designed to track the opinions of Americans over the last four decades.

Other databases we will use in the book include the following:

- The Centers for Disease Control and Prevention (CDC) conducts the Behavioral Risk Factor Surveillance System (BRFSS) as a health-related telephone survey to measure American residents' health conditions, health behaviors, and use of preventative services.[2]

[1] Tom W. Smith, Peter Marsden, Michael Hout, and Jibum Kim. General Social Surveys, 1972–2012 [machine-readable data file]/Principal Investigator, Tom W. Smith; Coprincipal Investigator, Peter V. Marsden; Coprincipal Investigator, Michael Hout; Sponsored by National Science Foundation. – NORC ed. – Chicago: National Opinion Research Center [producer]; Storrs, CT: The Roper Center for Public Opinion Research, University of Connecticut [distributor], 2013. 1 data file (57,061 logical records) + 1 codebook (3432 pp.). -- (National Data Program for the Social Sciences, No. 21).

[2] Centers for Disease Control and Prevention (CDC) (2013). *Behavioral Risk Factor Surveillance System Survey Data*. Atlanta, Georgia: U.S. Department of Health and Human Services, Centers for Disease Control and Prevention.

- Association of Religion Data Archives (ARDA) presents a series of databases on a variety of religion topics from the sociological perspective. In addition to other databases, the ARDA presents GSS databases on special modules (sets of questions) relevant to religion. By visiting the ARDA (www.thearda.com), you can peruse the codebook for the latest GSS file (www.thearda.com/Archive/ GSS.asp) to get a fuller sense of the types of questions a general survey asks. You can also visit the ARDA's "Learning Center" to take a survey that allows you to compare yourself to a larger national profile. The "Compare Yourself to the Nation" survey allows you to see how you compare to others based on the results from the 2005 Baylor Religion Survey (addressing religious identity, beliefs, experiences, paranormal views, etc.).

RESEARCH DESIGN

Researchers who write statistics books have a dilemma with respect to research design. Typically, statistics and research design are taught separately in order for students to understand each in greater depth. The difficulty with this approach is that the student is left on their own to synthesize the information; this is often not done successfully.

Colleges and universities attempt to manage this problem differently. Some require statistics as a prerequisite for a research design course or vice versa. Others attempt to synthesize the information into one course, which is difficult to do given the eventual complexity of both "sets" of information. Adding somewhat to the problem is the approach of multiple courses in both domains.

I do not offer a perfect solution to this dilemma. My approach focuses on an in-depth understanding of statistical procedures for actual research problems. What this means is that I cannot devote a great deal of attention in this book to research design apart from the statistical procedures which are an integral part of it. (You may wish to consult a separate book on research design I authored with my colleague Jennifer McKinney, *Understanding and Applying Research Design*, 2013.)

I try to address the problem in two ways. First, wherever possible, I connect statistics with specific research designs. This provides an additional context in which students can focus on using statistics to answer research questions. The research question drives the decision about which statistical procedures to use; it also calls for discussion of appropriate design in which to use the statistical procedures. We will cover essential information about research design in order to show how these might be used.

Second, I have an online course in research design that can be accessed to continue your exploration from this book. In addition to databases and other research resources, you can follow the web address in the preface to gain access to the online course as additional preparation in research design.

FOCUS ON INTERPRETATION

I call attention to problem solving and interpretation as the important elements of statistical analysis. It is tempting for students to focus so much on using statistical procedures to create meaningful results (a critical matter!) that they do not focus on what the results mean for the research question. They stop after they use a formula and decide whether or not a finding is statistically significant. I strongly encourage students to think about the findings in the context and words of the research question. This is not an easy thing to do because the meaning of the results is not always cut and dried. It requires students to think beyond the formula.

Statisticians and practitioners have devised rules to help researchers with this dilemma by creating criteria for decision making. For example, as we will see in Chapter 11, squaring a correlation yields the "coefficient of determination," which represents the amount of variance in one variable that is accounted for by the other variable (this is known as "effect size," a topic which we will spend a great deal of time with in this book). But the next question is, how much of the "accounted for variance" is meaningful? This consideration is key to understanding how to use and make decisions on the basis of big data.

In many ways, interpretation of results is an art undergirded by the cannons of science. Much of the ability to develop expertise in interpretation comes by long hours of tutelage with researchers who have done it for many years. We cannot hope to emerge from our study with this expertise, but through constant focus on interpretation, we can become aware of the acceptable ways of understanding and using statistical results.

Statisticians have suggested different ways of helping with interpretation. For example, when dealing with the "accounting of variance" example presented earlier, statisticians have created criteria that determine 0.01 (1%) of the variance accounted for is considered "small" while 0.05 (5%) is "medium" and so forth. (And, much to the dismay of many students, there are more than one set of these criteria.) Therefore, if we determine that the correlation between two variables reach these criteria levels, we can feel secure in sticking to good interpretation guidelines. Problems exist however in how to view these statistical results within the context of the research problem.

For example, if a research question is, "Does class size affect math achievement?" and the results suggest that class size accounts for 1% of the variance in math achievement, many researchers might agree the results represent a small and perhaps even inconsequential impact. However, if a research question is, "Does drug X affect Ebola survival rates?," researchers might consider 1% of the variance to be much more consequential than "small!" This is not to say that math achievement is any less important than Ebola survival rates (although that is another of those debatable questions researchers face), but the researcher must consider a range of factors in determining meaningfulness: the intractability of the research problem, the discovery of new dimensions of the research focus, whether or not the findings represent life and death, and so on. The material point is that statistical criteria are important for establishing meaningfulness of results, but overall interpretation involves the larger context within which the research takes place.

I have found that students have the most difficult time with these matters. Using a formula to create numerical results is often much preferable to understanding what the results mean in the context of the research question. Students have been conditioned to stop after they get the right numerical answer. They typically do not get to the difficult work of what the right answer *means* because it isn't always apparent.

I emphasize "practical significance" (effect size) in this book as well as statistical significance. In many ways, this is a more comprehensive approach to uncertainty, since effect size is a measure of "impact" in the research evaluation. It is important to measure the likelihood of chance findings (statistical significance), but the extent of influence represented in the analyses affords the researcher another vantage point to determine the relationship among the research variables.

Coverage of Statistical Procedures

The statistical applications we will discuss in this book are "workhorses." This is an introductory treatment, so we need to spend time discussing the nature of statistics and basic procedures that allow you to use more sophisticated procedures. We will not be able to examine advanced procedures in much detail. I will provide some references for students who wish to continue their learning in these areas. Hopefully, as you learn the capability of SPSS and Excel, you can explore more advanced procedures on your own, beyond the end of our discussions.

Some readers may have taken statistics coursework previously. If so, my hope is that they are able to enrich what they previously learned and develop a more nuanced understanding of how to address problems in educational research through the use of SPSS and Excel. Whether readers are new to the study or experienced practitioners, my hope is that statistics becomes meaningful as a way of examining problems and debunking prevailing assumptions in the social and health sciences.

Often, well-intentioned people can, through ignorance of appropriate processes, promote ideas that may not be true. Further, policies might be offered that would have a negative impact even though the policy was not based on sound statistical analyses. Statistics are tools that can be misused and influenced by the value perspective of the wielder. However, policies are often generated in the absence of compelling research. Students need to become "research literate" in order to recognize when statistical processes should be used and when they are being used incorrectly.

2

DESCRIPTIVE STATISTICS: CENTRAL TENDENCY

When I teach statistics, I typically begin by offering a series of questions that emphasize the importance of statistics for solving real research problems. Statistical formulas and procedures are logical and crucial, but the primary function for statistical analyses (at least, in my mind) is to bring clarity and understanding to a research question. As I discussed in a recent book dealing with statistics for program evaluation (Abbott, 2010), statistical procedures are best used to discover patterns in the data that are not directly observable. Bringing light to these patterns allows the student and the researcher to understand and engage in problem solving.

WHAT IS THE WHOLE TRUTH? RESEARCH APPLICATIONS (SPURIOUSNESS)

Finding the "truth" is a laudable goal and one that should inform all research efforts. However, in statistics, it is not likely that we will ever really discover ultimate truth. The nature of statistics is that we strive to observe as fully as possible what relationships exist among variables so that we can understand likely causal linkages. Does poverty "cause" crime? Is longevity affected by access to health care? These questions intimate valid relationships between the research variables. However, one of the first lessons in statistics and research is that valid and meaningful relationships are not always easily visible. Certainly most realities in contemporary life are much

Using Statistics in the Social and Health Sciences with SPSS® and Excel®, First Edition.
Martin Lee Abbott.
© 2017 John Wiley & Sons, Inc. Published 2017 by John Wiley & Sons, Inc.

more complex than can be explained by two variables. We therefore must be able to "see" patterns among data using both numerical and visual means that underlie seemingly simple relationships.

As we will discuss in Chapter 11, there is a big difference between "correlation" and "causation." This statistical adage helps to point out the complexity of understanding the patterns among variables. Just because two variables are strongly statistically related does not mean that there is a causal relationship between them. Causality is difficult to prove. In order to understand the apparent causal relationship more fully, we must look at other variables that might have a meaningful but "hidden" relationship with both "visible" variables. Researchers use the term "spuriousness" to describe whether an apparent relationship between two variables might be the influence of variables not in the analysis. An example of spuriousness is the relationship between ice cream consumption and crime.[1]

There is a positive relationship between rates of ice cream consumption and crime; when one increases, so does the other. Should we conclude then that ice cream consumption leads to criminal behavior in a causal way? Spuriousness means that there may not a true or genuine relationship between factors even if it looks like there is. Some unobserved or unnoticed variable may be related to both of the variables we can "see" (in this example ice cream consumption and crime), which may make it appear that the "visible" variables have a cause–effect relationship.

In this example, ice cream consumption increases as crime increases; and, consequently, when crime increases, so does the consumption of ice cream. These two variables appear to be consistently related to each other. They probably do not have a causal relationship, however, since both ice cream consumption and crime are related to a third factor: temperature. When temperatures rise, ice cream consumption increases (people eat more ice cream in the summer than winter). Also, when temperatures rise, crime increases. If we include these additional relationships in our study, then we can see that the apparent causal relationship between ice cream consumption and crime is probably really more an issue of the weather; both of the variables are "linked" by temperature.

Without considering spuriousness, some might be tempted to explain why there is a causal relationship between ice cream consumption and crime. For example, does ice cream lead to feelings of grandeur or a propensity for aggression, which causes people to commit crime? Or is it that good ice cream is so expensive that people commit crimes in order to support their ice cream habit? Which makes most sense? Although we could come up with several reasons (mostly fanciful) why one of these variables might be causally related to the other, we need to be cautious.

This situation leads to one of the most profound lessons in social science: *objectivity is necessary to pursue knowledge dispassionately*. If we assume there is a relationship between things without using objective means of assessing the truth of the situation, then we are simply imposing a subjective understanding of the situation that is not "anchored" in science. Some call this the "procrustean exercise" referencing the mythological figure who forced people to an iron bed by either stretching them to

---

[1] This example and explanation are discussed in Abbott and McKinney (2013).

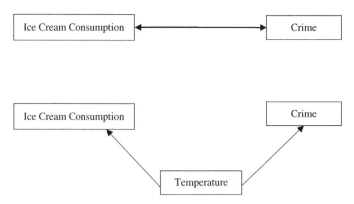

Figure 2.1   The possible spurious relationship between ice cream consumption and crime.

fit or cutting off the excess. Thus, by not taking an objective stance, we may have a tendency to make apparent reality "fit" our mental picture or subjective assumptions.

Figure 2.1 shows how the possible relationships among ice cream consumption, crime, and temperature. The top panel shows the apparent relationship between ice cream consumption and crime, with a two-way line connecting the variables indicating that the two are highly related to one another. The bottom panel shows that, when the third variable (temperature) is introduced, the apparent relationship between ice cream consumption and crime disappears, as indicated by the absence of a line connecting them.

Identifying potentially spurious relationships is often quite difficult and comes only after extended research. The researcher must know their data intimately in order to make the discovery. An example of this is a study I conducted in a study of industrial democracy several years ago. It was generally accepted in industry at the time that, if workers were given the ability to participate in decision making, they would have higher job satisfaction (JS). This was a reasonable assumption, given similar findings in the research literature. However, the more I examined my own data from workers in an electronic industry, the more I questioned this assumption and decided to explore the matter further.

I noticed from interviews that many workers did not want to participate in decision making, even though they had the opportunity to do so. I therefore analyzed the original "participation–job satisfaction" but this time added variables that measured workers' attitudes toward their work and a desire for management. Through a series of analyses, I found a number of surprising results that "modified" the original assumption of a direct (and causal) relationship between participation and JS. One of these findings was that a worker's attitude toward management had a lot to do with their eventual satisfaction levels. Those workers who participated in decision making and who had a positive view of management showed stronger satisfaction than those workers who did not such a positive view of management. Thus, a third variable (view of management) that was not originally included in the simple relationship (participation–satisfaction) had an impact on the findings. This subsequent analysis discovered a pattern in the data that was not "visible" at the outset.

The popular press often presents research findings that are somewhat bombastic but might possibly be spurious. Is student achievement really just a matter of ethnicity, or are there other factors involved (e.g., family income)? Do lifestyle choices directly impact longevity, or are there other considerations that need to be taken into account (e.g., social class)? The value of statistics is that it equips the student and researcher with the skills necessary to debunk simplistic findings.

DESCRIPTIVE AND INFERENTIAL STATISTICS

Statistics, like other courses of study, is multifaceted. It includes "divisions" that are each important in understanding the whole. Two major divisions are descriptive and inferential statistics. Descriptive statistics are methods to summarize and "boil down" the essence of a set of information so that it can be understood more readily and from different vantage points. We live in a world rich with data; descriptive statistical techniques are ways of making sense of it. Using these straightforward methods allows the researcher to detect numerical and visual patterns in data that are not immediately apparent.

Inferential statistics are a different matter altogether. These methods allow you to make predictions about attitudes, behaviors, and patterns on a large scale based on small sets of "sample" values. In real life, we are presented with situations that cannot provide us with certainty: Would a national training method improve patients' satisfaction ratings of their physicians? Can we predict workers' health scores or longevity in a variety of industries based on their job positions? Inferential statistics allow us to infer or make an observation about an unknown value from sample values that are known. Obviously, we cannot do this with absolute certainty – we do not live in a totally predictable world. But we can do it within certain bounds of probability. Hopefully, statistical procedures will allow us to get closer to certainty than we could get without them.

THE NATURE OF DATA: SCALES OF MEASUREMENT

The first step in understanding complex relationships like the ones I described earlier is to be able to understand and describe the nature of what data are available to a researcher. We often jump into a research analysis without truly understanding the features of the data we are using. Understanding the data is a very important step because it can reveal hidden patterns and it can suggest custom-made statistical procedures that will result in the strongest findings.

One of the first realizations by researchers is that data come in a variety of sizes and shapes. That is, researchers have to work with available information to make statistical decisions and that information takes many forms. Students are identified as either "qualified" or "not qualified" for free or reduced lunches:

1. Workers either "desire participation" or "do not desire participation."
2. Job satisfaction is measured by worker responses to several questionnaire items asking them to "Agree Strongly," "Agree," "Neither Agree nor Disagree," "Disagree," or "Disagree Strongly."

3. Medical researchers measure workers' physical health by how many days during the last month their physical health was good.

Nominal Data

The first example shows that data can be "either–or" in the sense that they represent mutually exclusive categories. If a worker indicates that they "desire participation" on a survey instrument, for example, they would not fit the "do not desire participation" category. Other examples of "categorical" data are sex (male and female) and experimental groups (treatment or control).

This type of data, called "nominal," does not represent a continuum, with intermediate values. Each value is a separate category only related by the fact they are categories of some larger value (e.g., male and female are both values of sex). These data are called nominal since the root of the word indicates "names" of categories. They are also appropriately called "categorical" data.

The examples of nominal data just mentioned can also be classified as "dichotomous" since they are nominal data that have only two categories. Nominal data also include variables with more than two categories such as schooling (e.g., public, private, homeschooling). We will discuss later that dichotomous data can come in a variety of forms also, like "true dichotomies" in which the categories naturally occur like sex, and "dichotomized variables" that have been created by the researcher from some different kind of data (like satisfied and not satisfied workers). In all cases, nominal data represent mutually exclusive categories. Educators typically confront nominal data in classifying students by gender or race, or, if they are conducting research, they classify groups as "treatment" and "control."

In order to quantify the variables, researchers assign <u>numerical values</u> to the categories. For example, "treatment groups" might be assigned a value of "1" and "control groups" might be assigned a value of "2." In these cases, the numbers are only categories; <u>they do not represent actual measurements</u>. Thus, a control group is not twice a treatment group. The numbers are only a convenient way of identifying the different categories.

Because nominal data are categorical, we cannot use the mathematical operations of addition, subtraction, multiplication, and division. It would make no sense to divide the number of Jeeps in a parking lot (one category) by the number of Teslas in the same parking lot (second category) to get a single measure of the automobiles. In order to get an idea of the automobiles n the parking lot, researchers would need to identify the categories of automobiles and find the percentage of each category in the parking lot. Thus, we might say that there are 15% Jeeps, 2% Teslas, 29% Toyotas, and so on in the parking lot.

Ordinal Data

The second example listed in the previous section (THE NATURE OF DATA: SCALES OF MEASUREMENT) indicates another kind of data: ordinal data. These are data with a second characteristic of meaning, position. There data are also categories, as in nominal data, but with the <u>categories related</u> by "more than" and "less than." Some categories are placed <u>above in value or below in value</u> of some other category.

Medical researchers typically find ordinal data in many places: county surveys regarding citizens' health and preference for treatment options, for example. In these cases, one person's response can be more or less than another person's on the same measure. According to our earlier discussion, JS can be measured by a question that workers answer about their work like the following:

"I am happy with the work I do."

1. Agree Strongly (SA)
2. Agree (A)
3. Neither Agree nor Disagree (N)
4. Disagree (D)
5. Disagree Strongly (SD)

As you can see, one worker can be quite happy, which indicates "Agree Strongly," while another can report that they are a little less happy by indicating "Agree." Both workers are reporting different levels of happiness with some being more or less happy than others.

Figure 2.2 shows another example of ordinal data categories; this example from the BRFSS Codebook in which medical researchers assigned numbers to respondents' reported health.[2]

As you can see in Figure 2.2, the response categories ("Excellent," "Very good," etc.) are still categories, but they are linked by "gradual amounts" of agreement.

Variable Name: GENHLTH

Description: Would you say that in general your health is:

Value	Value Label	Frequency	Percentage	Weighted Percentage
1	Excellent	85,532	17.39	18.66
2	Very good	159,104	32.35	31.68
3	Good	150,548	30.61	31.11
4	Fair	66,700	13.56	13.31
5	Poor	27,909	5.68	4.76
7	Don't know/not sure	969	0.20	0.18
9	Refused	1,004	0.20	0.29
BLANK	Not asked or missing	7		

Figure 2.2   The BRFSS GENHLTH variable values.

[2]Centers for Disease Control and Prevention (CDC). *Behavioral Risk Factor Surveillance System Survey Questionnaire.* Atlanta, Georgia: U.S. Department of Health and Human Services, Centers for Disease Control and Prevention, 2013.

TABLE 2.1 Typical Ordinal Response Scale

SA	A	N	D	SD
1	2	3	4	5

According to the data shown, 17.39% of the respondents reported that they would rate their health was excellent, while 5.68% of respondents rated their health as poor.

These examples of survey data are the stock-in-trade of social scientists because they provide such a convenient window into people's thinking. Medical, health, and social researchers use them constantly for gaining insight into, and making decisions about, policies in health care, urban planning, worker democracy, education, and other related arenas.

There is a difficulty with these kinds of data for the researcher however. Typically, the researcher needs to provide a <u>numerical</u> referent for a person's response to different questionnaire response categories in order to examine and describe the set of responses. Therefore, they assign numbers to the response categories as shown in Table 2.1.

The difficulty arises when the researcher treats the numbers (1–5 in Table 2.1) as <u>integers</u> rather than <u>ordinal indicators</u>. If the researcher thinks of the numbers as integers, they typically create an average rating on a specific questionnaire item for a group of respondents. Thus, assume, for example, that four people responded to the questionnaire item above ("I am happy with the work I do") with the following results: 2, 4, 3, 1 (i.e., person one "Agrees," receiving a 2 for "Agree"; person two "Disagrees," person 3 is "Neutral," and person 4 "Strongly Agrees"). <u>The danger is in averaging these</u> by adding them together and dividing by four to get 2.5 as follows $(2 + 4 + 3 + 1)/4$. This result would mean that on average, all four respondents indicated an agreement halfway between the 2 and the 3 (and therefore halfway between "Agree" and "Neutral"). This assumes that each of the numbers has an equal distance between them, that is, that the distance between 4 and 3 is the same as the distance between 1 and 2. *This is what the scale in Table* 2.1 *looks like if you simply think of the numbers as integers.*

However, an ordinal scale makes no such assumptions. Ordinal data only assumes that a 4 is greater than a 3, or a 3 is greater than a 2, *but not that the distances between the numbers are the same*. Table 2.2 shows a comparison between how an ordinal scale <u>appears</u> and how it might <u>actually be represented in the minds</u> of two different respondents.

According to Table 2.2, respondent 1 is the sort of person who is quite certain when they indicate SA. This same person, however, makes few distinctions between

TABLE 2.2 Perceived Distances in Ordinal Response Items

Scale Categories	SA	A	N	D	SD
The way it appears	1	2	3	4	5
Respondent 1 *perception*	1	2	3		4 5
Respondent 2 *perception*		1 2 3		4	5

A and N and between D and SD (but they are certain that any disagreement is quite a distance from agreement or neutrality). Respondent 2, by contrast, doesn't make much of a distinction between SA, A, and N, but seems to make a finer distinction between areas of disagreement, indicating stronger feelings about how much further SD is from D.

Hopefully this example helps you to see that the numbers on an ordinal scale do not represent an objective distance between the numbers, but they are only indicators of ordinal categories and can differ between people on the same item. The upshot, for research, is that you cannot add the numbers and divide by the total to get an average because the distances between the numbers may be different for each respondent! Creating an average would then be based on different meanings of the numbers and would not accurately represent how all the respondents, as a group, responded to the item.

Interval Data

The majority of the procedures we will study in this book use interval data. These data are numbers that have the properties of nominal and ordinal data, but add another characteristic, equal distance between the numbers. Interval data are numbers that have equal distance between them, so that the difference between 90 and 91 is the same as the distance between 103 and 104; in both cases, the difference is one unit. The value of this assumption is that you can use mathematical operations (multiplication, addition, subtraction, and division) to analyze the numbers because they have equal distances. Interval data are also "continuous" since an interval variable is expressed through a large number of equal distance measures.

An example of an interval scale is a standardized assessment test such as an intelligence quotient (IQ) test. A standardized test is one that meets strict criteria for testing and can ensure strong validity and reliability. These tests are benchmarked by having been used with a number of different sets of respondents under the same directions, with the same materials, time, and general conditions. They also typically have published norms so that researchers can have an objective measure for which to compare the results of the respondents of their own study.

While psychologists and educational researchers disagree about what IQ really represents, nevertheless, the numbers share the equal distance property. With IQ, or other standardized tests, the respondent indicates their answers to a set of questions designed to measure the characteristic or trait studied. Since the IQ measure has been used and benchmarked with so many different groups of people over the decades, the scores come to have the property of equal intervals between IQ quotients.

JS is another example. Respondents usually indicate that they strongly agree, agree, etc., with a series of items measuring their attitudes toward their job. The Job Diagnostic Survey (JDS) (Hackman and Oldham, 1980) includes the following item as part of the measurement of JS: "I am generally satisfied with the kind of work I do in this job" (response scale is "Disagree Strongly," "Disagree," "Disagree Slightly," "Neutral," "Agree Slightly," "Agree," and "Agree Strongly"). The measurement of JS uses a series of these kinds of questions to measure a worker's attitude toward their job.

What makes this kind of data different from ordinal data, which uses a similar response scale, is that the JDS and similar JS indexes use a standardized approach to measurement, as noted in the discussion earlier. The JDS items measured JS among managerial, clerical, sales, machine trade, and other workers. With such wide application, the *set* of items comprising the JS index comes to represent a consistent score. In fact, there are specific statistical procedures that measure the extent to which the scores are consistent across usage.

The result of repeated, standardized use of these kinds of instruments is that the response scales come to be accepted as interval data. The distance between units comes to have meaning as equivalent distances. Thus, even though they may be based on the same kind of ordinal response scales, as we discussed earlier, the set of measures can be multiplied, divided, added, and subtracted with consistent results. This is the way interval measures are typically used by social and health researchers. Whether or not we truly understand what one unit of IQ represents, nevertheless, we can proceed with measurement using recognized statistical procedures.

Treating Ordinal Data as Interval A difficulty in research is that all kinds of items might be thrown together by someone unaware of the nature of research to yield a "scale" that is then used in statistical procedures for problem solving. For example, a hospital administrator may wish to understand the attitudes of health-care practitioners regarding the sanitization policy governing the use of scopes used for colonoscopies. She might ask other hospital administrators if they have conducted similar studies, or she may simply sit down and compose a few questions that she believes measures the policy elements accurately. Typically, this might involve her creating a series of items with response categories like those illustrated in Table 2.1. Leaving aside the issue of whether the items are written correctly, she might then distribute the questions to her health-care practitioners and record the results. As you might imagine, she might compile the results by *assigning numbers to the response categories* (as in Table 2.1) and then create averages to each item across all the respondents.

The difficulty with this procedure is, I hope, now obvious. Rather than averaging the response scores, the administrator should simply report the frequencies of the practitioners who report each category. Consider the example in Table 2.3 in which five practitioners respond to an administrator-created item like "We should change the sanitation policy . . . ." As you can see, the practitioners indicated their attitudes by their choices using an "x" under the appropriate response scale category. If the administrator were to average the responses (thereby treating the data as interval), the five practitioners would indicate a 3.2 average, or slightly above neutral. However, if the administrator treated the data as ordinal, she would report the frequencies in the bottom row of Table 2.3. According to this report, 60% of the practitioners who responded to the item were in agreement, while 20% were strongly unfavorable and 20% were neutral. Using the data differently indicates different views of the practitioners' responses.

This example illustrates several characteristics of numbers that we will discuss in subsequent chapters. However, I point out here that statistics students and researchers need to be careful to understand what kind of data they have available and how to treat it for answering a research question.

TABLE 2.3   Comparison of Interval and Ordinal Scales

	1	2	3	4	5	
	SD	D	N	A	SA	Avg.
Respondent 1	x					1
Respondent 2				x		4
Respondent 3			x			3
Respondent 4				x		4
Respondent 5				x		4
	20%	0	20%	60%		3.2

In the course of actual research, evaluators often treat ordinal data as if it were interval data. While, from a purist standpoint, this is not strictly accurate, nevertheless, researchers use this assumption, especially with a survey instrument they, or other researchers, have used repeatedly. Standardized instruments like IQ or some JS measures are widely accepted and used as interval data. Regardless, students and researchers need to carefully consider the nature of the items of any instrument used to measure attitudes and decide how most accurately to represent the results.

Confidence with this assumption increases with well-written items. The interested student should seek research publications that discuss the criteria for creating survey items. Our book on research design (Abbott and McKinney, 2013) is one such resource that provides a thorough set of guidelines for creating appropriate questions. Creating items that conform to rules such as these provides a stronger foundation for treating these kinds of ordinal data as interval. Students and researchers should still exercise caution, especially with self-generated instruments.

Ratio Data

It is hard to imagine a worker with *no* satisfaction! Even if they are not completely enthralled with their work, or totally hate it, they have some attitude. Even "neutral" attitudes indicate a sort of ambivalence in which there are some positive and some negative aspects of the job. The fact is it is difficult to imagine the *absolute absence* of some concepts, attitudes, and behaviors, even IQ. Someone low on the IQ scale still *has* an IQ, even if their IQ "score" is zero.

There are other variables that can be said to have the possibility of absolute zero: the amount of money in your pocket, the distance between two lines, number of credits of math, number of friends, age, and so on. In such cases, a "0" value means *none*. Percentages can have a meaningful zero, as in the case of what percentage of students go on to medical school once they graduate from college or what percentages of students pass the MCAT.

Often, interval scale measures have zeros, but they are not "true" zeros in the sense of absolute nothing! The statistical value of ratio scales is that they have absolute zeros. This enables researchers to make ratios, hence the derivation of the name. If there is a fixed and absolute zero, then two things can be referenced to one another since they have a common benchmark. Nurse A with four patients can have *twice* the number of patients as nurse B who has two patients, for example. If you express this relationship in a number, you can divide the four patients (of nurse A) by the two patients of nurse B to get 2, or twice the number of patients. Of course you can also express the ratio the other way by saying nurse B has only half the patients as nurse A (or $\frac{1}{2}$). Or we can speak of hospital X showing twice the patient load as hospital B (assuming both hospitals count patients in the same way).

Choosing the Correct Statistical Procedure for the Nature of Research Data

An important rule to remember about statistics is to use appropriate statistical tools with the different kinds of data. In the following chapters we will learn about different methods for solving a particular problem using the approach that fits the available information. In this sense, statistics is like a collection of tools that we can use. We typically do not remove a screw with a sledge hammer (although I have been tempted at times!); we assess what particular tool works best with the screw that has to be removed. In the same way, we have to assess what statistical tool works best with the data we have available. Scales of measurement help us to classify the data in order to determine what the next steps might be to analyze it properly.

In real life, research data come in many forms: nominal, ordinal, interval, and ratio scales. Hopefully, you will gain familiarity with these as we discuss them in this book. This primary step in statistics is often the one that confounds even experienced researchers. You cannot use certain methods with certain kinds of data – if you do, you will not get accurate or meaningful results. As I mentioned earlier, you cannot calculate a mean (you could, but it would be "meaningless") on nominal or ordinal data. And we shouldn't trust a mean calculated on the appropriate level of data (interval) if the data are of a certain kind that might show a "distortion" (e.g., income, housing values, etc.); more of this is discussed later in the book. It takes practice to recognize the scale of measurement, but it is a step that cannot be missed.

DESCRIPTIVE STATISTICS: CENTRAL TENDENCY

Descriptive statistics include numerical and graphical procedures to assist the researcher to understand and see patterns in data. Typically, a researcher gathers data, which, unexamined, exists as a series of numbers with no discernable relationship. By using descriptive statistical techniques, the researcher can present the data in such a way that whatever patterns exist can be assessed numerically and visually.

The best way to understand these procedures is to begin with a real example. The data shown in Table 2.4 are taken from the public school database in Washington. The scores represent a sample of schools ($N = 40$) that reported scores from the fourth-grade students' state achievement test a few years ago. Each case in Table 2.4 represents the aggregated scores for each school in which the given percentage of students passed the math achievement portion of the test.

**TABLE 2.4   Aggregated School Percentages
of Students Passing the Math Standard**

Math Percent Met Standard

38	59	35	50
37	74	73	79
46	50	69	89
63	62	66	50
51	25	24	42
30	53	34	73
36	63	40	56
50	72	58	10
40	50	49	56
41	77	28	27

Simply looking at the numbers is not the best way to understand the patterns that may exist. The numbers are in no particular order, so the researcher probably cannot discern any meaningful pattern. Are there procedures we can use to numerically understand these patterns?

Central tendency measures suggest that a group of scores, like those in Table 2.4, can be understood more comprehensively by using a series of numerical and graphical procedures. As these measures suggest, we can understand a lot about a set of data just by observing whether or not most of the scores cluster or build up around a typical score. That is, do the scores have a *tendency* to approach the middle from both ends? There will be scores spreading out around this central point (we will explore this variability topic in the next chapter), but it is helpful to describe the central point in different ways and for different purposes. The primary question the researcher asks here is, "can we identify a "typical" score that represents most of the scores in the distribution?" In this example, the researcher needs to know what math achievement passing score is typical for this sample of schools.

Mean

Perhaps the most basic statistical analysis for numerically describing the central tendency is the mean, or arithmetic average of a set of scores. Remember from our discussion of the levels of data that the researcher needs at least interval data to create a mean score. This is because you need to use mathematical procedures like add, subtract, multiply, and divide in order to calculate it. If you have less than interval data, it would not make sense to use these arithmetic operations since you could not assume the intervals between data points are equal. Thus, for example, you could not get an average gender (nominal) or an average opinion about the value of constructivist teaching (ordinal, unstandardized survey question).

Calculating the mean value uses one of the most basic formulas in statistics, the average: $\dfrac{\sum X}{N}$.

This formula uses the "$\sum$" symbol which means "sum of." Therefore, the average, or mean value, can be calculated by adding up the numbers (designated by "X" for raw score), or summing them, and then dividing by how many numbers there are in the set (designated by "N"). Using the values in Table 2.4, we can calculate the mean by summing the 40 numbers to get 2025. If we divide this number by 40, the amount of numbers in the set, we get 50.63:

$$\frac{\sum X}{N} = \frac{2025}{40} = 50.63$$

What does the mean of 50.63% indicate? If you inspect the data in Table 2.4 you will see that 10% of the students in one school passed the math assessment, while 89% of the students at another school passed. That is quite a difference! What is the *typical* percentage of students who passed the math assessment? That is, if you had to report one score that most typified all the scores, which would it be? This is the mean, or average value. It expresses a central value (toward the middle) that characterizes all the values.

Median

Another measure of central tendency is the median, or middle score among a set of scores. This is not a calculation like the mean, but rather it identifies the score that lies directly in the middle of the set of scores when they are arranged large to small (or small to large). In our set of scores, the median is 50. Since we have an equal number of values, we would rank order the set of scores by listing them small to large and then average the values of the two middle ranks. This procedure would yield the direct middle score of the set of scores. In the example, the twentieth (50) and twenty-first (50) numbers are in the middle of the list. In order to identify the direct middle score, you would have to average these two numbers. In this case the middle of these two values is 50 $\left(\frac{50+50}{2}\right)$. An equal number of scores in the group of scores are above and below 50.

The median is important because <u>sometimes, the arithmetic average is not the most typical score in a set of scores</u>. For example, if I am trying to find the typical housing value in a given neighborhood, I might end up with a lot of houses valued at a few hundred thousand and five or six houses valued in the millions. If you added all these values up and divided by the number of houses, the resulting average would not really characterize the <u>typical</u> house because the influence of the million-dollar homes would present an inordinately high value.

To take another example, the values in Table 2.5 are similar to those in Table 2.4 with the exception of seven values. In order to illustrate the effects of "extreme scores," I replaced each score over 70 with a score of 98 (thereby creating extreme scores). If you calculate an <u>average</u> on the adjusted values in Table 2.5, the resulting value is 54.35.

Changing seven values resulted in the mean changing from 50.63 to 54.35. But what happens to the <u>median</u> when we make this change? Nothing. The median remains 50, since it represents the middle of the group of scores, not their average

TABLE 2.5   Adjusted School Percentages

Math Percent Met Standard

38	59	35	50
37	98	98	98
46	50	69	98
63	62	66	50
51	25	24	42
30	53	34	98
36	63	40	56
50	98	58	10
40	50	49	56
41	98	28	27

value. In this case, which is the more *typical* score? The mean value registers the influence of these large scores, thereby "pulling" the average away from the center of the group. The median stays at the center.

This small example shows that only a few extreme scores can exert quite an influence on the mean value. It also shows that the median value in this circumstance might be the more typical score of all the scores since it stays nearer the center of the group. Researchers should be alert to the presence of extreme scores since they oftentimes strongly affect the measure of central tendency. This is especially true anytime the values reflect money, like housing values, household income, and so on.

Mode

The mode is the most frequently occurring score in a set of scores. This is the most basic of the measures of central tendency since it can be used with virtually any set of data. Referring to Table 2.4, you can arrange the scores and discover that 50 is the most frequently occurring score in the set. The mode is a typical score or category since data most often "mass up" around a central point, so it makes sense that the mode, at the greatest point of accumulation in the set, represents the most prevalent score.

Central Tendency and Levels of Data

Earlier, I stated that statistics are like tools and the researcher must use the most appropriate tool with the data available for their research. This is true with representing central tendency as well.

The mean is used with interval (or ratio) data since it is a mathematical calculation that requires equal intervals. The median and mode can be used with interval as well as "lower levels" of data (i.e., ordinal and nominal), whereas a mean cannot. Using either median or mode with interval data does not require a mathematical calculation; it simply involves rank ordering the values and finding the middle score or the most frequently occurring score, respectively. The mean cannot be used with ordinal or nominal data since we cannot use mathematical calculations involving addition, subtraction, multiplication, and division on these data, as I discussed earlier.

The median is a better indicator of central tendency than the mean with "skewed" or imbalanced distributions. We will have more to say about skewed (extreme) sets of scores, but for now, we should recognize that a set of scores can contain extreme scores that might result in the mean being unfairly influenced and therefore not being the most representative measure of central tendency. Table 2.5 shows this situation as we discussed in "Median" section. Even when the data are interval (as, i.e., when the data are dealing with monetary value, or income), the mean is not always the best choice of central tendency despite the fact that it can use arithmetic calculations.

The mode, on the other hand, is helpful in describing when a set of scores fall into more than one distinct cluster ("bimodal distribution"). Consider Table 2.6 in which I "adjusted" just a few scores to illustrate the situation in which a set of scores has more than one most frequently occurring value. If you look closely, you will see that there are now two modes: 50 and 73.

In this situation, what is the most appropriate measure of central tendency? The data are interval, so we could calculate a mean. The mean for these adjusted scores is 50.80, just slightly higher than the mean (50.63) of the data in Table 2.4. However, would the resulting mean value truly be the most characteristic, or typical, score in the set of scores? No, because the scores in the set illustrated in Table 2.6 no longer cluster around a central point; they cluster around two central points.

Figure 2.3 shows how this looks graphically. As you can see, the math achievement values along the bottom axis show that there are two most common scores: 50 and 73 (the chart identifies this value as 75 because I used class intervals – values between 70 and 75). Clearly, this distribution does not look like a smooth "balanced" curve. Rather, there are two bars that are much higher than the other bars, which makes it problematic to define with just one characteristic value. In this case, if we reported that the mean value of students who pass math in the set of schools to be 50.8%, you can see that it is not the most characteristic score and would therefore be misleading.

These are real educational data. If we were using the data to describe the sample of schools' achievement, for example, we might report that the set of schools contain

TABLE 2.6   Math Achievement Percentages
Demonstrating a Bimodal Distribution of
Scores

Math Percent Met Standard

38	59	35	50
37	74	73	79
46	50	72	89
63	62	73	50
51	25	24	42
30	53	34	73
36	63	40	56
50	73	58	10
40	50	49	56
41	73	28	27

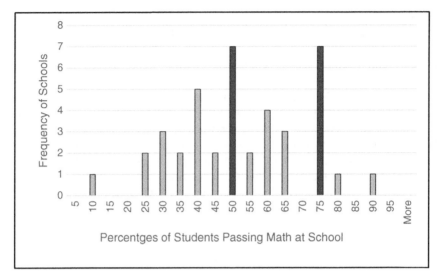

Figure 2.3 Graph of bimodal distribution.

two separate groups. Several schools performed at around 50% met standard for math achievement, whereas another group performed around 73%. If this were the case, we might want to investigate the characteristics of the different groups of schools to see why they might perform so differently.

We examine in the following text the graphing procedures we used to create Figure 2.3 (in Excel). First, we will examine how to use SPSS® and Excel to calculate central tendency values, which with these two tools is straightforward and simple.

The BRFSS includes several variables that we can use as examples for this exercise. I chose to take a random sample of the entire database (over 490,000 cases) on the GENHLTH question we examined from Figure 2.2. The question to respondents was, "Would you say that in general your health is". ... The resulting samples of 50 cases (listed in two columns) are listed in Table 2.7.[3] You can calculate the central tendency values manually and then follow the instructions in the following sections to use SPSS and Excel for the same calculations.

USING SPSS® AND EXCEL TO UNDERSTAND CENTRAL TENDENCY

Before you proceed with the following topics, and with those throughout the book, you need first to examine the two appendices (Appendices A and B) in the back of the book because they discuss the general features of both SPSS and Excel. If you

---

[3]Centers for Disease Control and Prevention (CDC). *Behavioral Risk Factor Surveillance System Survey Data*. Atlanta, Georgia: U.S. Department of Health and Human Services, Centers for Disease Control and Prevention, 2013.

**TABLE 2.7   BRFSS Responses to the
General Health Question**

GENHLTH

4	1
1	3
2	1
3	2
2	3
2	2
2	3
1	1
3	3
2	1
2	4
3	1
2	2
2	4
2	3
1	3
5	5
2	5
4	4
1	3
4	2
2	5
3	3
2	3
1	2

spend a bit of time with the discussions there, you will be ready to use these tools to help you with all the statistical procedures we cover in the book.

SPSS®

As I mentioned earlier in this chapter, in the course of actual research, evaluators often treat ordinal data as if it were interval data. While from a purist standpoint this is not strictly accurate, nevertheless, researchers use this assumption, especially with a survey instrument they, or other researchers, have used repeatedly. I will use the GENHLTH data shown in Table 2.7 to illustrate the use of SPSS for obtaining central tendency despite the fact that it represents a typical ordinal scale.

Figure 2.4 shows the SPSS data screen that I imported from the Excel file. (As you can see, only the first twenty cases or so are shown in the interest of space.) The drop-down menus from the Analyze menu provide a range of choices from which I specified "Descriptive Statistics" and "Frequencies" in secondary drop-down menus. You will also notice that there is another choice we could make if we wished to

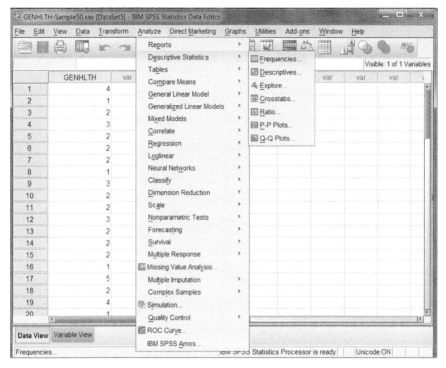

Figure 2.4   Descriptive frequencies menus in SPSS®.

obtain descriptive statistics: "Descriptives" the choice immediately below Frequencies. Choosing Frequencies enables me to specify percentages of cases in the categories of the variable, while Descriptives provides the calculated central tendency measures. I will show both processes in the following.

"Descriptive – Frequencies"   Figure 2.5 shows the SPSS submenu screens that result from choosing Frequencies. The first screen that appears allows you to specify which variable you wish to use in the analyses. Use the arrow in the middle of the screen to select and move the variable into the "Variable(s)" window. The second screen comes from choosing "Statistics" in the Frequencies submenu. You can see this button just to the right of the "Variable(s)" screen. This second screen enables you to select Mean, Median, and Mode (among other analyses) as shown in Figure 2.5.

When you make these selections for GENHLTH, SPSS generates an output file showing the results of your request, as shown in Figure 2.6. The output file lists the measures of central tendency we requested in the top panel of the output. The bottom panel of output in SPSS includes a frequency table in which each raw score value is listed along with the number of times it appears in the data ("Frequency") and the

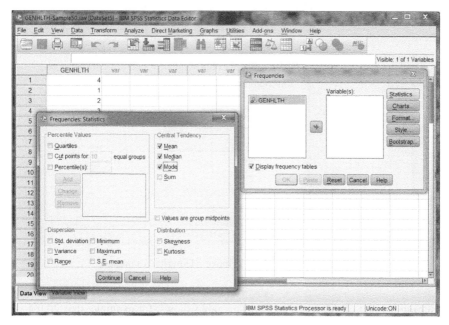

Figure 2.5 Frequencies submenus in SPSS®.

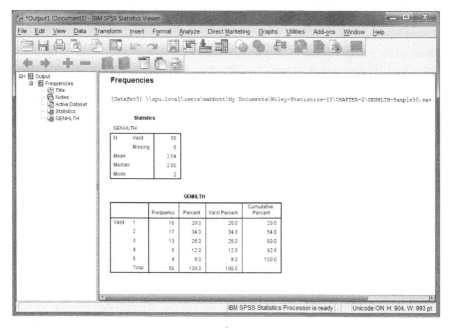

Figure 2.6 SPSS® frequency output.

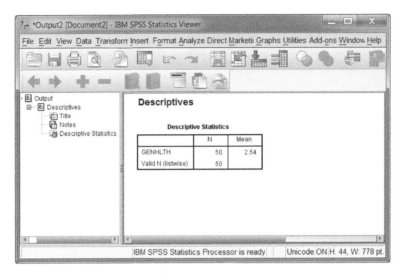

Figure 2.7   SPSS® Descriptive – Descriptives output.

resulting percent of the set of scores. This table shows, for example, that 20.0% of the sample cases were for a GENHLTH value of "1."

With large data sets, SPSS output may note "multiple modes," with the entire set of data. Depending on how you are treating the data, this warning may help you to understand the way the data are distributed so that you can decide how to report the findings.

"Descriptive – Descriptives"   Figure 2.4 shows another choice in the drop-down menus for calculating central tendency. Just below "Frequencies" in the right panel drop-down menu shown is "Descriptives." This choice results in direct calculations of central tendency as interval-level data, but only reports the mean value, as shown in Figure 2.7. There are several other choices for analysis in this submenu that we will discuss later.

Excel

Figure 2.8 shows a simple Excel spreadsheet listing the GENHLTH values from Table 2.7 (the spreadsheet contains only the first 15 cases for space consideration). You will see at the top of the spreadsheet a menu ribbon for several choices in Excel, one of which, "Data," is highlighted in the figure. This choice yields a secondary menu ribbon just below, the right part of which is "Data Analysis."

Figure 2.9 shows the resulting submenu when you select "Data Analysis." In this submenu, you can see several analysis tools available for statistical procedures, among which is "Descriptive Statistics" that we can use to calculate central tendency values. Selecting Descriptive Statistics results in a further drop box that you will use to specify your analysis, as shown in Figure 2.10.

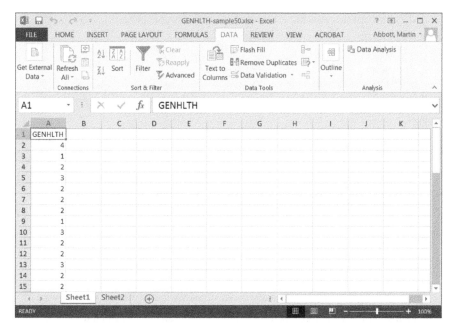

Figure 2.8 Excel spreadsheet showing GENHLTH data.

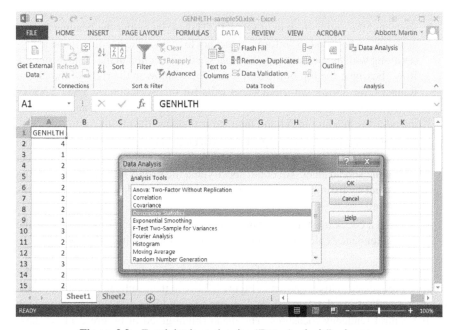

Figure 2.9 Excel database showing "Data Analysis" submenu.

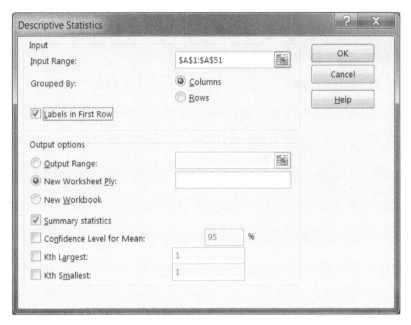

Figure 2.10   "Descriptive Statistics" drop box for calculating central tendency.

There are several features to observe in Figure 2.10:

1. I selected the entire column of GENHLTH data, including the heading for the analyses, so I needed to "inform" Excel not to include the heading in the analyses along with the percentages. You can see this selection in the "Labels in First Row" box near the top of the drop box. The window to the right of the "Input Range:" row shows the spreadsheet cells for this selection – "$A$1:$A$51" which indicates that I chose the cells from A1 to A51 for my analysis. This includes the <u>heading</u> in A1 and then the percentage data from A2 to A41.

2. Near the middle of the drop box, I selected "New Worksheet Ply:". This instructs Excel to present the results of the analyses on a <u>separate</u> worksheet within the spreadsheet. We could specify that the results be placed in the <u>same</u> worksheet by listing the appropriate location in the window to the right of this selection.

3. I placed a check mark in the "Summary Statistics" option. This will create the central tendency calculations on a separate worksheet within the spreadsheet.

When I select "OK" Excel provides a separate worksheet with the results of the analysis I requested. This is shown in Figure 2.11 with the results in a separate worksheet ("Sheet3") from the data values. You can see a column of results among which are the central tendency measures. The mean (highlighted in Figure 2.11) is 2.54, and the median and mode are both 2. The mean value is the same as that calculated in SPSS shown in Figure 2.7. There are many other calculated values as well that we

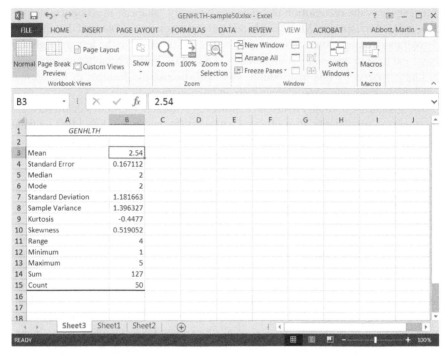

Figure 2.11   Descriptive statistics results worksheet.

will discuss in subsequent chapters. You should note that Excel does not make it clear if there is more than one mode.

DISTRIBUTIONS

The purpose of descriptive statistics, like the measures of central tendency we have discussed thus far, is to explain the features of a set of values that are helpful in response to a research question. We used the sample of general health values shown earlier to identify a <u>typical</u> score among a set of scores, for example. In the next chapter, we will explore visual ways of describing the same data.

Data in the real world presents itself to the researcher in patterned ways. We know from experience that people's attitudes and behaviors are fairly predictable. This doesn't mean that our actions are predetermined or fixed. Rather, it suggests that human beings approach life and experience in similar ways, with similar results. I discuss this assumption in more detail in my earlier book on the nature of patterns embedded in data (Abbott, 2011). In my classes, I stress the point that *statistics cannot achieve certainty; it can only increase our understanding of uncertainty*. Researchers focus their analyses at discovering the patterns of likelihood for certain actions and beliefs.

I will not belabor these points here, but I do want to point out that, because behavior and attitudes are somewhat predictable, we can study them scientifically. Part of this study is the recognition that data are typically "shaped" in recognizable patterns called *distributions*. Most people recognize the concept of "normal distribution" where data mass up around some middle value and taper off to the left and right (or above and below) this value. A great many, if not most, human behavior and attitudes are characterized by this distribution. (We will discuss the features of the normal distribution much more comprehensively in later chapters.)

Not all data are normally distributed, however. Although the values distributed are patterned and predictable, they often take many different shapes depending on what they measure. For example, a "Poisson" distribution, which measures the likelihood of rare events with large numbers of people (e.g., rare diseases across the United States), does not always have the appearance of the normal "bell"-shaped distribution. There are many other distributions that you can study in advanced mathematical statistics if you are interested. In this course, we will base our statistical analyses on the normal distribution.

Think of the distribution as values being "dealt out" along some scale of values. The more values there are to be dealt out, the more the values pile up around a central value with fewer values falling above and below the central point. Figure 2.12 shows an example of a normal distribution. You can see the "hump" in the middle with "tails" in the ends of the distribution of values. When we calculated the mean, median, and mode values earlier, we were calculating the values of the distributed data that represented the best characterization of all the values taken together. If the mean, median, and mode all fell on the same value, we could observe that the total set of values achieve a certain symmetry with the data arranged in the familiar bell shape. Statistically, we could speak of a "perfect" normal distribution where there are known percentages of values distributed under the curve compared to the normal distribution created by mathematical formulas. If the central tendency measures were the same, then there would be only one mode, the median would be the exact middle of the set

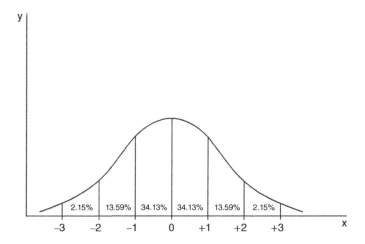

Figure 2.12   Example of the normal distribution of values.

of scores, and the mean value would not reflect extreme scores that would imbalance the set of scores in one or the other direction.

DESCRIBING THE NORMAL DISTRIBUTION: NUMERICAL METHODS

We can learn a great deal about the normal distribution by seeing it graphically with a set of actual data. I will show how to create a visual distribution by using the frequency information calculated in SPSS. Before we enter that discussion, however, I want to point out several ways to describe the normal distribution using numerical calculations.

Central Tendency

We have already discussed these calculations (i.e., mean, mode, and median), but there are other ways to capture a characteristic central point among a set of values. In advanced statistics courses, you might learn some of these additional measures of central tendency. You may learn to create the "harmonic mean," the "geometric mean," or the "quadratic mean," depending on the nature of your data. In this course, we will describe how the data from a distribution of scores "clusters up" using the arithmetic mean.

Skewness

Skewness is a term that describes whether, or to what extent, a set of values is not perfectly balanced but rather *trails off* to the left or right of center. I will not discuss how to calculate skew, but it is easy to show. Figure 2.13 shows scores in an example database that appear to be "imbalanced." The scores appear to trail to the right of the mean. In this case, we can say that the distribution is positively skewed (SK+) since the values trail to the right. The distribution would be negatively skewed (SK−) if the scores trailed away to the left.

Both SPSS and Excel provide calculations for skewness. Figure 2.14 shows the output from SPSS. As you can see, the skewness statistic is 0.519, and this value is accompanied by the "Std. error" of 0.337. This latter value is the standard error of skewness, which as we will discuss later is a value that helps to create a better estimate of skewness used in predicted values.

Figure 2.11 shows the output from Excel. As you can see from the figure, the skewness value is the same as that reported by SPSS, 0.519. Excel does not provide the standard error of the estimate for skewness.

The interpretation of skewness helps to understand the shape of a distribution of values. A skewness value of zero indicates perfect balance, with the values in the distribution neither trailing excessively to the left or right of the center. Positive values indicate values trailing to the right, and negative values indicate left trailing. As you can see from the tables in both Figures 2.11 and 2.14, the skewness value of 0.519 is a positive number, and therefore the values of GENHLTH will trail to the right.

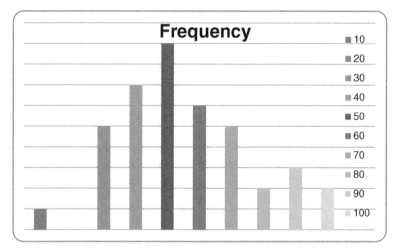

Figure 2.13 Illustration of a positively skewed distribution.

The important question researchers must ask is, "how far from zero is considered excessive" for the skewness value? That is, how big can the skewness number get with the distribution still retaining the general shape of a normal distribution? The SPSS output in Figure 2.14 is helpful because it provides the standard error value for skewness. We will discuss this value in greater depth in later chapters, but for now, you can use the standard error value to establish a general rule of thumb for excessive skew. When you divide the skewness value (0.519) by the standard error of skewness (0.337), the result (1.54) is a sort of skewness *index*. If this index number does not exceed values from 2.50 to 3.00 or so (either positively or negatively), depending on the number of values in the distribution, the distribution is considered "normal" and balanced. You can use the sign (positive or negative) of the skewness value to indicate which way the skew tends (i.e., left for negative values and right for positive values), but the index magnitude indicates whether or not the skewness is excessive.

The skewness index of 1.54 is closer to 2.50 than it is to "0" so you could expect that a graph showing the distribution of GENHLTH values would trail to the right of the mean value. This may result in a distribution that appears imbalanced, but it can be considered normally distributed for statistical purposes, according to the rule above of 2.50–3.00 for excessive skewness.

I mentioned earlier that the *number of values in the distribution* affects the skewness index. While this will become clearer in a later chapter, I mention here that the Std. error of skewness reported by SPSS will be *smaller* with larger numbers of values in the distribution. So, larger data sets (200–400) might have very small Std. error of skewness numbers and result in the overall skewness index being very *excessive* (since dividing by a smaller number yields a larger result). Small data sets (30–50) will typically have large Std. error of skewness numbers with resulting smaller skewness indexes.

In light of these issues, the researcher needs to consider the *size of the distribution* as well as the *visual evidence* to make a decision about skewness. In the example

Descriptive Statistics

	N	Minimum	Maximum	Mean	Std. Deviation	Skewness		Kurtosis	
	Statistic	Statistic	Statistic	Statistic	Statistic	Statistic	Std. Error	Statistic	Std. Error
GENHLTH	50	1	5	2.54	1.182	.519	.337	-.448	.662
Valid N (listwise)	50								

Figure 2.14 SPSS® output showing descriptive statistics including skewness.

shown in Figures 2.11 and 2.14, a skewness number of 0.519 seems nonexcessive, since it has a Std. error of skewness of 0.337 and a resulting skewness index of 1.54 (and therefore lower than our rule of thumb of ±2.5–3.00). However, if we were to add several more cases to the distribution, the Std. error of skewness would likely shrink resulting in a larger skewness index. If we use a large data set, I might view the visual evidence alone as a better measure of overall balance. Smaller data sets are more problematic, even though the skewness indexes are within normal bounds. *Use both the visual and numerical evidence to help you decide upon the overall shape of skewness.*

There is another way to help assess the extent of skewness using the three measures of central tendency we discussed (mean, median, and mode). If a distribution of scores is "balanced," with most of the scores massing up around a central point, the mean, median, and mode will all lie on the same point. The mean is typically the most "sensitive" indicator and will get pulled toward the direction of the skew more readily than the median and the mode. You can use both the numerical results and the visual inspection to see if this method helps.

The output shown in Figure 2.11 show that the mean of the GENHLTH values is 2.54, while both median and mode are 2.0. While this appears to be a slight discrepancy, the three values are very close to one another. Since the mean, the most "sensitive" indicator of central tendency, is larger than both the median and mode, the resulting distribution will show a positive skew.

Kurtosis

Kurtosis is another way to help describe a distribution of values. This measure indicates how "peaked" or flat the distribution of values appears. Distributions where all the values cluster tightly around the mean might show a very high point in the distribution since all the scores are pushing together and therefore upward. This is known as a "leptokurtic" distribution. Distributions with the opposite dynamic, those with few scores massing around the mean and the other values spread out left and right, are called "platykurtic" and appear flat. "Perfectly" balanced distributions show the characteristic pattern like the distribution in Figure 2.12 where the distribution appears being neither too peaked nor too flat.

Making a determination of the extent of kurtosis is similar to the method with evaluating skewness. You can see from Figure 2.14 that SPSS reports both kurtosis and "Std. error" of kurtosis, while Figure 2.11 shows only the kurtosis value from Excel. Like skewness, dividing the kurtosis by the standard error of kurtosis (creating a kurtosis index) will provide a helpful measure for interpretation. You can use the same rule of thumb we discussed earlier for interpreting skewness (i.e., ±2.50–3.00). Thus, kurtosis index values greater than 2.50–3.00 are considered excessive and out of the boundaries for a normal distribution. In this example, the GENHLTH values show a kurtosis value of −0.448 with a standard error of kurtosis of 0.662. These result in a kurtosis index of −0.677, which does not indicate an excessive value for kurtosis. The sign of kurtosis indicates which direction (platykurtic or leptokurtic) the values in the distribution appear to take: positive kurtosis values that are excessive are considered leptokurtic, whereas negative kurtosis values that are excessive are platykurtic. It is also important to use visual evidence with kurtosis values as it is for interpreting skewness.

DESCRIPTIVE STATISTICS: USING GRAPHICAL METHODS

Up to now, we have discussed *numerical* ways of deciding upon the shape of distributions. As I mentioned in the discussion of skewness earlier, it is also important to be able to describe data *visually*. Many students and researchers, as well as consumers of statistical reports, are experienced in viewing a variety of visual expressions of data. Therefore, it is important to be able to inspect and analyze the distribution of values by visual means in order to understand better the nature of the data and to communicate the results effectively.

The simplest way to visually describe data is simply to rank order it from high to low or from low to high. Beyond this are several ways of displaying data to see its underlying patterns. The frequency distribution is a common way of showing the array of data.

Frequency Distributions

Frequency distributions are tables that describe a distribution by showing groups of values. We can use the GENHLTH values in Table 2.7 to demonstrate the method of creating a frequency distribution and how to view the results. Table 2.8 shows these values in two columns (because of the large number of values, the columns include only the first and last sets of 10 values). The "Unordered" column shows the values as they originally were recorded, without ranking or other ordering processes. The "Ordered" column shows all of the values ranked and presented from smallest to largest values.[4]

You can use a frequency distribution to help visualize potential patterns in the data, and then from the frequency distribution, you can create a visual depiction of the GENHLTH values through a histogram. The graphical capabilities of SPSS and Excel enable the researcher to show both of these processes.

Before this, you must first decide the size of the groups within which each of the GENHLTH values will be placed. Some people call these groups "buckets" since it is similar to taking each value from the original set of values and tossing it into a bucket of a certain size or position. Excel, for example, creates the frequency distribution using "bins" or categories according to a set of values the user wishes to use.

Since there are five response categories for GENHLTH, we can create 5 bins in which to capture each of the values. Table 2.9 shows how Excel creates a table with 5 bins and the number of (unordered) GENHLTH values (total of 50 values) that fit into each bin. Thus, for example, Bin 2 shows that there are 17 GENHLTH values with a response of "2." This frequency distribution shows that there are more GENHLTH

---

[4]The two columns in Table 2.8 are not "linked." That is, the ordered values in the second column represent all the values in the database sorted and reported as lowest ("1") to highest ("5"). Thus, there are 10 values (shown) that are 1's in the raw data and four 5's in the original data.

TABLE 2.8   GENHLTH Responses as Unordered and Ordered

GENHLTH (Unordered)	GENHLTH (Ordered)
4	1
1	1
2	1
3	1
2	1
2	1
2	1
1	1
3	1
2	1
…	…
3	4
5	4
5	4
4	4
3	4
2	4
5	5
3	5
3	5
2	5

TABLE 2.9   Frequency of GENHLTH Responses in Five Bins

Bins	Frequency
1	10
2	17
3	13
4	6
5	4
More	0

values in the first three bins than there are in the last two bins. How would these values look if we graphed the frequency numbers?

"Column Charts" in Excel

In order to portray the distribution of GENHLTH values graphically, we can use the "Histogram" feature of Excel. Figure 2.9 shows the "Data Analysis" submenu choice

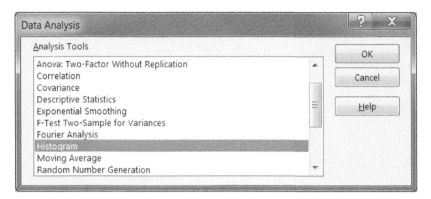

Figure 2.15 Excel output showing the Histogram specification and the data columns.

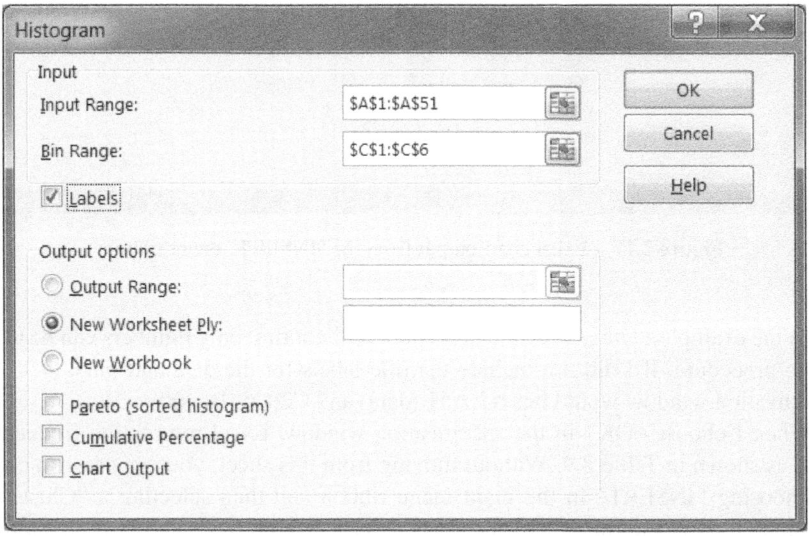

Figure 2.16 Excel output showing the Histogram specification and the data columns.

when you select "DATA" from the top menu ribbon. In the present case, we can choose "Histogram" instead of "Descriptive Statistics" (as shown in Figure 2.9).

Figure 2.15 shows the first step in creating a histogram in Excel. Choosing the Data Analysis button from the Data menu results in the submenu in which I can select Histogram. Selecting the Histogram tool results in a specification window that allows the user to identify the location of data and where to place the resulting output. This specification window is shown in Figure 2.16.

As you can see in Figure 2.16, I specified cells A1:A51 in the "Input Range" window to identify the table of data and cells C1:C6 to indicate the "Bin Range." Remember we created five bins to be used to categorize our data. Be sure to check the "Labels" box (as shown in Figure 2.16) if you include the variable labels (A1 and

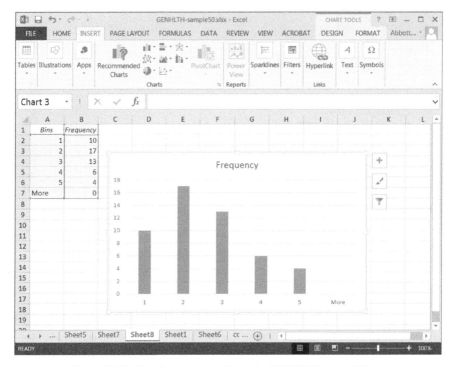

Figure 2.17   Excel chart output from the "INSERT" menu ribbon.

C1 in the example). Otherwise, the procedure will not run; only numbers can be used in the procedure. If I did not include the title labels for the data and bins, then the specification window would be: A2:A51 (data) and C2:C6 (Bins).

When I choose "OK" in the specification window, Excel returns the frequency table as shown in Table 2.9. Without moving from this sheet, you can create a chart by choosing "INSERT" in the main menu ribbon and then selecting a "Clustered Column" icon at the top left of the chart choices. Figure 2.17 shows the resulting column chart. You can use the various menu choices in the separate menu ribbon to edit, label, or specify the chart further. Finally, you can cut and paste this chart into a separate document.

You can see that the general shape of the distributed values in the chart is roughly normal, but with a skew to the right. Taken together with the numerical analyses discussed in the earlier sections (skewness and kurtosis values, size and similarity of mean, median, and mode), this indicates that the data in this set are positively skewed, but still within the bounds of a normally distributed set of values.

"Bar Charts" and "Histograms"

Excel results in a column chart of values as shown in Figure 2.17. SPSS allows the user to create both column charts (called "Bar Charts" in SPSS) and histograms. Before we examine the SPSS charts, we need to make a distinction between bar charts and histograms. Bar charts are designed for "categorical" data (see earlier discussion of categorical data in this chapter). Essentially, this means that each vertical bar represents the values in a particular category. The chart shows each bar as separated from the other bars, indicating that the data used to generate the graphic were not "continuous" data. In our previous example, we used the numbers 1–5 to represent each possible response to the GENHLTH survey question. This means that our resulting Excel column chart made no assumptions that the categories were numerically "ordered."

Histograms are different from bar (or column) graphs. Essentially, histograms are designed for continuous data (e.g., interval or ratio). The bars are connected to indicate that the categories are numerically linked. You can see from the category axis of a histogram that the bars are labeled according to the nature of the data. In our GENHLTH example, we only had five categories, so the bars would be labeled 1–5, assuming that the data are continuous. However, if our data were percentages of students passing a math test, for example, then the bars might represent intervals, or groups of values. In this case, we might have a bar representing 0–10% passing, then 11–20% passing, and so forth.

Bar Charts and Histograms in SPSS®

You can also create histograms in SPSS by using the "Graphs" menu. When you select Graphs from the top menu ribbon, SPSS returns a series of submenus as shown in Figure 2.18. As you can see, Graphs allows you to choose from a series of graph templates, among which is "Legacy Dialogs." This gives you a list of classical graph

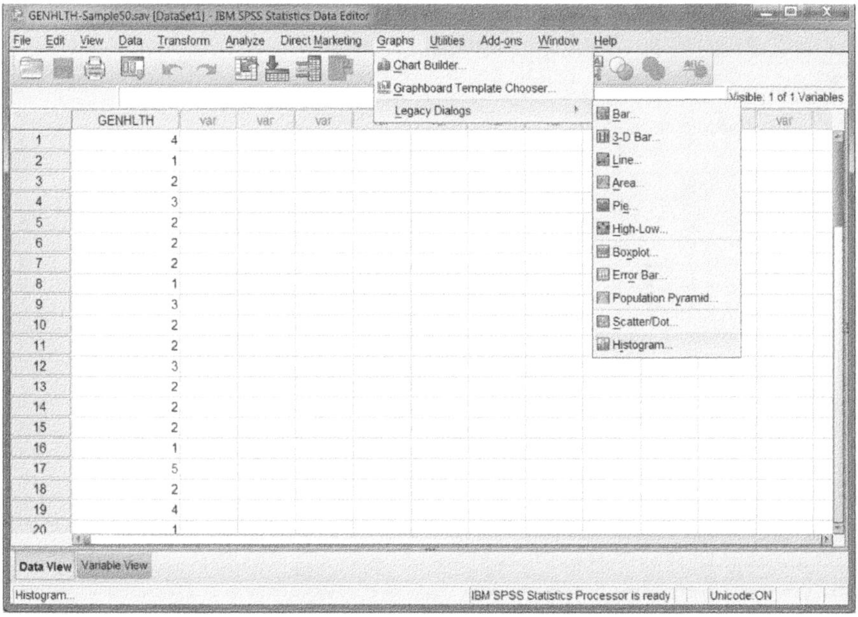

Figure 2.18 SPSS® procedure for creating the histogram.

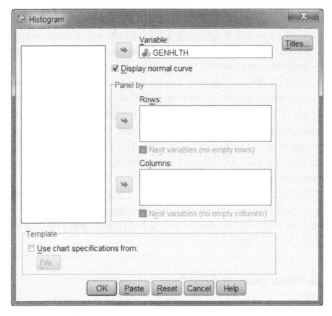

Figure 2.19 SPSS® procedure for specifying the features for the histogram.

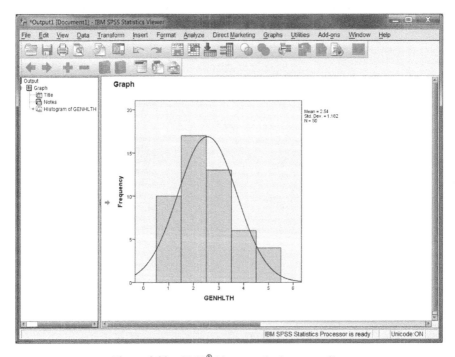

Figure 2.20 SPSS® histogram in the output file.

designs including the histogram. (Note that this submenu also gives you the oppor-tunity to create the bar graph by choosing the first option.)

Choosing the Histogram option results in a drop box appearing in which you can specify the features of the histogram, as shown in Figure 2.19. As you can see, you can call for a line showing the normal curve superimposed on the histogram bars by checking the box "Display Normal Curve."

The final result of these procedures is shown in Figure 2.20, the output file that includes the histogram. You can double-click on the histogram and copy it so that you can include it in a word processing file or other report format. You can also change the format features (axis intervals, titles, etc.) by double-clicking in the graph area. When you do this, you are presented with several dialog boxes that include several tools in which you can produce custom histograms.

Note that the graph in Figure 2.20 from SPSS presents a similar "picture" of the data as the Excel column graph in Figure 2.17. The added feature in Figure 2.20 is the superimposition of the normal curve so that you can compare the "raw data" distribution (i.e., the distribution of actual values) to the "ideal" normal curve. As noted previously, the numerical findings suggested a distribution slightly positively skewed, but within the bounds of the normal distribution. In this case, the graphical information and numerical information coincide.

TERMS AND CONCEPTS

Bimodal:	A set of data with two modes.
Categorical data:	Objects or subjects that are classified into different mutually exclusive groups. An example might be hospital patients who have had their appendix removed versus those patients who have their appendix. Categorical variables can have more than two categories. See Nominal data.
Central tendency:	One of the ways to describe a set of data is to measure the way in which scores "bunch up" around a mean, or central point of a distribution. Mean, median, and mode are typical measures of central tendency.
Continuous data:	Data obtained from an interval variable, which can be expressed through a large number of equal distance measures.
Descriptive statistics:	The branch of statistics that focuses on measuring and identifying data in such a way that the researcher can discover patterns that might exist in data not immediately apparent. In these processes, the researcher does not attempt to use a set of data to refer to populations from which the data may have been derived, but rather to gather insights on the data that exist at hand.

Data distributions: The patterned shape of a set of data. Much of statistics for research uses the "normal distribution" which is a probability distribution consisting of known proportions of the area between the mean and the continuum of values that make it up.

Frequency distributions: Tabular representations of data that show the frequency of values in groupings of data.

Histograms: Graphical representations of frequency distributions used with continuous data. Typically these are in the form of graphs in which bars represent groups of numerical values.

Inferential statistics: The branch of statistics that uses procedures to estimate and make conclusions about populations based on samples.

Interval data: Data with the qualities of an ordinal scale, but with the assumption of equal distances between the values and without a meaningful zero value.

Kurtosis: The measurement of a distribution of scores that determines the extent to which the distribution is "peaked" or flat. Data distributions that have excessive kurtosis values may be overly peaked ("leptokurtic") or overly flat ("platykurtic").

Mean: Average value in a set of data.

Median: Middlemost score in a set of data.

Mode: The most commonly occurring value in a set of data.

Nominal data: Data that exist as mutually exclusive categories (e.g., homeschooling, public schooling). These data can also refer to "categorical data," "dichotomous variables" (when there are two naturally occurring groups like male/female), or "dichotomized variables" (when two categories are derived from other kinds of data like rich/poor).

Ordinal data: Data that exist in categories that are ranked or related to one another by a "more than/less than" relationship like "Strongly Agree, Agree, Disagree, Strongly Disagree."

Procrustean exercise: A tendency to make apparent reality "fit" our mental picture or subjective assumptions, thereby denying the objectivity required to understand a reality. This concept references the mythological figure who forced people to an iron bed by either stretching them to fit or cutting off the excess.

Ratio data: Interval data with the assumption of a meaningful zero constitute ratio data. An example might be the amount of money people have in their wallets at any given time. A zero in this example is meaningful!! The zero allows the researcher to make comparisons between values as "twice than" or "half of" since the zero provides a common benchmark from which to ground the comparisons. Thus, if I have 2$ in my pocket and you have 4$, I have half of your amount.

Scales of measurement: The descriptive category encompassing different classes of data. Nominal, ordinal, interval, and ratio data differ according to the information contained in their scales of values. Also known as "levels of measurement."

Skewness: A measurement of a data distribution that determines the extent to which it is "imbalanced" or "leaning" away from a standard bell shape (in the case of a normal distribution).

Spuriousness: A condition in which an assumed relationship between two variables may be explained by another variable not in the analysis.

Standardized test: A test that meets strict criteria for testing and can ensure strong validity and reliability. These tests are benchmarked by having been used with a number of different sets of respondents under the same directions, with the same materials, time, and general conditions. They also typically have published norms so that researchers can have an objective measure for which to compare the results of the respondents of their own study.

DATA LAB AND EXAMPLES (WITH SOLUTIONS)

In this section, I will provide a couple of example problems so you can practice calculating and understanding central tendency. The first problem is shorter so that you can try to do the calculations manually. (You can even try to create a graph manually as well. Use SPSS or Excel to check your work.) The second problem is longer and is designed to help you become familiar with both SPSS and Excel. You can try to do the problem manually once you get the results from the software tools.

Problem 1

The data in Table 2.10 represents the job satisfaction (JS) ratings of assembly workers at a software company. These scores represent a JS index where higher values indicate greater JS and range from a possible score of "1" (lowest JS) to "10" (highest JS).

Using the data in Table 2.10:

1. Find the mean, mode, and median values for these JS scores.

2. Create a graph that shows the distribution of the scores.

**TABLE 2.10   Job Satisfaction
Ratings of Assembly Workers**

Job Satisfaction Ratings

3
7
8
4
6
5
6
6
8
7
5
7
5
4
6
9

Problem 2

Table 2.11 shows the first exam scores in an anatomy and physiology class. There are 100 points possible on the exam.

**TABLE 2.11   Exam
Scores in an AP Class**

AP Scores

10	56
24	58
25	59
27	62
30	63
34	63
36	66
38	69
40	72
44	75
45	78
46	79
49	82
50	89
51	91
53	

Using the data from Table 2.11:

1. Create a data file in both SPSS and Excel.

2. Obtain central tendency results.

3. Note and discuss skewness and kurtosis results.

4. Create a graph showing the distribution of AP scores.

5. Provide a summary or interpretation of the findings.

DATA LAB: SOLUTIONS

Problem 1

Mean: 6.00
Mode: 6.00
Median: 6.00

Distribution Graph (SPSS) (Figure 2.21):

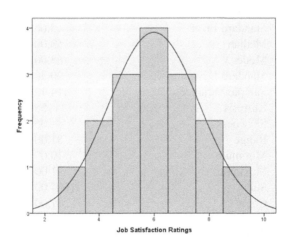

Figure 2.21   SPSS® histogram showing the distribution of JS scores.

Problem 2

1. Create a data file in both SPSS and Excel.

2. Obtain central tendency results.

Figures 2.22 and 2.23 show central tendency results for the AP scores in SPSS and Excel (respectively). Both sets of results agree that:

Statistics

AP Scores

N	Valid	31
	Missing	0
Mean		53.68
Median		53.00
Mode		63
Skewness		−.059
Std. Error of Skewness		.421
Kurtosis		−.577
Std. Error of Kurtosis		.821
Minimum		10
Maximum		91

Figure 2.22   SPSS® (Frequency) central tendency results for AP scores.

AP Scores	
Mean	53.68
Standard Error	3.66
Median	53.00
Mode	63.00
Standard Deviation	20.36
Sample Variance	414.49
Kurtosis	−.58
Skewness	−.06
Range	81.00
Minimum	10.00
Maximum	91.00
Sum	1664.00
Count	31.00

Figure 2.23   Excel (Frequency) central tendency results for AP scores.

Mean = 53.68, median = 53.00, and mode = 63.00.

3. Note and discuss skewness and kurtosis results.

Both SPSS and Excel results show figures for skewness and kurtosis (see Figures 2.22 and 2.23). Only SPSS provides the standard errors for skewness and kurtosis that you can use to determine whether or not the data "conform" to a normally distributed set of scores. Using Figure 2.22 results, you can see that the overall skewness would be −0.14 (determined by dividing −0.059 by 0.421). Thus, the distribution of values should not appear to be "unbalanced" since this number (−0.14) is less than the 2.5–3.0 range we discussed earlier in the chapter as being a criterion for a roughly normal distribution. Likewise, by this same criterion, the overall kurtosis result for this set of scores is −0.70 (determined by dividing −0.577 by 0.821), which would be considered a roughly normal distribution.

4. Create a graph showing the distribution of AP scores.

Figures 2.24 and 2.25 show the distribution of AP scores in SPSS and Excel, respectively. Note that in both cases, the graphs show roughly balanced distributions of scores.

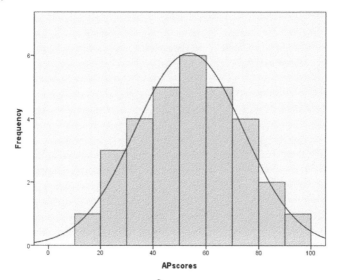

Figure 2.24   SPSS® histogram of AP scores.

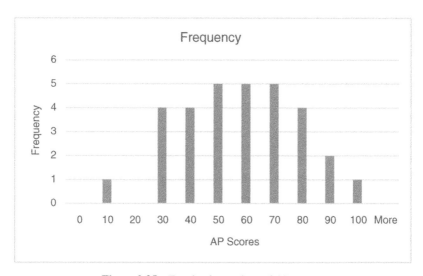

Figure 2.25   Excel column chart of AP scores.

5. Provide a summary or interpretation of the findings.

Taken together, the numerical and visual evidence suggest that AP scores on the first exam appear to be roughly normally distributed with an average score (53.68) that can be considered typical of the group.

3

DESCRIPTIVE STATISTICS: VARIABILITY

In Chapter 2, we examined several aspects of central tendency in the attempt to describe a set of data. In addition to mean, median, and mode, we discussed skewness and kurtosis as measures of the balance of a distribution of values. SPSS® and Excel provided visual descriptions as well as numerical results to help make assessments of the likely normal distribution of a set of data. The frequency distribution and histogram are effective ways of communicating the shape and features of the distribution.

I will continue to explore descriptive statistics in this chapter. This time, we will examine the extent to which scores spread out from the mean of a distribution of values. It is important to understand the characteristic score or value of a distribution, as we saw with central tendency, but it is also important to understand the extent of the *scatter* of scores away from the center. How far away do scores fall, and what is the average distance of a score from the mean? The answers to these and similar questions will help us to complete our description of the distribution of values.

This chapter thus deals with *variability* or *dispersion* of scores. Several measures of variability are important to grasp since we will use them throughout the book in virtually all the statistical procedures we cover.

RANGE

The first way to measure variability is the simplest. The range is simply the numerical difference between the highest and lowest scores in the distribution and represents a helpful global measure of the spread of the scores. But remember it is a

Using Statistics in the Social and Health Sciences with SPSS® and Excel®, First Edition.
Martin Lee Abbott.
© 2017 John Wiley & Sons, Inc. Published 2017 by John Wiley & Sons, Inc.

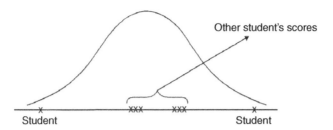

Figure 3.1   The characteristics of the range.

global measure and will not provide extensive information. Look at Figure 3.1. If two students score on the extremes of the distribution of achievement scores and everyone else scores near the mean, the range will provide a distorted view of the nature of the variation. The range represents the "brackets" around the scores, but it cannot tell you, for example, how far the "typical" score might vary from the mean.

Nevertheless, the range contains important information. It provides a convenient shorthand measure of dispersion and can provide helpful benchmarks for assessing whether or not a distribution is generally distributed normally (I will develop this benchmark later in this chapter).

There are several ways of "dividing up" the distribution of scores in order to make further sense of the dispersion of the scores. Some of these are rarely used, but others are quite important to all the procedures we will explore in this book.

PERCENTILE

The percentile or percentile rank is the point in a distribution of scores below which a given percentage of scores fall. This is an indication of *rank* since it establishes a score that is above the percentage of a set of scores. For example, a student scoring in the 82nd percentile on a math achievement test would score above 82% of the other students who took the test.

Therefore, percentiles describe where a certain score is in relation to the others in the distribution. The usefulness of percentiles for educators is clear since most schools report percentile results for achievement tests. The general public also sees these measures reported in newspaper and website reports of school and district progress.

Statistically, it is important to remember that percentile ranks are ranks and therefore not interval data. Figure 3.2 shows the uneven scale of percentile scores along the bottom axis of values in the frequency distribution.

As Figure 3.2 shows, the distance between the 30th and 40th percentiles is not the same as the distance between the 10th and 20th percentiles, for example. The 30–40 percentile distance is much shorter than the 10–20 percentile distance. That is because the *bunching up* of the total set of scores around the mean and the tailing off of the scores toward either end of the frequency distribution result in uneven percentages along the scale of the distribution. Thus, a greater percentage of the scores lay closer to the mean, and a lesser percentage of the scores lay in the tails of the distribution.

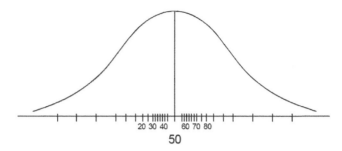

Figure 3.2   The uneven scale of percentile scores.

Many researchers have fallen into the trap of assuming percentiles are interval data and using them in statistical procedures that require interval data. The results are somewhat distorted under these conditions since the scores are actually only ordinal data. The US Department of Education developed the normal curve equivalent (NCE) score as a way of standardizing the percentile scores. This results in a scale of scores along the bottom axis of the frequency distribution that has equal distances between values. This transforms rank scores to interval scores enabling the educational researcher to use the values in more powerful statistical procedures.

SCORES BASED ON PERCENTILES

Educational researchers use a variety of measures to help describe how scores relate to other scores and to show rankings within the total set of scores. The following are some of these descriptors based on percentiles:

  Quartiles – These measures divide the total set of scores into four equal groups. This is accomplished by using three "cut points" or values that create the four groups. These correspond to the 25th, 50th, and 75th percentiles.

  Deciles – These measures break a frequency distribution into 10 equal groups using 9 cut points (the 10th, 20th, 30th, 40th, 50th, 60th, 70th, 80th, and 90th percentiles). They are called deciles since they are based on groups of 10 percentiles.

  Interquartile range – This measure represents the middle half of a frequency distribution since it represents the difference between the first and third quartiles (the 75th minus the 25th percentiles). This is a global descriptor for the variability of a set of scores since the other half of the scores would reside in both of the tails of the distribution.

USING SPSS® AND EXCEL TO IDENTIFY PERCENTILES

SPSS® Procedures

The example I use to illustrate these processes consists of the database from problem question 2 of Chapter 2, AP scores. The first example uses SPSS with the

"Analyze – Descriptives – Frequencies" command. The second example in Excel uses some of the drop-down formulas in the "FORMULAS" main command ribbon.

The procedure to identify a percentile value is straightforward using SPSS. Selecting the Frequencies procedure, as I described in Chapter 2 (see Figure 2.4), I can specify a percentile value that will *indicate at what score in the distribution below which a given percent of the scores fall* (i.e., by definition, the percentile). To take an example, suppose we want to identify the AP score below which 46% of all the AP scores fall. This means that we want to know the score value that identifies the 46th percentile.

Figures 3.3 and 3.4, respectively, show how to use SPSS to identify a score below which 46% of scores in the distribution fall (using the "Statistics" button in the "Frequencies" window). The output shows the result of 50.72. This indicates that 46% of the AP scores lie below 50.72 in this distribution of scores.

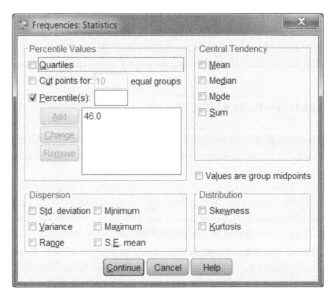

Figure 3.3   Specifying a percentile with SPSS® "Frequencies: Statistics" functions.

Statistics

AP Scores

N	Valid	31
	Missing	0
Percentiles	46	50.72

Figure 3.4   SPSS® output for percentile calculation.

Excel Procedures

Excel uses drop-down menus to identify percentile values. The top menu choice "FORMULAS" button allows the user to specify which function is needed from a list of formulas. Figure 3.5 shows the Excel screen specifying the procedure for identifying the percentile value for the score of 46, which we used in the SPSS example previously. As you can see, I selected the button from the top menu ribbon "FORMULAS" and then "More Functions" to obtain the "Statistical" functions. From this menu, I choose "PERCENTILE.EXC."

You will see in the list of formulas that there are several ways of identifying percentiles, depending on what you need. In my example, I chose "PERCENTILE.EXC"

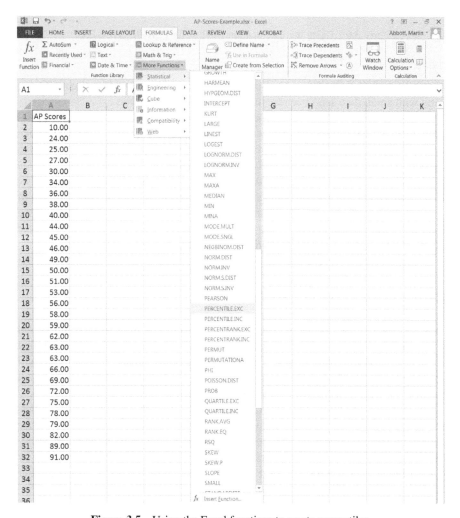

Figure 3.5 Using the Excel functions to create percentiles.

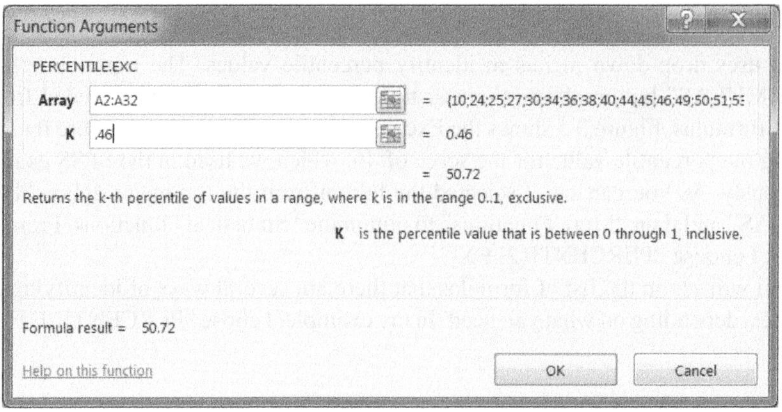

Figure 3.6   Using the specification window for PERCENTILE.EXC.

but "PERCENTILE.INC" would also be appropriate. The two differ slightly (especially with small data sets) because of slightly different formulas.

Figure 3.6 shows a specification menu from choosing PERCENTILE.EXC. In this example, I called for the value that identifies the score in the distribution below which 46% of the AP scores will fall, the same example I used with SPSS (i.e., the 46th percentile). Figure 3.6 shows the 46th percentile in the "K" window. Notice that you must specify the 46th percentile as "0.46," which is in the form of a percentage. The "Array" window shows all the values in the distribution we selected from the list of data (A2:A32). Selecting "OK" results in the value 50.72, which is the score in the distribution below which 46% of the AP scores fall. This value is also shown in the specification window itself in the third row of figures.

STANDARD DEVIATION AND VARIANCE

The range and percentiles that we discussed previously are helpful ways to understand the distribution of a set of raw scores. However, researchers use further measures that are more precise for calculation and understanding of statistical procedures we will cover in this book. Make sure you have a level of comfort with what they represent and how to calculate them before you move on to the further topics we discuss.

The standard deviation (SD) and variance (VAR) are both measures of the dispersion of scores in a distribution. That is, *these measures provide a view of the nature and extent of the scatter of scores around the mean*. So, along with the mean, skewness, and kurtosis, measures of dispersion (i.e., the SD and VAR) provide a fourth way of describing the distribution of a set of scores. With these measures, the researcher can decide whether a distribution of scores is normally distributed.

Figure 3.7 shows how scores in a distribution spread out around the mean value. Each score can be thought to have a "deviation amount" or a distance from the mean. Figure 3.7 shows these deviation amounts for four raw scores (X_1, X_2, X_3, and X_4).

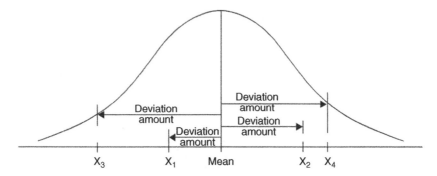

Figure 3.7 The components of the SD.

The VAR is by definition the square of the SD. Conceptually, the VAR is a *global measure of the spread of scores* since it represents an average squared deviation. If you summed the squared distances between each score and the mean of a distribution of scores (i.e., if you squared and summed the deviation amounts), you would have a global measure of the total amount of variation among all the scores. If you divided this number by the number of scores, the result would be the VAR, or the *average squared distance from the mean.*

The SD is the square root of the VAR. If you were to take the square root of the average squared distances from the mean, the resulting figure is the *standard deviation.* That is, it represents a *standard* distance between the mean and each score in the distribution (not the average *squared* distance, which is the VAR). We refer to this as *standard* since we created a standardized unit by dividing it by the number of scores, yielding a value that has known properties to statisticians and researchers. We know that if a distribution is perfectly normally distributed, the distribution will contain about six SD units, three on each side of the mean.

Both the SD and the VAR provide an idea of the extent of the spread of scores in a distribution. If the SD is small, the scores will be more alike and have little spread. If it is large, the scores will vary greatly and spread out more extensively. Thus, if a distribution of test scores has an SD of two, it conceptually indicates that *typically* the scores were within two points of the mean. In such a case, the overall distribution would probably appear to be quite "scrunched together," in comparison to a distribution of test scores with an SD of 5, depending on the range of the scores.

Conceptually, the SD is a standardized measure of how much all of the scores in a distribution vary from the mean. A related measure is the "average deviation" (AD), which is actually the *mean of all the absolute values of the deviation scores* (the distances between each score and the mean). So, in a practical way, the researcher can report that the average achievement test score (irrespective of sign) among a group of students was two points away from the mean, for example.

CALCULATING THE VARIANCE AND STANDARD DEVIATION

I will discuss two ways of calculating the SD, which can then be squared to provide the VAR: the deviation method and the computation method. Both methods have merit: the first is helpful to visualize how the measure is created, and the second is a simpler calculation.

The Deviation Method

The deviation method allows you to "see" what is happening with the numbers. In this formula, the "X" values are raw scores, "M" is the mean of the distribution, and "N" is the total number of scores in the distribution:

$$SD = \sqrt{\frac{\sum (X - M)^2}{N}}$$

As you can see, the formula uses deviation scores in the calculation (the "$X - M$" portion between the parentheses in the formula). Thus, the mean is subtracted from each score to obtain the deviation amount. These "$X - M$" values in the formula represent the deviation values shown in Figure 3.7. The deviation scores are squared, summed, and divided by the number of scores. Finally, the square root is taken to yield the SD. (If the square root were not taken, the resulting value would be the VAR.)

One curious aspect of the formula is that the deviation scores are *squared* and then the *square root* is taken of the entire calculation! This appears pointless until you consider some of the features of deviation scores that become important to later statistical procedures.

An example may help to illustrate the features of this formula and the process for calculating SD using the deviation method. Table 3.1 shows the example AP scores we used earlier in this chapter to discuss percentiles. (The data are also listed in Table 2.11.) As you can see, I placed the raw scores (AP scores, "X") in a column along with separate columns for the deviation scores $(X - M)$ and the squared deviation scores $(X - M)^2$. I included the mean values for each column.

You can see that the mean value for the deviation scores is "0.00" since, in a set of normally distributed values, there will be equal numbers of values that lay to the left and to the right of the mean. Adding them up in effect creates a zero total since there will be as many negative as positive values. Therefore, it is necessary to square all the values to avoid the effects of the negative and positive signs. Once the values are squared and divided by N, the formula puts everything under the square root sign to remove the earlier squaring of values. The formula thus provides a neat solution to avoid the negative and positive deviation values adding to zero.

Table 3.1 also shows the sum of the squared deviation scores to be 12,434.774 (see the last row of the table). Creating the final calculation shows the SD to be 20.028 for this sample of AP scores. Therefore, the typical AP test score in this class deviates 20.028 points from the mean of 53.68. The largest positive deviation value is 37.32 and the largest negative deviation is −43.68:

$$SD = \sqrt{\frac{\sum (X - M)^2}{N}} = \sqrt{\frac{12,434.774}{31}} = \sqrt{401.122} = 20.028$$

TABLE 3.1   Using the Deviation Method to Calculate SD

AP SCORES (X)	X – M	(X – M)²	
10	–43.68	1907.942	
24	–29.68	880.902	
25	–28.68	822.542	
27	–26.68	711.822	
30	–23.68	560.742	
34	–19.68	387.302	
36	–17.68	312.582	
38	–15.68	245.862	
40	–13.68	187.142	
44	–9.68	93.702	
45	–8.68	75.342	
46	–7.68	58.982	
49	–4.68	21.902	
50	–3.68	13.542	
51	–2.68	7.182	
53	–0.68	0.462	
56	2.32	5.382	
58	4.32	18.662	
59	5.32	28.302	
62	8.32	69.222	
63	9.32	86.862	
63	9.32	86.862	
66	12.32	151.782	
69	15.32	234.702	
72	18.32	335.622	
75	21.32	454.542	
78	24.32	591.462	
79	25.32	641.102	
82	28.32	802.022	
89	35.32	1247.502	
91	37.32	1392.782	
53.68	0.00	401.12	MEANS
		12434.774	SUM OF (X – M)²

The Average Deviation

I mentioned that the AD is the mean of the absolute values of the deviation scores. In this example, if we created a mean from the absolute value of each of the school ratios, the AD would equal to 16.57. (You can compute this in Excel by using the Formula menu and then choosing "Statistical" and then "AVEDEV.")

Why the discrepancy between the AD (16.57) and the SD (20.028)? There is a long answer and a short answer. The short answer is that the SD is based on calculations of the perfect normal distribution with known mathematical properties of the curve and based on large sample values. That is why the SD is known as standardized deviation to make use of these known properties and characteristics. The AD does not make reference to these properties; rather, it is simply the average (absolute) deviation from the mean of a distribution of values. Generally, it yields a slightly different value than the SD to account for the properties of the perfect normal distribution.

The Computation Method

The second method for calculating the SD is using the computation formula. It looks more complex than the deviation method, but it is much easier computationally since it does not involve creating the deviation values. The formula is as follows:

$$SD = \sqrt{\frac{\Sigma X^2 - \frac{(\Sigma X)^2}{N}}{N}}$$

Computing the SD with this formula involves only two columns, the column of values and the column of squared values. Table 3.2 shows the same AP scores with a second column of those scores squared. I included the second column as "X^2," indicating that each of the AP scores was squared. The bottom rows include some important results that allow us to use this computation formula:

Mean – This is the average of the AP scores.

(ΣX) – This value is simply adding up the AP scores.

$(\Sigma X)^2$ – This value is squaring the summed AP scores, or squaring the preceding value (ΣX).

ΣX^2 – This is the sum of the column of scores that have each been squared.

The values of $(\sum X)^2$ and $\sum X^2$ are quite different. The first value $(\sum X)^2$ is squaring the *sum of all the raw score values themselves (1664)*, yielding 2,768,896 (i.e., $1664^2 = 2{,}768{,}896$).

The second value $(\sum X^2)$ is obtained by adding up the values of *each of the raw scores that have already been squared*, yielding 101,754 (the sum of the "X^2" column).

When you use the values in the formula, you compute the same SD as you did with the deviation formula (with slight differences due to rounding):

$$SD = \sqrt{\frac{\Sigma X^2 - \frac{(\Sigma X)^2}{N}}{N}} = \sqrt{\frac{101{,}754 - \frac{(1664)^2}{31}}{31}} = \sqrt{\frac{12{,}434.78}{31}} = \boxed{20.028}$$

The Sum of Squares

The top part of both the deviation and computation formulas, under the radical sign, is known as the "sum of squares" since it is a global measure of all the variation in a distribution of scores. These measures will be important for later procedures that

TABLE 3.2 Using the Computation Method to Calculate SD

AP SCORES (X)	X^2
10	100
24	576
25	625
27	729
30	900
34	1156
36	1296
38	1444
40	1600
44	1936
45	2025
46	2116
49	2401
50	2500
51	2601
53	2809
56	3136
58	3364
59	3481
62	3844
63	3969
63	3969
66	4356
69	4761
72	5184
75	5625
78	6084
79	6241
82	6724
89	7921
91	8281

MEAN	**53.68**		
SUM OF X or (ΣX)	**1664**	**SUM OF X^2 or ΣX^2**	**101754**
SUM OF (X)^2 or (ΣX)^2	**2768896**		

analyze the differences between sets of scores by comparing VAR values. Remember these are equivalent formulas, with the second being an algebraically equal (computation) approach:

$$\sum(X-M)^2 \quad \text{or} \quad \sum X^2 - \frac{\left(\sum X\right)^2}{N}$$

POPULATION SD AND INFERENTIAL SD

I will have much more to say about this difference in later chapters when I discuss inferential statistics. For now, it is important to point out that computing SD for an entire set of *sample* values, as we did with the AP scores, will yield a different value depending on whether we understand the distribution of data to represent a complete set of scores by itself (i.e., as the entire population of AP scores) or as a sample set taken from an entire set of AP scores from all AP classes and used to make attributions about what the overall population SD should be (we designate this latter value as the inferential SD since we are using it to estimate the overall or population SD).[1]

Remember that inferential statistics differs from descriptive statistics primarily in the fact that, with inferential statistics, we are using sample values to make inferences or decisions about the populations from which the samples are thought to come. In descriptive statistics, we make no such attributions; rather, we simply measure the distribution of values at hand and treat all the values we have as the complete set of information (i.e., its own population). When we get to the inferential statistics chapters, you will find that *in order to make attributions about populations based on sample values, we typically must adjust the sample values since we are making estimates about what the populations look like.* To make better estimates of population values, we adjust the sample values.

Neither SPSS nor Excel distinguishes inferential or descriptive computations of SD in their typical outputs. Therefore, they present the *inferential* SD as the default value. Figure 3.8 shows the descriptive statistics output for our AP variable (from Excel). As you can see, the mean value (53.68) is the same as that reported in Table 3.1. However, the SD (the fifth shaded values from the top of the first column) is 20.36 according to this output. In our computations of the data, we calculated the SD to be 20.028. Thus, there is a discrepancy between our calculation of the population SD (which assumed the AP scores to be their own population) and the inferential SD result reported by Excel (which assumed that the AP scores were only a sample set of values that we can then use to estimate the entire set of AP scores in all AP classes, which is not possible to obtain).

You can obtain the population SD by using the formula menus of Excel as shown in Figure 3.9. As you can see, I have highlighted the "STDEV.P" choice of statistical functions which is the "SD of the population." This will calculate an SD based on all of a set of scores as if they constituted the entire population of scores. This value will be equivalent to the SD calculations we discussed previously. The Excel default value for the SD (the inferential SD) is also available in the list of functions as "STDEV.S."

---

[1] Some refer to the SD of a complete set of values by themselves as the "sample SD." This assumes that the sample values are NOT used to estimate a population SD. I try to remove some of the confusion by referring to this as the population SD. When this sample set (i.e., entire set of values) is used to estimate an unknown population value, it becomes an inferential SD.

AP Scores	
Mean	53.68
Standard Error	3.66
Median	53.00
Mode	63.00
Standard Deviation	20.36
Sample Variance	414.49
Kurtosis	−0.58
Skewness	−0.06
Range	81.00
Minimum	10.00
Maximum	91.00
Sum	1664.00
Count	31.00

Figure 3.8 The Excel descriptive statistics output for AP scores.

OBTAINING SD FROM EXCEL AND SPSS®

I demonstrated how to obtain the SD from Excel in the preceding section. Obtaining the SD from SPSS is straightforward, but, like Excel, it returns the inferential SD as the default value. Figure 3.10 shows the menu screens and options for creating descriptive statistics, including the SD. You can obtain the SD through the SPSS menus for Descriptive – Frequencies that we discussed in the previous sections regarding percentiles. Figure 3.3 showed how to use the Frequencies menus to obtain percentiles and included options for SD and means, among other measures. Figure 3.10 shows how to obtain the SD using the "Descriptive Statistics – Descriptives" menu.

Figure 3.11 shows the output from this procedure. As you can see, the listed SD is 20.359, the same (inferential SD) value reported in Excel (see Figure 3.8). Since this is the default inferential SD, you can use the Excel "SDEV.P" to calculate the population SD value or you can convert the inferential SD to the population SD using the following formula:

$$SD_{(Population)} = SD_{(Inferential)}\sqrt{\frac{N-1}{N}}$$

$$SD_{(Population)} = 20.359\sqrt{\frac{30}{31}} = 20.028$$

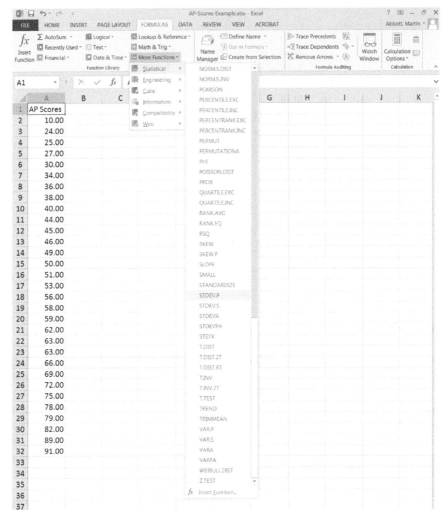

Figure 3.9   Using the Excel functions to calculate the "actual" SD.

Conversely, you can calculate the inferential SD <u>from</u> the population SD as follows:

$$SD_{(Inferential)} = SD_{(Population)} \sqrt{\frac{N}{N-1}}$$

Note the other descriptive statistics reported in Figure 3.11. The skewness and kurtosis values, when divided by their respective standard errors, are within bounds of a normal distribution (−0.14 and −0.70, respectively). The visual evidence suggests that the distribution of AP scores will appear close to a normally distributed set of data, which is confirmed by the histogram shown in Figure 3.12.

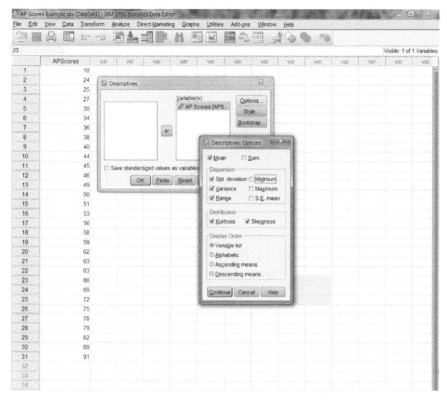

Figure 3.10   Using the "Descriptives" menus in SPSS®.

Descriptive Statistics

	N	Range	Mean	Std. Deviation	Variance	Skewness		Kurtosis	
	Statistic	Statistic	Statistic	Statistic	Statistic	Statistic	Std. Error	Statistic	Std. Error
AP Scores	31	81	53.68	20.359	414.492	−.059	.421	−.577	.821
Valid N (listwise)	31								

Figure 3.11   The Descriptive Statistics output from SPSS®.

A rule of thumb is that you cannot calculate an SD or VAR less than 0 or "negative variability." You can have small variation, or even no variation (e.g., where every score is the same), but never less than zero. This is one way to check whether you are calculating the VAR and SD correctly.

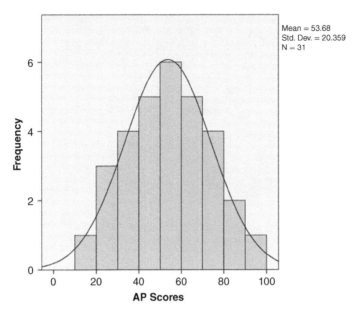

Figure 3.12   The AP score histogram from SPSS®.

TERMS AND CONCEPTS

Average deviation: The average deviation represents the mean of the absolute values of the deviation scores in a distribution.

Deciles: These measures break a frequency distribution into 10 equal groups using 9 cut points based on the 10th, 20th, 30th, 40th, 50th, 60th, 70th, 80th, and 90th percentiles.

Interquartile range: These scores represent the middle half of a frequency distribution since they represent the difference between the first and third quartiles (the 75th minus the 25th percentiles).

Normal curve equivalent (NCE) scores: These are transformed percentile scores that yield values with equal distances.

Percentile (or percentile rank):   Percentiles represent the point in a distribution of scores below which a given percentage of scores fall.

Population SD: This is the SD calculated on all the scores of a distribution of values and not used to estimate the SD of a larger sampling unit. The "actual" SD of a set of scores.

Quartiles: These are measures that divide the total set of scores in a distribution into four equal groups using the 25th, 50th, and 75th percentiles.

Range:	The range is the numerical difference between the highest and lowest scores in the distribution and represents a helpful global measure of the spread of scores.
Inferential SD:	The SD from a sample used to estimate a population SD. This is used in inferential statistics and is different from an SD used to represent *only* the values of the sample distribution of values ("population SD").
Standard deviation (SD):	The SD represents a *standard* distance between the mean and each score in the distribution. It is the square root of the variance (VAR).
Variance (VAR):	The variance is the average squared distance of the scores in a distribution from the mean. It is the squared SD.

DATA LAB AND EXAMPLES (WITH SOLUTIONS)

The following two problems will help you continue practice in central tendency. As with the practice problems in Chapter 1, the first is shorter so that you can try to do the calculations manually (use SPSS or Excel to check your work), and the second is designed to help you become familiar with both SPSS and Excel.

Problem 1

Table 3.3 shows an example of a combined rating of neighborhood characteristics among a sample of low-income housing residents. The ratings include respondents' perceptions of road quality, traffic flow, access to groceries, crime, and related perceptions. The ratings are measured from 1 to 100, with 100 as the highest.

TABLE 3.3   Neighborhood Characteristics Ratings Sample

Neighborhood Characteristics

33
72
81
45
64
53
63
64
80
70
54
70
56
47
62
91

Using the data from Table 3.3, respond to the following questions:
1. What are the population and inferential SD values?

Problem 2

Table 3.4 presents partial data from a housing survey I conducted some years ago. The Quality of Life Index was a compiled value that included residents' perceptions of health services, recreational opportunities, air quality, community involvement, fear of crime, and related measures.

TABLE 3.4   Housing Survey Data: Quality of Life Index

Quality Index (Modified)		
8	30	37
11	30	37
14	31	37
16	31	38
16	31	38
17	31	38
19	32	38
19	32	39
20	32	39
20	32	40
21	32	40
22	32	40
23	33	40
23	33	40
23	33	41
24	33	41
24	33	42
25	34	42
25	34	42
26	34	42
26	34	43
26	35	43
27	35	43
27	35	43
27	35	43
27	35	44
27	36	44
28	36	45
28	36	45
28	36	46
29	36	48
29	36	49
30	37	50
30	37	51
30	37	53

Conduct analyses in SPSS and Excel that provide the following:

1. Mean, SD, variance, skewness, and kurtosis

2. Population and inferential SD values

3. Histogram

4. Comment on your results from the previous analyses.

DATA LAB: SOLUTIONS

Problem 1

1. What are the population and inferential SD values?

Figure 3.13 shows the values used to calculate the population SD and inferential SD figures, which are both listed at the bottom of the table. You can calculate

Ratings	X^2
33	1089
72	5184
81	6561
45	2025
64	4096
53	2809
63	3969
64	4096
80	6400
70	4900
54	2916
70	4900
51	2601
62	3844
91	8281

MEAN	63.53		
SUM OF X OR	953	**SUM OF X^2**	63671
(ΣX)		**OR ΣX^2**	
SUM OF (X)^2	908209		
OR (ΣX)^2			
SD (POP)	14.4308		
SD (Inferential)	14.937		

Figure 3.13 The solution for Problem 1.

Descriptive Statistics

| | N | Range | Minimum | Maximum | Sum | Mean | Std. Deviation | Variance | Skewness | | Kurtosis | |
	Statistic	Statistic	Statistic	Statistic	Statistic	Statistic	Statistic	Statistic	Statistic	Std. Error	Statistic	Std. Error
Quality of life index-Modified	105	45	8	53	3475	33.10	8.839	78.125	-.339	.236	.085	.467
Valid N (listwise)	105											

Figure 3.14 The SPSS® output for Problem 2.

the inferential SD from the population SD using the formulas shown in the section "OBTAINING SD FROM EXCEL AND SPSS®."

Problem 2

In what follows, I provide SPSS and Excel figures for responding to Problem 2 questions (from data shown in Table 3.4).
1. Mean, SD, variance, skewness, and kurtosis
   Figures 3.14 and 3.15 show the SPSS and Excel output (respectively) for this part of the question. As you can see, the answers are shown in the shaded areas of the two output figures.

Quality of Life Index	
Mean	33.10
Standard Error	0.86
Median	34.00
Mode	32.00
Standard Deviation	8.84
Sample Variance	78.13
Kurtosis	0.08
Skewness	-0.34
Range	45.00
Minimum	8.00
Maximum	53.00
Sum	3475.00
Count	105.00

Figure 3.15   The Excel output for Problem 2.

2. Population and inferential SD values
   The (inferential) SD is 8.839.
   The (population) SD is 8.797.

3. Histogram Figure 3.16 shows the SPSS histogram for the Quality of Life data.

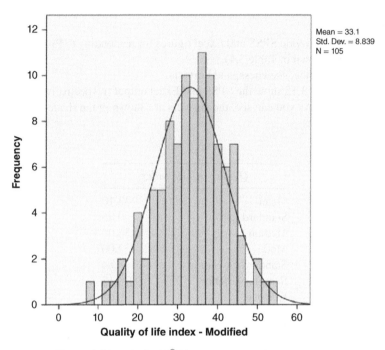

Figure 3.16   The SPSS® histogram output for Problem 2.

4. Comment on your results from the previous analyses

The results of the analyses we conducted indicate that the Quality of Life data can be assumed to be normally distributed, based on the variability, skewness, and kurtosis figures. The histogram provides a visual depiction of the data, which appears to generally confirm the numerical findings.

4

THE NORMAL DISTRIBUTION

Thus far, we have discussed how to describe distributions of raw scores graphically and in terms of central tendency, variability, skewness, and kurtosis. We will continue to perform these calculations since most all of the statistical procedures we will discuss in subsequent chapters require that data be normally distributed. Using what we have learned with calculating these descriptive statistics, we can confirm whether our data are normally distributed or if we must use different procedures. Often, even if the variables are not strictly or exactly normally distributed, we can still use them since many statistical procedures are "robust" or able to provide meaningful and precise results even if there are some violations of the normal distribution assumptions.

THE NATURE OF THE NORMAL CURVE

The normal distribution, as I explained earlier, is very common in social science and health sciences research, so we need to deepen our understanding of some of the properties of the normal *curve*. I call the normal distribution a curve since the histogram forms a curve when the top midpoints of the bars are joined together. Technically, this is called a *frequency polygon*. If you look back to Figure 3.12, you will see the SPSS® histogram for the AP score distribution of raw scores we discussed. In the figure, SPSS overlaid the normal curve on top of the histogram, so you can see the extent to which the data approximate a normal distribution. As you can see from that figure, if you were to connect the top midpoints with a line, it would not be the

Using Statistics in the Social and Health Sciences with SPSS® and Excel®, First Edition.
Martin Lee Abbott.
© 2017 John Wiley & Sons, Inc. Published 2017 by John Wiley & Sons, Inc.

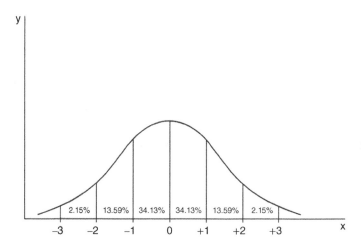

Figure 4.1   The normal curve with known properties.

smooth line you see but rather a more jagged line. However, as a database increases its size, the histogram approximates the smooth normal curve in variables that are normally distributed; the jagged line becomes filled in as more cases are added.

When we speak of the normal distribution and how our sample data set is normally distributed, we actually speak about our data *approximating* a normal distribution. We refer to the *perfect* normal distribution as an ideal so that we have a model distribution for comparison to our actual data. Thus, the normal curve is a kind of perfect ruler with known features and dimensions. In fact, we can mathematically chart the perfect normal curve and derive a picture of how the areas under the curve are distributed. Because of these features, we refer to the perfect normal distribution as a *standard normal distribution*.

Look at Figure 2.12, which is reproduced here as Figure 4.1. As you can see, the perfect normal curve is represented as having known proportions of the total area between the mean and given standard deviation (SD) units. A standard normal curve (also known as a *z distribution*) has a mean of 0 and an SD of 1.0. This is always a bit puzzling until you consider how the mean and SD are calculated. Since a perfect distribution has equal numbers of scores lying to the left and to the right of the mean, calculating the mean is akin to adding positive and negative values resulting in 0. Dividing 0 by N, of whatever size, will always equal to 0. Therefore, the mean of a perfect standard normal distribution is equal to 0.

The standard normal distribution has an SD equal to 1 unit. This is simply an easy way to designate the known areas under the curve. Figure 4.1 shows that there are six SD units that capture almost all the cases under the perfect normal curve area. (This is the source of the rule for the range equaling six times the SD in a raw score distribution.) This is how the standard normal curve is "arranged" mathematically. So, for example, 13.59% of the area of the normal curve lies between the first (+1) and second (+2) SD on the right side of the mean. Since the curve is symmetrical, there is also 13.59% of the area of the curve between the first (−1) and second (−2) SD on the left side of the curve and so on.

Remember that this is an ideal distribution. As such, we can compare our actual data distributions to it as a way of understanding our own raw data better. Also, we can use it to compare two sets of raw score data since we have a perfect measuring stick that relates to both sets of "imperfect" data.

There are other features of the standard normal distribution we should notice:

- The scores cluster in the middle and "thin out" toward either ends.
- It is a balanced or symmetrical distribution, with equal numbers of scores on either side of the middle.
- The mean, median, and mode all fall on the same point.
- The curve is "asymptotic" to the *x*-axis. This means that it gets closer and closer to the *x*-axis but never touches since, in theory, there may be a case very far from the other scores – off the chart, so to speak. There has to be room under the curve for these kinds of possibilities.
- The *inflection point* of the standard normal curve is at the point of the (negative and positive) first SD unit. This point is where the steep decline of the curve slows down and widens out. (This is a helpful visual cue to an advanced procedure called *factor analysis*, which uses a *scree plot* to help decide how many factors to use from the results.)

THE STANDARD NORMAL SCORE: *Z SCORE*

When we refer to the standard normal deviation, we speak of the "z score," which is a very important measure in statistics. *A z score is a raw score expressed in SD units.* Thus, a z score of 0.67 would represent a raw score that is two-thirds of one SD to the right of the mean. These scores are shown on the *x*-axis of Figure 4.1 and represent the SD values that define the areas of the distribution. Thus, +1 SD unit to the right of the mean contains 34.13% of the area under the standard normal curve (from the mean), and we can refer to this point as a z score of +1. So, if a given AP test score had a z score of 3.5, we would recognize immediately that this school would have an inordinately high raw score, relative to the other values, since it would fall three and

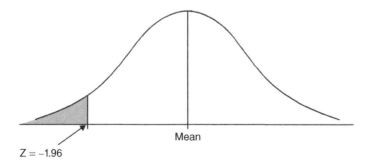

Figure 4.2 The location of $z = (-)1.96$.

one-half SDs above the mean where there is only an extremely small percent of the curve represented.

Because it has standardized meaning, the z score allows us to understand where each score resides compared to the entire set of scores in the distribution. It also allows us to compare one individual's performance on two different sets of (normally distributed) scores. It is important to note that z scores are expressed not just in whole numbers but as decimal values, as I used in the example earlier. Thus, a z score of -1.96 would indicate that the raw score is slightly less than two SDs below the mean on a standard normal curve as shown in Figure 4.2.

THE Z SCORE TABLE OF VALUES

Statisticians use a table of values to help researchers understand how various scores in the standard normal distribution relate to the total area under the curve. Consider the (partial) table in Figure 4.3. This is the first half of the Z Score Table you will find in Appendix C. (The entire table is in two pages with z score values of 0.06–0.09.) The Z Score Table has an initial column for the "root" of the z score (i.e., the z score in tenths) and separate panels for adding hundredths in various amounts to the root. There are two columns in each of these panels to help locate the percentages in reference to the mean (first column graph) and in reference to the tail of the distribution (second column graph).

This table of values is based on *proportions of the area under the normal curve relative to the mean and various z scores.* Since the total proportion of the area under the normal curve is 1.0 and the total area is 100%, you can interpret the values in the table as *percentages* of the area within the distribution. The shaded graphs at the top of each column of the panels indicate the proportion of the curve in relationship to specific z score values.

As you can see, the table is laid out in such a way that you can locate the relevant proportions for given z scores under the curve. The set of z scores represented in Figure 4.3 in the last panel (with shaded values) is a z score of "0.05" since it combines the "root" of 0.0 (in the far left column) with the 0.05 column of proportions in the hundredths panel to represent a z score of 0.05 (0.00 + 0.05 = 0.05).

Each z score has two reference panels illustrated by two shaded graphs at the top (hundredths). In the left part of the "0.05" panel, each z score value is represented in the table in such a way that you can identify the percent of the area in the normal curve

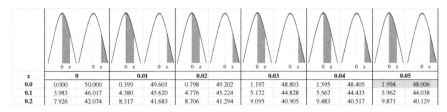

z	0		0.01		0.02		0.03		0.04		0.05	
0.0	0.000	50.000	0.399	49.601	0.798	49.202	1.197	48.803	1.595	48.405	1.994	48.006
0.1	3.983	46.017	4.380	45.620	4.776	45.224	5.172	44.828	5.567	44.433	5.962	44.038
0.2	7.926	42.074	8.317	41.683	8.706	41.294	9.095	40.905	9.483	40.517	9.871	40.129

Figure 4.3   The (partial) Z Score Table of Values.

that is <u>between a given z score and the mean of the distribution</u>. As you can see, the graph shows this in the shaded region to the right of the mean up to the z score in question. The table reports this value as 1.994 for a z score of 0.05. Thus, 1.994% of the area of the standard normal curve lies between the mean and a z score of 0.05.

The right graph of the two data columns in the panel shows the percent of the area of the curve that lies in the "tail" of the distribution or the percent of the area that lies <u>beyond</u> the given z score. In the 0.05 z score panel, this would mean that 48.006% of the area under the normal curve lies beyond (i.e., to the right) a z score of 0.05.

It is important to note that the proportions in the table are <u>symmetrical</u>. That is, z scores of -0.05 (i.e., negative) have the same proportions as z scores of 0.05 (i.e., positive) except that they have references on the left side (negative) of the curve. The sign of negative or positive does not affect the location of the value in the table since the values in the table are symmetrical; they apply to both "sides" of the distribution equally. The sign is crucial to remember, however, since it indicates the *direction of the score in relation to the mean*. Negative scores are located to the left of the mean, as shown in Figure 4.2, and positive scores are located to the right of the mean.

To take the example shown in Figure 4.2 (where $z = -1.96$), you would find the "tenths" part of the score (1.9) in the first column of the Z Score Table of Values, titled "z," and then follow that row across until you found the "hundredths" part of the score (in the "0.06" column). When combined, the score of -1.96 (i.e., $1.9 + 0.06$) indicates a value of "47.50" (or 47.50%) in the left column of the 0.06 panel. This number indicates the percent of the curve between the mean and the z score of -1.96. Since -1.96 is almost 2 SDs below the mean, you can do a quick mental check to see if this is reasonable by looking at Figure 4.1.

Since there is 34.13% between the mean and the first SD and another 13.59% between the first and second SDs, then the combined total of 47.72% (adding the percentages together) shows the percent of the curve between the mean and the second SD. This value is very close to the table value (47.50%) for $z = -1.96$.

Alternatively, the second column of the 0.06 panel shows a value of 2.500, which indicates that 2.500% of the area under the curve lies beyond (in this case, to the left) a z score of -1.96. Note that adding the left and right columns of numbers (47.50 and 2.50) yields 50%, or half of the entire curve. This is because the table applies equally to both halves of the curve to yield a total 100% of the area under the curve.

NAVIGATING THE Z SCORE DISTRIBUTION

It is a good idea to familiarize yourself with the z score table since you may need to visualize where certain scores are in relation to one another in the z distribution. You can also use the table to create "cumulative proportions" of the normal curve at certain z score values. Cumulative proportions are simply the summed percentages or proportions of the area in the normal distribution. Percentiles represent one such proportion measure since they are by definition the percent of the scores below a given score. You can also calculate cumulative proportions that exist *above* given z scores in the same fashion using the z score table. Here is an example.

If you are interested in the percentage of scores that lie below a given score (as you would in the calculation of a percentile), you can use the z score table to help you. *What percentage of the standard normal curve lies below a z score of 1.96?*
Before you consider your answer in detail, try to create a "ballpark" solution:

- We are looking for a score almost two SDs <u>above</u> the mean (1.96).
- The percentage distribution in the standard normal curve (see Figure 4.1) is 34.13% between the mean and SD 1 and 13.59% between SD 1 and SD 2.
- Therefore, about 47.72% of the curve (34.13% + 13.59%) lies between the mean and a z score of 1.96.
- Since the score is to the right of the mean, you will need to add 50% (the other half of the distribution) to 47.72% to get an approximate of 97.72% of the curve lying below $z = 1.96$.

Now, compare this ballpark answer to a more precise method of using the z score table.

- Locate 1.96 in the table of values as we did earlier using the table in Figure 4.3. The value is 47.50% of the distribution which lies between the mean and the score of 1.96 (shown in the first column of the 0.06 panel). Remember 47.50% *IS NOT THE ENTIRE AMOUNT OF THE CURVE BELOW* 1.96. It is only the amount of the curve that lies between the mean and the z score of 1.96.
- Add 50% (the other half of the curve) to the table value to yield 97.50% of the distribution lying below a z score of 1.96. Remember, because the curve is symmetrical, each side contains 50.00 (50%). Therefore, you must add the 50.00% from the left half of the curve to the 47.50% from the right half. This would yield a total of 97.50% of the curve below a z score of 1.96.
- This percentage (97.50%) is slightly less than the <u>estimated</u> percentage (97.72%) since the target score is slightly less than 2 SDs (i.e., 1.96 SDs versus 2.00 SDs).
- Figure 4.4 shows this identification.

The process is the same for negative z score values. Take the example of -1.96. *What percent of the curve lies below a z score of -1.96?* Using the ballpark estimate method:

- We know from the standard normal curve that a score 2 SDs from the mean (either above or below) contains about 47.72% of the distribution (i.e., 34.13% between the mean and SD 1 plus 13.59% between SD 1 and SD 2).
- Since we need the percent of the distribution <u>below</u> -1.96, we need to subtract 47.72% from 50%, the total area in the left half of the distribution.
- This results in <u>approximately</u> 2.28% of the distribution below $z = -1.96$.

Now, using the Z Score Table of Values, create a more precise calculation of the percent of the distribution below $z = -1.96$.

- Locate 1.96 in the table of values using the Z Score Table of Values in Appendix C. The value is 47.50% of the distribution which lies between the mean and the score of 1.96 (since the table identifies the percentages for either positive or negative values).
- Subtract this amount from 50% (the left half of the curve) to get 2.50% of the distribution lying below a z score of -1.96. Since you are not interested in the percentage of the distribution that lies above the score of -1.96, you must "subtract it out" of the entire half of the distribution (50%) to see what percentage lies below the given scores.
- This percentage (2.50%) is slightly greater than the estimated percentage (2.28%) since the target score is slightly closer to the mean, leaving a greater area to the left of the target score of -1.96.
- Figure 4.5 shows this identification.
- Note that you can also identify this same amount (2.50%) using the second column of the panel in the 0.06 panel in the Z Score Table of Values since this proportion is in the "tail" of the distribution to the left of the score (i.e., below a negative z score). Since the table is symmetrical, you can see that the percent of the area in the right (positive) tail would be equivalent to the area in the left (negative) tail, which is the area you sought to solve the problem.

CALCULATING PERCENTILES

You will notice that the two examples in Figures 4.4 and 4.5 show how to identify a *percentile.* This is a special feature of using the cumulative proportions in the standard normal distribution and one that we will revisit in subsequent sections.

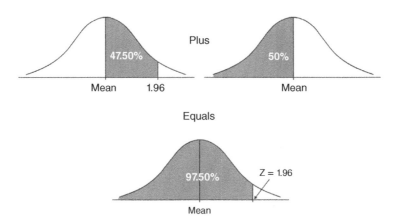

Figure 4.4 Using the Z Score Table to identify the percent of the distribution below a z score.

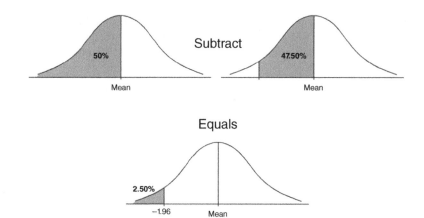

Figure 4.5   Using the Z Score Table of Values to identify the percent of the distribution below $z = -1.96$.

CREATING RULES FOR LOCATING Z SCORES

Some statisticians and researchers like to create rules for the operations we discussed earlier. Thus, for example, we might create the following rules:

1. For locating the percent of the distribution lying below a positive z score, add the tabled value to the 50% from the other half of the distribution.
2. For locating the percent of the distribution lying below a negative z score, subtract the tabled value from the 50% of the left half of the distribution.

While these may be helpful to some students, they can also be confusing since there are so many different research questions that could be asked. Generating a rule for each question would present an additional burden for the student to remember! Here is another example that illustrates this point. *What percent of the standard normal curve lies between a z score of −1.96 and −1.35?*

Look at Figure 4.6, which illustrates the solution to this problem.

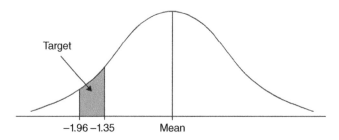

Figure 4.6   Identifying the area between z scores.

Visualizing the distribution is helpful so that you can keep the "order of operations" straight.

- Using the Z Score Table of Values, you find that 47.50% of the curve lies between the mean and −1.96.
- The Z Score Table of Values identifies 41.15% of the area between the mean and −1.35.
- Subtracting these areas yields 6.35% as the total area of the distribution that lies between z scores of −1.96 and −1.35 (i.e., 47.50% − 41.15% = 6.35%).

Figures 4.7 and 4.8 show the visual progression that will enable you to answer this question. Figure 4.7 shows the areas between the mean and the different z scores (i.e., the tabled values), and Figure 4.8 shows how to treat the two areas to respond to the question.

If we created a rule for this operation, it would be something like "in order to identify the area between two negative z scores, subtract the tabled values of the two scores." Again, this might be useful but adds to the list of rules we already generated earlier.

Other situations for which we would need to generate rules would be as follows:

- Identifying the area between two positive z scores
- Identifying the area between one positive z score and one negative z score
- Identifying the area that lies above a negative z score
- Identifying the area that lies above a positive z score

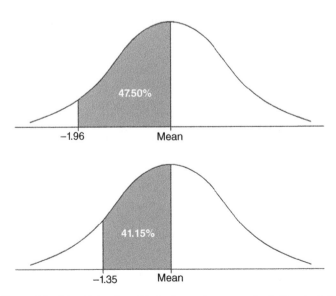

Figure 4.7   Identifying the tabled values of z scores of −1.96 and −1.35.

There are many other potential rules as well. My overall point is that I think it is better to *visualize* the distribution and then highlight which area percentage you need to identify. In this method, there is only one rule: *Draw a picture of the curve and shade in the portion of the curve that you need to identify.*

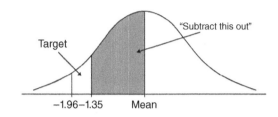

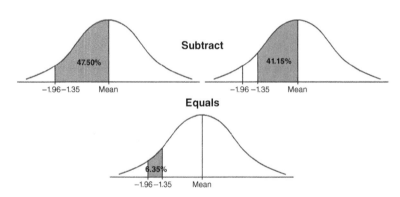

Figure 4.8   Subtracting the areas to identify the given area of the distribution.

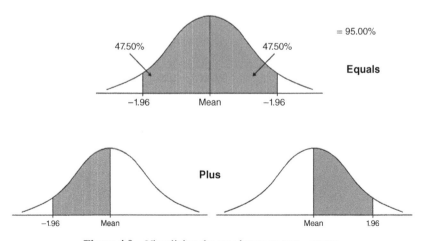

Figure 4.9   Visualizing the area between two *z* scores.

Here is an example for you to visualize. *What percentage of the distribution falls between the z scores of −1.96 and +1.96?* This one might be easy now that we have used these values before, but if you use the "visualization" method, simply draw a normal distribution freehand and shade in the target area (i.e., the percentage of the distribution you need to answer the question). It might look like the drawings in Figure 4.9.

Visualization provides the approach to answer any such question. Essentially, after drawing the figures, you can use the table of values to identify the shaded areas in any way you need to respond to the question. Memorizing all the possible rules for identification of percentages of areas seems to me to be more burdensome and complex.

CALCULATING Z SCORES

Z scores are important scores because they provide a perfect standard of measurement to compare raw score distributions that may not be perfectly normally distributed. Remember, the standard normal curve is a perfect curve. Real-life distributions make the assumption that the raw score data *approximate* a normal distribution.

Raw score distributions like the AP Scores example we discussed in Chapter 3 (see Figure 3.12) appeared to be near normally distributed but still not perfectly so. Because raw score distributions are not always perfectly distributed, you must perform numerical descriptive analyses to see if they are within normal boundaries. Thus, by looking at the skewness and kurtosis of a distribution, you can see if the raw score distribution is balanced and close to a normal shape; if the mean, median, and mode are on the same point that is another indication that the data approximate a normal distribution. Finally, we can use the visual evidence of the histogram and frequency polygon to help us understand the shape of the distribution.

Suppose a similar set of AP test scores from another semester have a mean of 100 and an SD of 15. Suppose that a student's score on the test is 120 and she calls

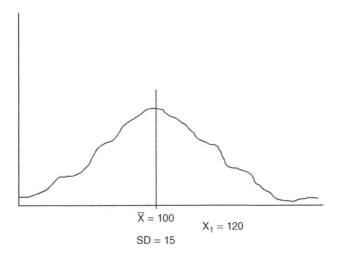

Figure 4.10   An example AP raw score distribution.

to inquire about how she performed on the test. What would you tell her? Look at Figure 4.10.

The distribution of raw scores is not perfect since it is based on scores derived from real life and probably not on a large group. For the purposes of the research and after assessing skewness, kurtosis, and so on, we might assume that the data are normally distributed. The difficulty is that, since it is not the standard normal curve with known proportions under each area of the curve, we cannot use the method we just described for computing a percentile (the percent of the scores that lie below the student's score). We can tell the student that she scored more than 1 SD above the mean, if that would be of value to her. What we really need, however, is to translate the student's raw score of 120 into a z score so that we can calculate a meaningful percentile.

Before we do this however, we might try our estimation skills just by looking at the raw score information. The student's score is 120, which is 20 points above the mean. Since the SD is 15, that means that the student's score of 120 is 1 and 1/3 SD above the mean (or approximately 1.33 SDs). Thus a ballpark estimate of a percentile is as follows:

- 50% (left half of distribution)
- +34.13% (distance between mean and SD 1)
- +4.48% (approximately 0.33 of the distance between SD 1 and SD 2)
- Total estimate = cumulative proportion of 88.61% or the 89th percentile

We can *transform* raw scores to z scores in order to understand where the scores in a raw score distribution fall in relation to the other scores by making use of the standard normal distribution. This process involves visualizing and calculating where a certain raw score would fall on a standard normal distribution. That is, we would "translate" the x (raw score) to a z (standard score) to enable us to understand where the raw score is in relation to its own mean and so on. (I like to think of this as "ecstasy" since we are transforming "x" values to "z" values: "x" to "z"!) In doing so we are using the standard normal curve as a kind of yardstick to help us compare information that we observe in real life.

The formula for transforming raw score values (x) to standard normal scores (z) is as follows, where X is the raw score, M is the mean, and SD is the standard deviation of the group of scores:

$$Z = \frac{X - M}{SD}$$

In the earlier example, we can use the standard normal distribution to transform the student's raw score of 120 to a z score that contains more accurate information. Thus,

$$Z = \frac{120 - 100}{15} = \frac{20}{15} = 1.33$$

With the Z of 1.33, the percentile is calculated as follows:

- Distance of Z score (1.33) from the mean = 40.824%.

- Add 50% from left half of z distribution.
- Percentile is 91st (90.824% of the curve lies below this point).

We can therefore report to the student that her score of 120 on the AP test is in the 91st percentile: not a bad result if you are comparing one student's performance to the others.

Here is another example using the AP test data from Chapter 3 (see Table 3.1). Consider a student who scores 50 on the AP test. You can identify where 50 falls in relation to the other test scores, but how many "SD units" above the mean does this score represent?

$$Z = \frac{X - M}{SD}$$

Using this formula and the data reported in Chapter 3 ($M = 53.68$, SD $= 20.028$), we can calculate the value of the z score:

$$Z = \frac{X - M}{SD} = \frac{50 - 53.68}{20.028} = (-)0.184$$

Mathematically, the formula transforms raw scores into SD units, which is the definition of a z score. Remember that z scores in the standard normal curve are expressed in SD units. The numerator $(X - M)$ identifies how far the raw score is from its mean or the deviation amount. When the deviation amount is divided by SD, the denominator, it transforms the deviation amount into SD units, since dividing something by a number creates a solution with the characteristics of that number. (It is like miles per hour created from the number of miles divided by time; the result is distance per unit of time.)

The raw score of 50 in our example translates to a z score of −0.184. Therefore:

- The raw score lies slightly below the mean and is therefore a negative value.
- Since it is a negative z score, you would use the Z Score Table of Values *as you would if it were positive since the table is symmetrical*: 7.142% of values lie between the z score and the mean, therefore 42.858% of scores lie below the score (50 − 7.142% = 42.858%).
- Note: Since the Z Score Table of Values identifies z scores to only two decimal places, round your target z score to two decimal places (i.e., for −0.184, use −0.18).
- Alternate use of the Z Score Table of Values: "Using the Tail column" of the z value of 0.18, you can see that 42.858% of the scores lie below the z score of −0.184).
- The raw score of 50 represents the 43rd percentile.

Figure 4.11 shows the histogram for the AP scores. The raw score distribution is not perfect, but transforming the raw score values to z scores allows you to more accurately describe the position of a given raw score relative to the other raw scores.

The bottom line of these examples is that we can use the standard normal distribution to help us understand our raw score distributions better. We can translate raw

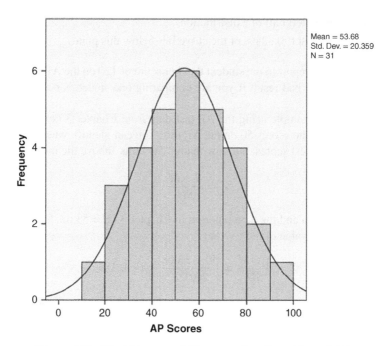

Figure 4.11   The histogram of AP score values (from Figure 3.12).

scores to z scores in order to see how they relate to the other scores in their own distribution. There are other uses of the standard normal distribution that we will examine in subsequent sections.

WORKING WITH RAW SCORE DISTRIBUTIONS

When you work with raw score distributions, just remember that in order to compare student scores, you need first to transform them to z scores so that you can use the perfection of the standard normal curve to help you understand the original raw scores. As is critical in an approach to using statistics for social and health sciences, consider what research question is being asked; what is the specific nature of the question? What ultimate outcome is required? Using the visualization and estimation processes we discussed ealier, you can proceed with z transformations and calculation of percentiles, if that is the desired outcome.

USING SPSS® TO CREATE Z SCORES AND PERCENTILES

Creating Z Scores

Using SPSS to create z scores is very easy using the "Descriptives – Descriptives" selection from the "Analyze" menu. Figure 4.12 shows the specification window in

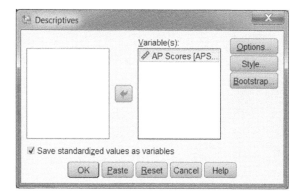

Figure 4.12   Using SPSS® to create z scores.

which I have identified the AP Scores from the data I used in Chapter 3. I can use the "Options" button to further specify mean, skewness, and a variety of other statistical procedures. However, I can create z scores by simply checking the box at the lower left corner of the Descriptives menu window shown in Figure 4.12 as the box "Save standardized values as variables." Checking this box results in a new variable being added to the data set, one consisting of the z score values corresponding to the raw score values of the (AP scores) variable selected. It is called "ZAPScores" in this case, which is simply the name of the original variable with a "Z" on the front to indicate that the values are z scores. Figure 4.13 shows the new variable besides the original. (Please remember that the z scores created in SPSS use the inferential SD, so they will be slightly different if you used the population SD.)

Creating Percentiles in SPSS®

There are a variety of ways to create percentiles in SPSS, but one way provides a broad transformation from the raw data. Since SPSS uses the inferential SD, however, the percentiles will not match exactly those you create using the population SD. Review the discussion in Chapter 3 (see Section "USING SPSS® AND EXCEL TO IDENTIFY PERCENTILES") to show how to use the SPSS procedure.

Figure 4.14 shows the specification menu for the "Analyze – Descriptive Statistics – Frequencies" procedure in which we can use SPSS more specifically for locating a percentile for a specific raw score. As you can see, just make sure that the box in the lower left of the menu entitled "Display frequency tables" is checked.

This procedure results in the output shown in Figure 4.15. As you can see, the table shown in Figure 4.15 lists the Cumulative Percent for each of the raw scores. By definition, this column of values identifies percentiles. In the earlier example, we identified the raw score of 50 as the 43rd percentile. You can see in Figure 4.15 that 41.9% of the scores lie below a raw score of 50, indicating that this raw score represents the 42nd percentile. (This represents a slight deviation from the 43rd percentile we calculated earlier, due to the precision of the Z Score Table of Values.)

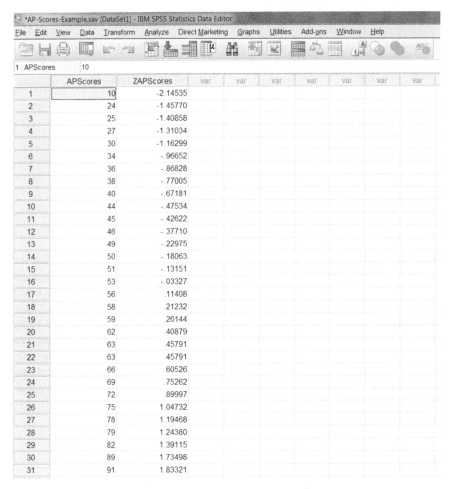

Figure 4.13 Creating a z score variable using SPSS® descriptive menu.

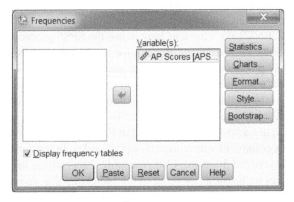

Figure 4.14 Using the SPSS® Frequencies menu to locate percentiles.

AP Scores

		Frequency	Percent	Valid Percent	Cumulative Percent
Valid	10	1	3.2	3.2	3.2
	24	1	3.2	3.2	6.5
	25	1	3.2	3.2	9.7
	27	1	3.2	3.2	12.9
	30	1	3.2	3.2	16.1
	34	1	3.2	3.2	19.4
	36	1	3.2	3.2	22.6
	38	1	3.2	3.2	25.8
	40	1	3.2	3.2	29.0
	44	1	3.2	3.2	32.3
	45	1	3.2	3.2	35.5
	46	1	3.2	3.2	38.7
	49	1	3.2	3.2	41.9
	50	1	3.2	3.2	45.2
	51	1	3.2	3.2	48.4
	53	1	3.2	3.2	51.6
	56	1	3.2	3.2	54.8
	58	1	3.2	3.2	58.1
	59	1	3.2	3.2	61.3
	62	1	3.2	3.2	64.5
	63	2	6.5	6.5	71.0
	66	1	3.2	3.2	74.2
	69	1	3.2	3.2	77.4
	72	1	3.2	3.2	80.6
	75	1	3.2	3.2	83.9
	78	1	3.2	3.2	87.1
	79	1	3.2	3.2	90.3
	82	1	3.2	3.2	93.5
	89	1	3.2	3.2	96.8
	91	1	3.2	3.2	100.0
	Total	31	100.0	100.0	

Figure 4.15   Using the SPSS® Frequencies output to locate percentiles.

USING EXCEL TO CREATE Z SCORES

In Chapter 3, I described how to use Excel to obtain percentiles. Please refer to that section to refresh your memory for that procedure. In this section, I show how to use Excel to create Z scores.

STANDARDIZE Function

This function, accessible in the same way as the other Excel statistical, makes use of the z score transformation formula we discussed earlier:

$$Z = \frac{X - M}{SD}$$

Figure 4.16 shows the specification of the values we are using in STANDARD-IZE to create a z score. Note that I chose a raw score (X) value of 50, in our earlier example, and I entered the mean (53.68) and the (population) SD (20.028). I chose to use the population SD (which I created using the STDEVP function and by calculation) rather than the default inferential SD used by Excel. Choosing the OK button results in the z score value being pasted into the cell I choose in the spreadsheet. However, you can see that the z score is also listed below the three input values as $z = -0.18374276$. You can calculate the same value using a calculator as I demonstrated earlier:

$$Z = \frac{X - M}{SD} = \frac{50 - 53.68}{20.028} = (-)0.184$$

The STANDARDIZE function therefore uses the z score transformation formula to return z scores from specified raw scores when you provide the mean and SD.

By the way, you can get the same outcome by *directly* entering the formula into a spreadsheet cell. If you look at Figure 4.17, you will see that I entered the formula directly into the cell (B15) adjacent to the value I want to transform to a z score (50) by selecting a cell outside the data and hitting the "=" key. This allows you to create

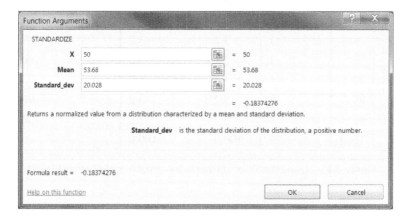

Figure 4.16   The Function Argument STANDARDIZE with AP score data.

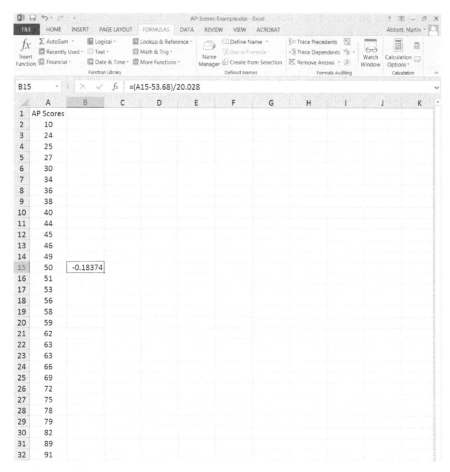

Figure 4.17   Entering formulas directly in Excel using the enter formula ("=") key.

the z score formula directly into the Excel spreadsheet. You can see the resulting formula in the formula window located in the band directly above the label row in the spreadsheet and just below the top menu ribbon as

$$(\text{“} = (A15 - 53.68)/20.028\text{”})$$

This formula shows the appropriate raw score location in the spreadsheet and the values (mean and SD) we calculated earlier. I entered the formula into a cell I selected adjacent to the column of data (in this case, I chose cell B15) and hit the "Enter" key, and Excel returned the value of (-0.18374), the z score transformation of the raw score value of 50.

As I discussed, using the equals sign notifies Excel that you are entering a formula. I did so in B15 (see Figure 4.17), but it is not listed since, for this example, I wanted to show how the value is returned and how Excel places the formula in the formula bar. If I make an error, I can make corrections in that band more easily than in the cell where I input the formula.

I used this example for another reason. You can use Excel to "replicate" actions by selecting and dragging cells. So, in the formula I created, I specified a cell location (B15) in the formula rather than inputting the raw score value of 50. If I choose, I could "drag" the formula in cell B15 down (or up) the B column. You can do this by selecting the cell with the formula (B15 in this example); when you move your cursor around that cell, you will see a variety of cursor styles. By hovering over the bottom right corner of the cell, you get a cursor style that looks like a "+" sign. By clicking and holding this cursor, drag the formula in cell B15 down the B column, and Excel will replicate the formula for each value in the adjacent data column (column A in this example). Figure 4.18 shows the results of this operation for the raw score values higher than an AP score of 50.

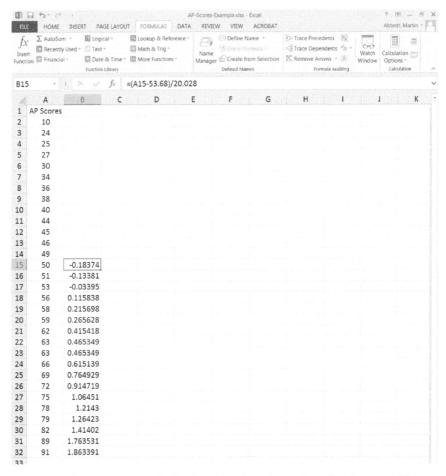

Figure 4.18 Entering formulas by dragging a formula to other values in a spreadsheet.

You can see the z scores in column B that correspond to the raw scores in Column A. For example, row 20, column A shows a raw score value of 59, and column B, row 20, shows this to be a z score of 0.265628. (Confirm this with your calculator.) Likewise, the raw score value of 53 (in column A, row 17) shows a transformation to a z score of −0.03395 (in column B, row 17). This procedure is a quick way to generate z score values from a set of raw scores in Excel.

USING EXCEL AND SPSS® FOR DISTRIBUTION DESCRIPTIONS

Excel has other ways of calculating z scores and cumulative proportions. I will review two of these later. The names of the functions are similar, so they may be confusing, but they are quite different. The NORM.S.DIST function calculates the cumulative proportion of the normal distribution below a given z score which you enter. The NORM.DIST function calculates the cumulative proportion of the normal distribution below a point that is calculated from the raw score, mean, and SD values (i.e., the data upon which a z score is calculated) which you enter.

NORM.S.DIST Function

This Excel function is quite helpful since it reports from an embedded z score table of values. It is quite simple to use. Figure 4.19 shows the NORM.S.DIST function submenu deriving from the Statistics formula menus. The user simply inputs a z score, and Excel returns the proportion of the standard normal distribution that lies below this value (essentially, the percentile).

As you can see from Figure 4.19, I entered a z score of −0.18374 from our earlier example. In this function, I specify "TRUE" in the "Cumulative" field to obtain the proportion of the distribution below the z score value. The value "0.427108714" is returned immediately below the two data windows. Thus, 0.427108714 proportion of the distribution lies below the given z score. It is therefore at the 43rd percentile. You can check the Z Score Table of Values to verify this number. There will be some differences due to the fact that the Table of Values only specifies a z score to two decimal places, whereas I input the entire z score field of −0.18374. (Give it a try with only −0.18 and the returned value in Excel is the same "42.858" in the Table of Values.)

The NORM.S.DIST function works with both positive and negative z scores. Our example in Figure 4.19 specifies a negative z score, and the returned value is less than the 0.50 proportion that lies at the mean of the z score distribution.

NORM.DIST Function

This Excel function is a bit different from the previous two I discussed. It is often confused with the NORM.S.DIST because of the similarity of the name. It produces similar information to both the previous functions. Figure 4.20 shows the function argument window that is produced by the NORM.DIST formula submenu. As you can see, I specified the first raw score value from our previous example (50.00) so

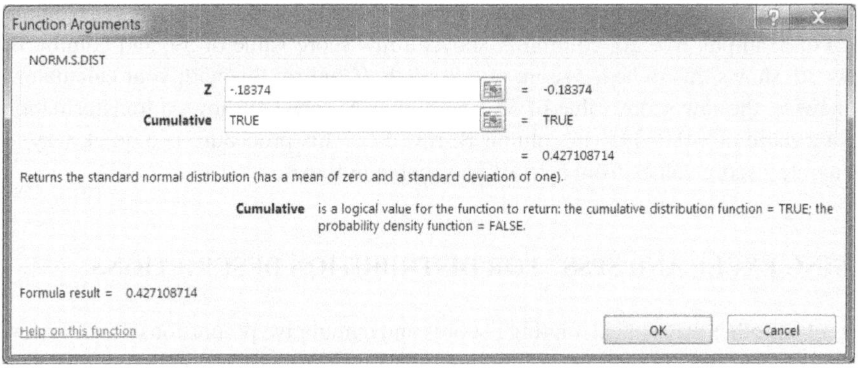

Figure 4.19   Using the Excel NORM.S.DIST function.

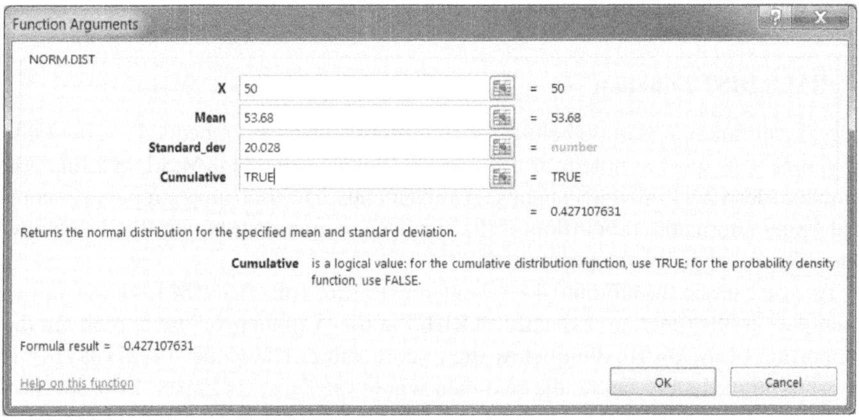

Figure 4.20   Using the Excel NORM.DIST function.

you can reference the output to our earlier example in Figure 4.17. As you can see in Figure 4.20, NORM.DIST returns the value "0.427107631" below the right hand "TRUE" entry. You will recognize this as the area of the standard normal distribution that lies below the raw score value of 50.00 and its z score equivalent of −0.18374.

Both STANDARDIZE and NORM.DIST create z scores from raw scores, and NORM.S.DIST calculates the cumulative proportion from the z score. NORM.DIST skips the step of reporting the z score by calculating the cumulative proportion directly from the raw score. The "Cumulative" information provided by the NORM.DIST function output can be either "TRUE" or "FALSE" depending on your needs. I input TRUE since I wanted the percentile (or the "cumulative distribution function"). I can use FALSE to calculate a different probability value for the given score, but that is the subject of a later chapter. We will return to this function.

TERMS AND CONCEPTS

Frequency polygon: A graph that is formed by joining the midpoints of the bars of a histogram by a line.

Standard normal distribution: A normal distribution that is "perfectly" shaped such that the percentages of the area under the curve are distributed in known and standard amounts around the mean. The mean has a value of 0 and the SD = 1. Also known as the "z distribution."

z Score: A raw score expressed in SD units. Also known as a "standard score" when viewed as scores of a standard normal distribution.

DATA LAB AND EXAMPLES (WITH SOLUTIONS)

Problem 1

Table 4.1 shows the hypothetical example of neighborhood characteristics ratings from a sample of low-income housing residents that we discussed in Chapter 3 (see Table 3.3). As you recall, the ratings include respondents' perceptions of road quality, traffic flow, access to groceries, crime, and related perceptions. The ratings are measured from 1 to 100, with 100 as the highest.

TABLE 4.1 Neighborhood Characteristics Ratings Sample

Neighborhood Characteristics
33
72
81
45
64
53
63
64
80
70
54
70
56
47
62
91

Using the data from Table 4.1, respond to the following questions:

1. Create the z score for the rating of 62 using both the SD population and SD inferential.

2. Can you identify a possible "extreme" z score? Discuss what this might mean.

Problem 2

Table 4.2 shows the Quality of Life Index data from Chapter 3 (see Table 3.4). As you recall, this index is a compiled value that included residents' perceptions of health

**TABLE 4.2   Housing Survey
Data – Quality of Life Index**

Quality Index (Modified)		
8	30	37
11	30	37
14	31	37
16	31	38
16	31	38
17	31	38
19	32	38
19	32	39
20	32	39
20	32	40
21	32	40
22	32	40
23	33	40
23	33	40
23	33	41
24	33	41
24	33	42
25	34	42
25	34	42
26	34	42
26	34	43
26	35	43
27	35	43
27	35	43
27	35	43
27	35	44
27	36	44
28	36	45
28	36	45
28	36	46
29	36	48
29	36	49
30	37	50
30	37	51
30	37	53

services, recreational opportunities, air quality, community involvement, fear of crime, and related measures.

1. Calculate z scores for each of the raw scores in SPSS (using the default SD inferential).

2. Using these results, can you identify possible extreme scores?

3. Calculate the z scores in Excel using the SD population using the Standardize function and "dragging" the formula.

4. Do you observe any extreme scores using the Excel function and the SD population?

5. Comment on your results from the previous analyses.

DATA LAB: SOLUTIONS

Problem 1

1. Create the z score for the rating of 62 using both the SD population and SD inferential.

   Using SD population:

   $$Z = \frac{X - M}{SD} = \frac{62 - 63.53}{14.431} = (-)0.106$$

   Using SD inferential:

   $$Z = \frac{X - M}{SD} = \frac{62 - 63.53}{14.937} = (-)0.102$$

2. Can you identify a possible "extreme" z score using the SD population? You can answer this question in two ways. First, by calculating all the z scores and seeing which, if any, exceed a z score value of 2.0 (both positively and negatively). Why? Because a z score of 2.00 exceeds almost 98% of the scores in the standard normal distribution. As we will discuss in later chapters, this is an important consideration for research problems, since we need to know at what point a score/value "distance itself" does from the other scores.

   A second way to answer the question is simply to double the SD (in this case, $2 * 14.431 = 28.86$) and see which scores in the distribution lie above or below this score in relation to the mean. Thus, on the negative side, $63.53 - 28.86 = 37.67$ or a score of 35. Since the score of 33 lies below this value, it might be considered "extreme" or of low likelihood. On the positive side, no scores exceed 92 ($63.53 + 28.86$), although the score of 91 is close ($z = 1.90$).

Problem 2

1. Calculate z scores for each of the raw scores in SPSS (using the default SD inferential). Use the "Descriptive Statistics – Descriptives" submenu, making sure to check the "Save standardized values as variables" box, as shown in Figure 4.21. This will add the z scores to your database.

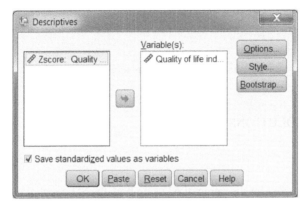

Figure 4.21   Using SPSS® to create z scores.

As a checking of your data, confirm the following z scores:
- Index Score of $33 = z$ score of -0.01077
- Index Score of $40 = z$ score of 0.78118

2. Using these results, can you identify possible extreme scores?
   - Quality Index Values of 8, 11, and 14 all exceed (negatively) a z score of -2.00.
   - Quality Index Values of 51 and 53 exceed (positively) a z score of 2.00.

3. Calculate the z scores in Excel using the SD population using the Standardize function and "dragging" the formula.Figure 4.22 shows the first 20 cases in which I dragged the formula from the first calculated z score (for the Quality Index value of 8 in Cell A2).

4. Do you observe any extreme scores using the Excel function and the SD population?
   - Negative z scores for 8, 11, 14, and possibly 16 could be considered extreme.
   - Positive z scores for 51, 52, and possibly 50 might be considered extreme.

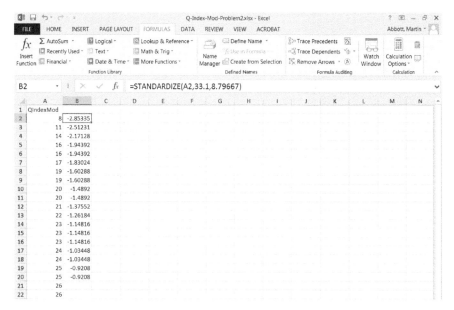

Figure 4.22 Using the Excel Standardize function to create z scores (using SD population).

5. Comment on your results from the previous analyses. Notice that as the number of cases increases, the disparity between the SD population and SD inferential decreases. The results from using both of these in the calculation of z scores earlier yield very similar results.

Most all respondents indicated Quality of Life Index scores according to a normal distribution, with only a few indicating more extreme (negative) views (three scores) or more positive views (two scores).

5

PROBABILITY AND THE Z DISTRIBUTION

Recently, a family was given a diagnosis of autism spectrum disorder (ASD) for their 3-year-old son. You may know that ASD currently affects about 1 in 68 children, an increasing incidence in recent years. The family had observed "autistic-like" behaviors (e.g., repetitive hand motions, lack of eye contact, etc.) but wanted to make certain that their child could in fact be classified as ASD, which would make it possible for the family to access resources to help them better parent their son.

Autism diagnoses are very complex and lengthy processes. Ordinarily, a child is given several initial screening tests by health-care providers, and then more formal diagnostic evaluations are performed by teams of professionals (often including psychologists, neurologists, speech therapists, etc.). One difficulty with these diagnostic procedures however is that they may not be perfect instruments to correctly identify the presence of ASD. While a great proportion of children tested would be correctly diagnosed (i.e., the test said ASD was present while it actually was), a slight proportion of the children tested could in fact be misdiagnosed (i.e., the test said ASD was present while it actually was not). This latter misdiagnosis can be referred to as a "false positive" since the test is positive for ASD but it is in fact not present.

In Chapter 1, I mentioned that Thomas Bayes was one of the earliest theorists who helped to establish statistics as a field. In fact, this eighteenth-century Presbyterian minister founded one of the most important theorems in statistics that is still used widely today, the Bayes theorem. In effect, this theorem allows a researcher to assign the likelihood (or probability) of a certain event given additional information about the event beyond what is initially known.

Using Statistics in the Social and Health Sciences with SPSS® and Excel®, First Edition.
Martin Lee Abbott.
© 2017 John Wiley & Sons, Inc. Published 2017 by John Wiley & Sons, Inc.

We will return to this discussion later when we discuss "conditional probability," but we must understand first the matter of probability generally.

THE NATURE OF PROBABILITY

Human actions are rarely, if ever, determined. However, it is also the case that human action is fairly predictable. One has only to consider the many ways in which the things (we think) we choose to do are really those things that are expected. Marketing specialists have made billions of dollars on this principle by targeting likely purchases of millennials using electronic records of previous buying behavior. Insurance providers have used these same principles for years to project how likely it is that a driver of a given sex and age will get into an accident.

Sociologically, when people repeatedly act in society, they create patterns or ruts that are both helpful (in economizing action and energy) and potentially problematic (since it becomes difficult to act differently than the rut allows). The result is that human behavior can be characterized by "predictability."

What does this have to do with statistics? Plenty. We have already seen that behaviors, attitudes, and beliefs have a great deal of variability. Why is there such variability? Why do people not always believe the same thing, act the same way, and so on? In descriptive statistics, we learn the ways to understand the extent of the variability and whether the resultant distribution of behaviors and beliefs conforms to a normal distribution. But that does not explain the *why*.

Human actions and beliefs have many causes. We cannot understand all of them. The fact that variance exists may be due to our inability to understand the full range of forces acting on the individual at any particular moment. But it may also exist because we cannot fully explicate individual choice or action.

In trying to understand this complexity, we must recognize the importance of probability. *Probability involves the realm of expectation by measuring the extent to which a certain action/event is likely to occur.* By observing and measuring actions and behaviors over time, we develop expectations that can help us better predict outcomes. If we observe students struggling with a certain subject area among schools over time, we might eventually predict the same outcome on future occasions, if there are no changes in conditions. Our expectation, being based on observation, will help us predict more accurately. This still does not explain *why* the students struggle, but it does turn the scrutiny toward the potential conditions for the struggle. We may never discover all the reasons, but the study of probability gets us closer to a more comprehensive understanding.

ELEMENTS OF PROBABILITY

In this book, I focus on using an understanding of probability and related statistical process that use probability to make statistical decisions. Probability is a crucial concept for statistics but one that cannot be comprehensively covered in a book such as this.

In the health sciences, for example, researchers are interested in the likelihood of certain conditions occurring in the population, so they can establish baseline information for potential remediation efforts. If you know that a certain cancer occurs 5% of the time in the population, then you can use this information to gauge efforts to reduce its incidence by various interventions (e.g., chemical, physical, etc.).

However, events in the real world are often complex and interrelated, so measuring probability is difficult. As we will see, this complexity makes it difficult to <u>measure certainty</u>, making it necessary to <u>estimate uncertainty</u>. That really is the nature of research; how can we use statistical procedures to establish the level of certainty/uncertainty of a given outcome? Will research findings increase our certainty and reduce our uncertainty about the likelihood of a certain event?

Empirical Probability

Empirical probability is simply the number of occurrences of a specific event divided by the total number of possible occurrences. If a student announces "I am here" at the top of their lungs when they enter a classroom, you can calculate the empirical probability of this event by observing the number of times the student makes the declaration divided by the number of days they enter the classroom. Thus, if they declare their presence 10 times out of 18 days of class, the probability of their making the declaration is

$$\text{Probability} = \frac{\text{Occurrences}}{\text{Possible occurrences}} = \frac{10}{18} = 0.556$$

Therefore, if we wanted to predict whether they would make the declaration on the next possible occasion, we would have slightly better than equal chance (0.556 vs. 0.50) of predicting their behavior (i.e., that they would make the declaration). In this example, you can see how probability is measured: as a number between 0 (no likelihood) and 1.00 (complete likelihood). We can indicate these events as follows:

- p = the probability of the event occurring
- q = the probability of the event not occurring
- Therefore, $p + q = 1$, and $p = (1 - q)$.

Combining Probabilities

In what follows, I will first discuss some of the "building blocks" of probability for research and then how to measure it in the context of actual research data. Determining probabilities is rarely as "simple" as finding the probability of a single event. More often, it is important to determine "overlapping" or multiple probabilities. In this case, there are different rules that help to illustrate how best to use and understand probability for complex events.

TABLE 5.1   Soccer Injuries by Incidence

Injury	Area of Body	Percent
Cranium	Head	10
Sternum	Chest	10
ACL	Knee	30
Metatarsal	Foot	50

Combining Probabilities: Addition Rule

We start by examining the aspects of probability that pertain to those events that are mutually exclusive or those events that cannot be two (or more) things at once. For example, I either have a diagnosis of diabetes or I do not; I cannot be classified as owning a black car if my car is green. These are both examples of being mutually exclusive.[1]

The additive rule of combining probabilities concerns the probability of one or another event occurring. When combining the probabilities of many mutually exclusive events, add the separate probabilities to determine the probability of any of these events occurring. The way this looks using a formula is as follows:

$$\text{Probability } (A \text{ or } B) = P(A) + P(B)$$

Table 5.1 shows some typical injuries for soccer players.[2] Assuming that players receive only one diagnosis, we can treat them as mutually exclusive events. That is, if you are diagnosed with a cranium problem, you are not diagnosed with a foot injury, and so on.

As you can see it is generally more likely for a soccer player to suffer injuries to legs and feet than the upper body areas. The probability of sustaining an injury to the knee or to the foot is 0.8 (80%) as shown using the additive rule:

$$\text{Probability } (A \text{ or } B) = P(A) + P(B)$$

$$\text{Probability } (\text{knee or foot}) = P(0.3) + P(0.5)$$

$$\text{Probability } (\text{knee or foot}) = 0.8$$

Combining Probabilities: Multiplication Rule

Situations and questions different from the previous text can be solved by using the multiplication rule of combing probabilities. If, for example, we are interested in finding the probability that two *independent* events occur together, we

---

[1] However, I can be a diabetic who owns a green car because together these are not mutually exclusive groups.

[2] These percentages are obtained from various sources but are not necessarily accurate; I am using them as an illustration.

need to adapt the rules. Independence in this situation refers to the fact that the probability of one event happening is in no way connected to the probability of the other event happening.

Thus, using the soccer injuries in Table 5.1, we might ask about the probability of one player leaving a game due to a knee injury and a second player leaving due to a head injury. In this event we would multiply the separate (independent) probabilities in order to find out the probability of them occurring together. This is also known as the "joint probability," which is particularly appropriate in this case!

$$\text{Probability } (A \text{ and } B) = P(A) * P(B)$$

To use the example from Table 5.1, what is the joint probability of a player leaving the game with a knee injury and a second player leaving with a head injury?

$$\text{Probability } (A \text{ and } B) = P(A) * P(B)$$

$$\text{Probability (knee injury and head injury)} = P(0.3) * P(0.1)$$

$$\text{Probability (knee injury and head injury)} = 0.3$$

COMBINATIONS AND PERMUTATIONS

These are categories of probability that focus on ordered sequences of events. Without going into much detail, I will present here some examples to distinguish the two concepts and then move toward a general consideration of how probability is used in social and health sciences research.

Combination

A combination of elements is a calculation of the total outcome without concern about the ordering of the elements. Thus, in a group of 10 students, a *combination* is whether Jim and Suzie take the top two spots in a spelling bee. They can place as "Jim first – Suzie second" or "Suzie first – Jim second." The combination considers all possible ways a set of events can occur, whereas a permutation considers the order of the finish among the events.

Example of the combination rule: In a group of 10 students in a spelling bee, how many groups of top finishers (i.e., first, second, third place) are there?

Combination formula:
$$\text{Combinations} = \frac{N!}{r!(N-r)!}$$

- ○ "N" is the number of students in the bee
- ○ "r" is the number of finishers we are interested in observing
- ○ "!" is the symbol for "factorial" or the multiplication of the successive integers equal to or less than the number specified ($0! = 1$)

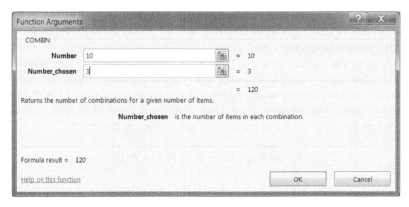

Figure 5.1   Specifying combinations using Excel "COMBIN" in the "Math & Trig" formulas.

$$\text{Combinations} = \frac{10!}{3!(10-3)!} = \frac{10*9*8*7*6*5*4*3*2*1}{(3*2*1)\,(7*6*5*4*3*2*1)}$$

$$= \frac{3,628,800}{(6)\,(5040)} = \frac{3,628,800}{30,240} = 120$$

Answer: There are 120 possible combinations of winners of the top three places, irrespective of who is first, second, or third.

Figure 5.1 shows how to specify the formula for combinations using Excel, which inserts a function from the "Math & Trig" group of "Formulas." As you can see, I used the same problem from the earlier example, and the correct answer is shown in the third row of values as 120.

Permutation

The permutation concerns the order of the events in a given combination; the order of finish is the focus. This refers to the fact that we are calculating the ordered sequence of events from a group. Thus, "Suzie first – Jim second" is a distinct permutation from "Jim first – Suzie second."

Example of the permutation rule: How many *unique arrangements* of winners of the top three spots in a spelling bee are possible with 10 entrants?

$$\text{Permutations} = \frac{N!}{(N-r)!} = \frac{10!}{(10-3)!} = \frac{3,628,800}{5040} = 720$$

Answer: There are 720 unique arrangements of the three top places in a spelling bee with 10 entrants.

Figure 5.2 shows how to specify the formula for permutations using Excel, which inserts a function from the "Statistical" group of "Formulas." As you can see, I used the same problem from the example earlier, and the correct answer is shown in the third row of values as 720.

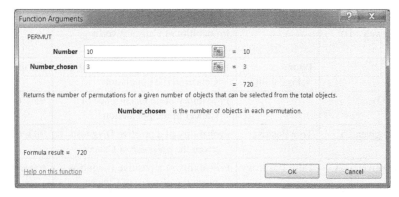

Figure 5.2   Specifying permutations using Excel "PERMUT" from "Statistical" functions.

CONDITIONAL PROBABILITY: USING BAYES' THEOREM

Probability is often based on "dependent" events since in the real world, things are tied together. So, in addition to understanding the probability of occurrence of a single event, we must consider the probability of an event happening GIVEN the fact that something else has already occurred. Thus, we "modify" the initial estimate of probability by adding new information.

Bayes' notion of conditional probability was essentially that initial estimates of an event could be revised, made more accurate, by adding information from known subsequent information about the event. Conditional probability is the likelihood that an event will take place given the fact that other events have taken place. In Bayes' theorem, which often involves events that have unknown prior events, we might distinguish between <u>prior probabilities</u>, which are likely occurrences of an event, and <u>posterior probabilities</u>, or revisions of the initial estimates of the event due to research or other information gathering.

As an example of this theorem, suppose researchers randomly test the population and discover that 5% of the population has a certain form of cancer. A new blood test is found to be 98% effective in detecting the cancer. Unfortunately, this test also detects that 6% of the subjects who do not have the cancer test positive (i.e., the test says they have it when in fact they do not). In terms of conditional probability, does the test increase our confidence in declaring that a person has the cancer?

Bayes' theorem helps us understand this problem by examining whether the new information (test results) increases our confidence in the presence of the cancer beyond the general rate of occurrence in the population.

Bayes' theorem looks daunting, but you can understand it as follows:

$$P(C \text{ given } + D) = \frac{P(+D \text{ given } C) \times P(O)}{[P(+D \text{ given } C) \times P(O)] + [P(+D \text{ given no } C) \times P(\text{no } O)]}$$

Table 5.2 shows the elements of this formula along with the percentages from the example problem expressed in decimal points. As you can see, there is a low

TABLE 5.2   Elements of the Bayes Theorem Problem

P(C given +D)		Probability of Cancer given a positive Diagnosis for cancer	
P(O)	Prior Probability	Probability of the Occurrence of the Cancer in the population	5% (.05)
P(no O)		Probability of no Occurrence of Cancer in the population	95% (.95)
P(+D given C)	True Positive	Probability of a positive Diagnosis given the *presence* of Cancer	98% (.98)
P(+D given no C)	False Positive	Probability of a positive Diagnosis given the *absence* of Cancer	6% (.06)

likelihood of occurrence in the population generally (0.05) with a test of 0.98 "accuracy" and a small likelihood of error (0.06). Following Table 5.2 is the use of Bayes' theorem to find the conditional probability:

$$P(C \text{ given} + D) = \frac{P(+D \text{ given } C) \times P(O)}{[P(+D \text{ given } C) \times P(O)] + [P(+D \text{ given no } C) \times P(\text{no } O)]}$$

$$= \frac{0.98 \times 0.05}{[0.98 \times 0.05] + [0.06 \times 0.95]}$$

$$= \frac{0.049}{[0.049] + [0.057]}$$

$$= \frac{0.049}{0.106}$$

$$= 0.462$$

From the result of 0.462, you can see that the initial random probability of having the cancer (0.05) is increased to 0.46 when using this test. Thus, using the Bayes formula resulted in adding information to the original estimate of having cancer.

Z SCORE DISTRIBUTION AND PROBABILITY

Thus far, we have discussed probability as the likelihood of certain events occurring. In the remainder of the book, we will continue to refer to probability as the likelihood of occurrence of certain events, but we will use the properties of the normal distribution to help us understand research problems dealing with problems in the social and health sciences which often use continuous data. Thus, researchers might ask about the probability of a certain intervention being successful among those with a serious disease or the likelihood that the attitudes of a sample of workers toward satisfaction at work would likely characterize all workers.

The z distribution that we discussed in Chapter 4 is very helpful to researchers because the features of the standard normal curve can be thought of as probabilities.

If you think about the normal curve, you will realize that human actions can take a number of different courses. Most responses tend to be clustered together, but there will be some responses that fall in different directions away from the main cluster. We can think of these normal curve features as a visual representation of the fact that we do not have certainty but probability in matters of such things as attitudes and buying behavior, test scores, and aptitude. That is, not all responses or choices will be the same; they will have different likelihoods of occurrence.

In inferential statistics, statisticians think of the normal curve in terms of probability. Since approximately 68% of the area (or a proportion of 0.68) of the normal curve lies between one standard deviation, positive or negative, for example, we can think of any given case having a 0.68 probability of falling between one standard deviation on either side of the mean.

The primary issue in this book is to recognize that the z score and probability are very much related, since they both can be characterized by the proportion of the area under the standard normal curve. *We can therefore think about certain kinds of problems as probability statements.* Knowing what we do of the distribution of area in the standard normal curve, we can observe that possible scores "beyond" 2 SDs (in either a positive or negative direction) are in areas of the distribution where there are very few cases. Thus, randomly selecting a score from a distribution in these small areas would have a much smaller probability than randomly selecting a score nearer the mean of the distribution. In a normally distributed variable, only 5% of cases or so will fall outside the ± 2 SD area. Therefore, with 100 cases, selecting a case randomly from this area would represent a probability of 0.05 (since $5/100 = 0.05$).

Since the standard normal distribution represents percentages (as proportions of the entire area in the distribution) and probabilities, it is easy to convert one to the other. You can convert percentages to probability simply by dividing the percentage by 100 (%) as follows:

$$\text{Probability}(p) = \frac{68\%}{100\%} = \frac{68}{100} = 0.68$$

The z distribution is very important to statistics since it provides an ideal model that we can use to understand the raw data distributions we create. In fact, in this book, the z distribution straddles both descriptive and inferential statistics, the "branches" of statistics I introduced earlier. We have seen how we can use the z distribution to understand raw scores by transforming them to z scores, and we have learned how to create and manage cumulative percentages. We will continue this discussion to complete our descriptive statistics section and then consider how the standard normal distribution can help us to understand inferential statistics.

Transforming a Raw Score to a Z Score: Statistical Testing

Chapter 4 discussed both z scores and cumulative percentages, focusing on how to use the Z Table to transform z scores. As you recall, the z score formula is as follows:

$$Z = \frac{X - M}{\text{SD}}$$

There are many uses for this formula, as you will see throughout the book. We have used it thus far to understand how to transform raw score information to z score, or standardized, information. As we will discuss shortly, variations of this formula are used to express how certain raw score sample data can be translated into estimated population data.

For now it is enough to know that sometimes you may have different kinds of information available, and you can use the formula to help you with various analyses of your data. You can actually use simple algebra to solve for the different parts of the formula. We will consider one such formula since it will become very important to our later statistical procedures.

Transforming a Z Score to a Raw Score: Estimation

In Chapter 4, we used the hypothetical example of a mother trying to understand the test score of her child. Using this same scenario, let us suppose that the student's mother was informed that on a certain test with a mean of 100 and a standard deviation of 15, her son received a z score of -1.64. Not being sophisticated in the interpretation of z scores, she may be interested in what the raw score was on the test. We can use the z score formula to calculate the raw score from the z score data and the descriptive information about the distribution.

What can we observe generally? Certainly, since z scores are expressed in standard deviation units on the standard normal distribution, the student probably did not perform highly on the test (i.e., since negative scores are on the left of the distribution – in this case more than one and $1/2$ SDs to the left of the mean). Consider the following formula, which is derived from the z score formula listed before:

$$X = Z(\text{SD}) + M$$

In this formula, the z score we need to transform to a raw score (X) is known, along with the SD and mean of the raw score distribution. Substituting the values we listed previously,

$$X = -1.64(15) + 100$$

$$= 75.40$$

So, we can inform the student's mother that her child received 75.40 on the test. Although we don't know how that might translate into a teacher's grade, it probably has more meaning to a parent who does not normally see z scores. To the researcher, however, the z score contains more information.

We will use variations of this same formula in the statistical procedures that follow to create estimates of population values if we only know sample values. Thus, if we survey a work group in the airline industry about their work satisfaction or productivity, we can use this information to estimate the attitudes of workers in the entire airline industry because we can never measure the attitudes of each individual worker.

Transforming Cumulative Proportions to *z* Scores

Another situation may arise in which we have cumulative proportions or percentiles available and wish to transform them to *z* scores. This is a fairly easy step since both are based on *z* scores.

In our previous example, the student's inquisitive mother would probably have been given a percentile rather than a *z* score since the educational system uses percentiles extensively as the means to make comparisons among scores. Here is a brief example, again using the mother. Suppose the student's mother was told that her son received a score that was at the 60th percentile. What would be the *z* score equivalent?

As we learned in previous sections, it might be good to first try to visualize the solution. Figure 5.3 shows how you might visualize this problem. In the top panel of Figure 5.3, you can see that a percentile score of 60 (or a cumulative percentage of 60%) would fall to the right of the mean by definition (i.e., since the score surpasses 60% of all the scores which is above the 50% mark).

Since the 60th percentile is 10% away from the mean (or the 50th percentile), we know that the percent of the distribution that lies between the mean and the target score is 10%. We know that the distance between the mean and the first SD on a *z* distribution contains about 34.13%, so our percentile score of 60 should represent an approximate *z* score of 0.29 (10% divided by 34.13%), using a ballpark estimate.

If you recall, knowing that the area of the distribution between the percentile score and the mean is 10% gives us additional information since this is what the *Z* Score Table of Values provides. We can now use the *z* score table *in reverse* to "finish" our visualization of the answer. If you locate the closest percentage to 10.00% that you can find in the table (among the first of the column "pairs" of percentages), you find 9.87% and 10.26%, corresponding to *z* scores of 0.25 and 0.26, respectively. Since 10.00% is closest to 9.87%, we can conclude that a percentile score with this distance

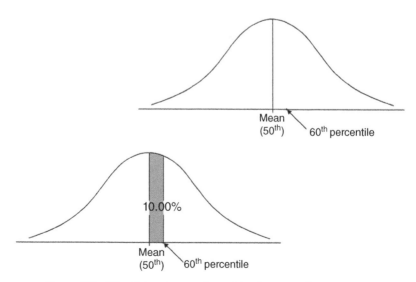

Figure 5.3   Visualizing the transformation of a percentile to a *z* score.

from the mean represents a z score of 0.25. (Locate 9.87% in the table, note the 0.2 in the first "z" column which is on the same row, and add the 0.05 from the z figure earlier in the z score numbered columns for a total of 0.25: i.e., $0.2 + 0.05 = 0.25$.)

A second method of arriving at the same z score of 0.25 is to use the second panel of the column pairs of percentages; those that are listed in the "tails" of the distribution. Knowing that the percentile score of 60 also creates a cumulative proportion of 40% in the tail, look for the closest value to 40.00% among the "tail" columns, and you will find the closest value is $z = 0.25$.

Deriving Sample Scores from Cumulative Percentages

This is another process that involves an understanding of the area in the standard normal distribution and how to transform scores. In essence, it simply combines the procedures we have already covered. Continuing with a similar example from before, we can consider how students fare on a test.

A certain class ($N = 40$ students) creates a mean test score of 50.16 and an (population) SD of 26.54 with the resulting raw score distribution appearing to be normally distributed according to the descriptive procedures we discussed earlier. Using this information, which student raw score would represent a cumulative percentage of 67% (i.e., fall at the 67th percentile) of this sample of data?

Using the admonition to try visualization before we use a formula, how can we represent the question? Figure 5.4 shows how you can "see" this with a graph of the distribution. As you see, the 67th percentile the "target" student score lies well above the mean. Since 34.13% of the distribution lies between the mean and SD 1, our target score should be approximately at the middle of this area (since 17%, the distance beyond 50%, the mean of the distribution, is about half of 34.13%), although a bit closer to the mean given the shape of the curve. Therefore, we can visualize a z score of about 0.5. With the z score, we can say the school score would be approximately 63, figured thus:

1. Our visual estimate of 0.5 z scores represents SD units; therefore the target score represents approximately 13.27, one-half of the sample score SD of 26.54.
2. This amount plus the mean of 50.16 equals approximately 63 (i.e., $13.27 + 50.16$).

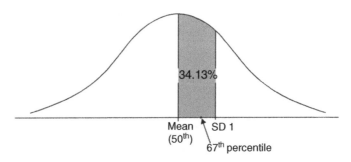

Figure 5.4 Visualizing the 67th percentile of the raw score test distribution.

Checking this visual calculation with the formula I presented previously, we can see how close we were to the actual sample score value. The 67th percentile falls at the z score of 0.44 (17% above the mean or 33% in the tail), so substituting the values in the formula, we find the sample score to be 61.84%. Therefore, a student with a score of 61.84% is at the 67th percentile of our data sample. Our estimate (63%) was not perfect, but it helped to check the analyses and try to see the relationship among all the various pieces of data:

$$X = 0.44(26.54) + 50.16$$
$$= 61.84\%$$

USING SPSS® AND EXCEL TO TRANSFORM SCORES

There are no established formulas or menus in SPSS® or Excel to make the transformations we discussed earlier in this chapter. Aside from the z score transformations from raw score distributions that we reviewed in Chapter 4, we are on our own to use both of these statistical programs to create appropriate transformations.

These are not difficult to do using the programs as elaborate "calculators." I already demonstrated how to create z scores using Excel. (Review "STANDARDIZE Function" section of Chapter 4.) You can easily use SPSS to do the same thing using the "Transform" menu and then selecting "Compute." Review the section in Chapter 4, "Using SPSS to Create Z Scores and Percentiles." In that section, I showed how to create z scores by simply checking a box on the "Analyze – Descriptive Statistics – Descriptives" menu choice (see Figures 4.12 and 4.13).

You can use SPSS to compute a <u>new</u> variable by entering the z score formula or other relevant formulas. For an example, I use the AP score data shown in Figure 4.13 since I used SPSS to show Z scores. To create a z score transformation by entering a formula, consider Figure 5.5, in which I use the "Transform" menu at the top of the page, and then, from that menu, choose "Compute Variable" which will yield the submenu shown in Figure 5.5.

As you can see, I created a new variable ("Target Variable") called "APScoreZ" in the upper left window. (I label the computed variable thus because SPSS used a default to create the variable "ZAPScores" when I used the process in Figures 4.12 and 4.13.)[3] Then, in the "Numeric Expression" window, I created the formula for calculating a z score from a raw score. I had to first include the existing raw score variable in the equation by selecting it from the "Type & Label" window and then moving it to the Numeric Expression window using the arrow button.

Hopefully, you will recognize this formula as simply the z score formula from earlier:

$$Z = \frac{X - M}{SD}$$

---

[3] Note that the z scores created by SPSS shown in Figure 4.13 are different than those created by the formula shown in Figure 5.5 because the former uses the inferential SD, while the equation we created in Figure 5.5 uses the population SD.

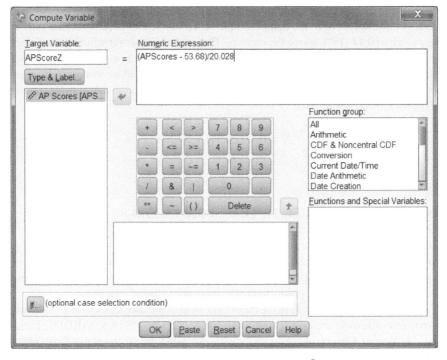

Figure 5.5 Using the Compute Variable menu in SPSS® to create z scores.

In SPSS, it looks like the Numeric Expression in Figure 5.5:

$$\text{APScoreZ} = \frac{(\text{APScores}-53.68)}{20.028}$$

I obtained the mean and (population) SD from the Descriptives procedure I used in earlier. Thus, I simply indicated in SPSS that I wanted to create a new variable that represents the raw score variable (X) minus the mean (53.68) and divided by the (population) SD (20.028). When I perform this operation, SPSS makes the calculations and creates z scores for each raw score. You will note, however, that the values for APScoreZ that I created using a formula are different from the ZAPScores that I obtained through the Descriptives menu because two different SD values were used: the inferential SD in the former and the population SD in the latter. Figure 5.6 shows these two z score variables in SPSS, so you can compare the differences.

The first variable shown in Figure 5.6 is the original raw score variable. The second variable is the new variable I created using the Transform – Compute process (APScoreZ). The third variable is the variable SPSS created through the Descriptives – Descriptives menu using the inferential SD. As you can see there are slight differences in the z scores depending on which SD is used.

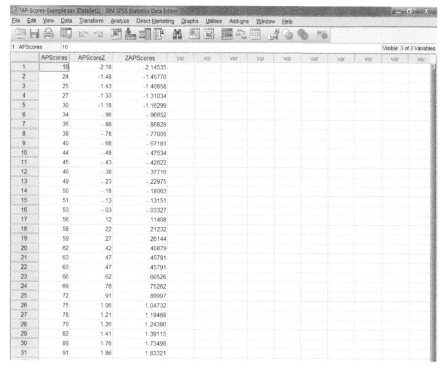

Figure 5.6   SPSS® data file with two z score variables.

USING THE ATTRIBUTES OF THE NORMAL CURVE TO CALCULATE PROBABILITY

Let us suppose that a manager for a group of aviation engineers was asked to select, at random, an engineer to represent the entire work group on a regional council for "innovative technology processes." Further, suppose that the manager has just administered a test of technology innovation to the engineers in the work group, and the distribution of results has a mean of 95 and a standard deviation of 12 (on a test with a top score that could possibly reach 140). What would be the probability of selecting at random from the work group an engineer who scored between 89 and 101 to represent the group on the council?

Using the procedures we learned in previous chapters, we can visualize the result and then calculate it specifically with the z score formulas.

1. Remember that probability statements are based on the same information as z scores.
2. Consider where you need to end, that is, what information must you have and how can you work backward to get it?
3. Draw or visualize a picture of the normal distribution with a shaded target area.

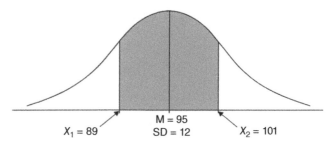

Figure 5.7   Visualizing the probabilities as a preliminary solution.

Figure 5.7 shows how you might visualize this problem. As you can see, with a mean of 95 and an SD of 12, the scores of 89 and 101 fall one-half an SD below and above the mean, respectively. Thus, both the lower and upper numbers are 0.5 z scores from the mean. With the distance from the mean to one SD (both positive and negative) at about 34.13%, the distance between 89 and 101 would occupy about 34% (17% below the mean and 17% above the mean would total 34%.). The probability would therefore be approximately 0.34 (34%/100%).

We can calculate the distances using the z score formula:

$$Z = \frac{X - M}{SD}$$

The raw scores of 89 (X_1) and 101 (X_2) would have z scores (Z_1 and Z_2) calculated as follows:

$$Z_1 = \frac{89 - 95}{12} = \frac{-6}{12} = -0.5$$

$$Z_2 = \frac{101 - 95}{12} = \frac{6}{12} = 0.5$$

From the Z Score Table of Values, we find that the area of the curve between the mean and z scores of 0.5 (positive and negative) is 19.15%. Therefore, 38.30% (i.e., 19.15% plus 19.15% = 38.30%) of the area of the distribution falls between scores of 89 and 101. This means that there is a probability of 0.38 of selecting at random an engineer whose score on the technology innovation test lies between 89 and 101.

Our visualization ($p = 0.34$) was lower than the calculated probability ($p = 0.38$) due to the shape of the curve. However, this exercise does point out how visualization can help you to "see" the dynamics and approximate solution to questions similar to this.

Calculating "Areas" of the Standard Normal Distribution

Oftentimes, researchers need to identify probabilities of cases that lie inside or outside sets of scores in a distribution. For example, we may be asked to identify the middle 90% of the students who take a specific test; or, conversely, we may be asked to identify the 10% that lie outside, in the extremes of the distribution (the two "tails" of the curve). In both cases, you can use the information you have already learned about the normal distribution to solve these problems.

Calculating these areas is very helpful to understand inferential statistics. Statisticians and researchers have created conventions about which z scores create "exclusion areas" that can be used to compare with the results of actual studies. When calculated values from statistical studies fall within or beyond these exclusion areas (defined by specific z scores), researchers can make statistical decisions about whether the findings are "likely," or "beyond chance."

Inclusion Area Example

Recall from our earlier example that a class of students ($N = 40$) showed a mean of 50.16 and an (population) SD of 26.54 on a certain test. What two raw scores "capture" (include) the middle 90% of the distribution?

Using the visualization shown in Figure 5.8, we can identify the middle portion of the distribution encompassed by 45% to the left of the mean and 45% to the right of the mean (since we want to identify the raw scores on both sides of the 90%). We know that the first 2 SDs contain about 47.72% of the distribution on either side of the mean (for a total of 95.44%) which is close to our 45% target area (i.e., the middle 90% of the scores) on either side of the mean. Therefore, our raw scores should fall inside the -2 SD mark and the $+2$ SD mark.

Now, <u>calculating</u> the raw score defining the area to the left (45%) of the distribution, $Z = 1.65$ (from the z table). Both Z values lie the same distance from the mean but on different sides. Therefore, $Z_1 = -1.65$ and $Z_2 = 1.65$. Using the formula from the section "Transforming a Z Score to a Raw Score: Estimation," we can use the z scores to identify raw scores on both sides of the mean of the distribution of raw scores that contain 90% of the sample of test scores. We use the formula two times, one with the negative z score (-1.65) and one with the positive z score (1.65):

$$X_1 = Z_1(\text{SD}) + M = -1.65(26.54) + 50.16 = 6.37$$

$$X_2 = Z_2(\textbf{SD}) + M = 1.65(26.54) + 50.16 = 93.95$$

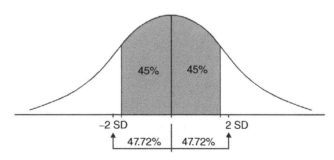

Figure 5.8   Visualizing the middle 90% area of the test scores.

Therefore, the middle 90% of the sample distribution of students' test scores is bracketed by the two raw scores of 6.37 and 93.95.

Exclusion Area Example

We can use a similar process to figure the <u>outside</u> portions of the distribution. This is the portion of the distribution that lies in the two "tails" of the distribution. As you will see, this is an important identification since much of how we will use probability will involve the "exclusion area" of scores in the tails of the distribution.

Using the same data as in the inclusion problem earlier, identify the two raw scores that cut off 5% of the distribution, and isolate it into the two tails. Recall that our sample students' test scores ($N = 40$) show a mean of 50.16 and an (population) SD of 26.54.

Figure 5.9 shows how this looks so you can practice the <u>visualization</u> of the solution. Picture the sample test score distribution with small shaded areas (5%) distributed in the two tails of the distribution (i.e., $5\%/2 = 2.5\%$ in each tail). We need to identify the raw score values that fall in these two areas combined. First, however, we need to use the z score table and calculations to help us.

Like the last example, we can use our knowledge about the standard normal distribution to help us with this visualization:

1. Two SDs (above and below the mean) contain about 95% of the distribution. Thus, the left (negative) side contains about 47.72%, and the right (positive) side contains about 47.72% of the distribution.
2. Since we are interested in the excluded portion of both sides, or about 2.5% in each of the "tails" of the distribution (i.e., one-half of 5% is 2.5%), we can observe that both sides will contain 95% of the distribution, leaving 47.50% on each sides of the distribution (i.e., $50\% - 2.5\% = 47.50\%$).
3. Therefore, our raw scores are going to lie close to z scores of ± 1.96 (the tabled value for 47.50% of the area between the mean and the tail).

Now we can <u>calculate</u> the raw score values using the same formula in the inclusion example. Since the distribution is symmetrical, the z score table identifies the same

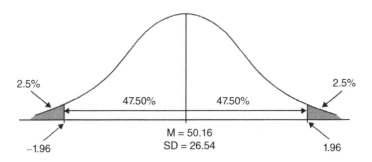

Figure 5.9   Visualizing the excluded 5% of the test score values.

z score on the left (negative value) and the right (positive value) of the distribution. Calculating the raw score defining the 2.5% in each side of the distribution,

$$Z_1 = -1.96 \text{ and } Z_2 = 1.96$$

$$X_1 = Z_1(SD) + M = -1.96(26.54) + 50.16 = -1.86$$

$$X_2 = Z_2(SD) + M = 1.96(26.54) + 50.16 = 102.18$$

Therefore, the scores of -1.86 and 102.18 identify the 5% area distributed in the two tails of the student score distribution. This is interesting because the scores range from 0 to 100. Why the discrepancy? <u>Because we are working with sample values that estimate population values</u>. Perhaps an easier way to identify the z score in this example using our z table of values is to find the z score that "creates" a tail of 2.50%. This value would be identified as the z score closest to a tail value of 2.50% from the tail panel of the z score table columns (i.e., 1.96).

"EXACT" PROBABILITY

Up to now, we discussed probability in terms of the area under the standard normal distribution. We have seen how to translate given areas (e.g., the percent of the distribution between the mean and first SD) into probability statements (e.g., $p = 0.34$, from the example earlier). We have thus converted a *range of scores* into a probability value.

Excel and SPSS provide this information, but they also report the *probability of exact values occurring* among a set of values. SPSS reports the exact probabilities for the results of statistical tests, while Excel can provide these through the NORM.DIST function that we reviewed in Chapter 4.

To show an example in Excel, recall our discussion in Chapter 4 regarding the NORM.DIST function using the distribution of AP scores. Figure 4.20 shows the example of calculating the cumulative distribution proportion for the score of 50. The value of 0.427 indicates that 42.7% of the distribution of AP scores falls below the score of 50. As you can see, I used the "TRUE" argument in the "Cumulative" window of the function to obtain the cumulative distribution proportion.

Figure 5.10 shows the same function window from Excel, except this time, I specified "FALSE" in the "Cumulative" window. As you can see, this returns the value of 0.019585799, the *exact probability* of the raw score of 50 occurring (known as the probability density function) in this distribution of values.

You can use Excel's "dragging" function to calculate the probabilities for each of the other scores as I discussed in Chapter 4 (see Figure 4.28). As you can see in Figure 5.11, I entered the NORM.DIST function formula in cell B2 adjacent to the AP score value of 10. The formula window directly above shows the specification window for this function that is shown in Figure 5.10, except that I specified the value for 10 (in cell A2) instead of 50 (in cell A15):

$$= \text{NORM.DIST}(A2, 53.68, 20.028, \text{FALSE})$$

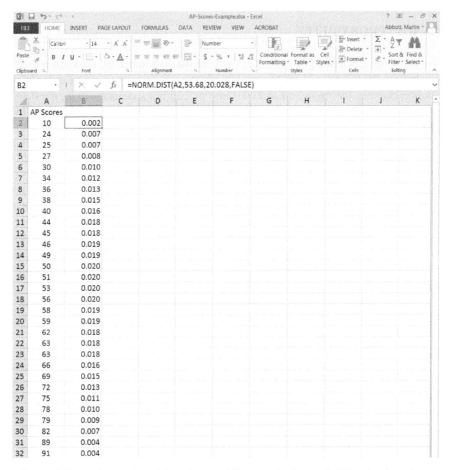

Figure 5.10 Using the Excel NORM.DIST function for exact probabilities (probability density function).

Figure 5.11 Using the Excel dragging capability to calculate probability density values.

When I received the value for the score of 10, I dragged the formula down the column of AP score values, and Excel calculated the probability density values for each raw score. You can compare the value for 50 shown in Figure 5.10 (as 0.019585799, or 0.02 when rounded) to the same value (0.02) in Figure 5.11.

Estimating "Exact" Probabilities

You can also *estimate* exact probability values using the Z Table of Values. Figure 5.12 shows how to do this using another example. Suppose a distribution of raw scores has a mean of 50.61 and a standard deviation of 17.45. What is the probability of a score of 37.70? Figure 5.12 shows the NORM.DIST specification that results in the value of 0.017388417, or 0.017 rounded.

Using the Z Table of Values, we can identify the approximate proportion of the normal distribution "occupied" by this value (37.7). You can see that in Figure 5.13, I identified the target point of 37.7, but I also identified two values very close to it. In

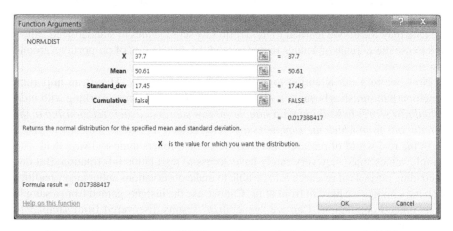

Figure 5.12   Excel NORM.DIST example for calculating exact probabilities.

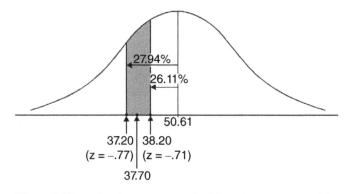

Figure 5.13   Estimating an exact probability using the *z* score table.

identifying raw score values $1/2$% to the left of the target (37.20%) and $1/2$% to the right (38.20%), I can create a rough estimate of the target point within one raw score percentage "band."

Using the z scores for these points (-0.77 and -0.71, respectively), you can calculate a percentage of 1.83 using the z score table as we have in past exercises (i.e., $27.94\% - 26.11\% = $ approximately 1.83). Transforming this percentage to a probability yields $p = 0.0183$. This is close to the probability identified in Figure 5.12 (0.017388417) but not exact. The probability of $p = 0.0183$ is the probability of a score occurring *between* raw scores of 37.20 and 38.20, not the exact probability of the raw score of 37.70. Nevertheless, you may see from this example what we mean by the calculation of an exact probability.

FROM SAMPLE VALUES TO SAMPLE DISTRIBUTIONS

Up to now, we have discussed and used examples of sets of raw scores to examine descriptive statistics. We concentrated on how to use statistical procedures to better describe data and to do it in such a way that we will gain a fresh perspective on what the data may mean. We learned to transform raw score values to standardized values and to use the Z Table of Values to understand the distribution of proportions around given scores.

Now, we turn our attention to a different level of inquiry. This is an important benchmark in statistics because it requires a shift of thinking from working with *individual raw scores* to working with *samples of raw scores and their relationship to the populations from which the samples supposedly came*.

In the real world of research and statistics, practitioners almost always deal with sample values since they very rarely have access to population information. But one overriding purpose of research is to be able to make observations about larger realities than the samples we have in front of us. Can we use the insights gained from a sample to its related population? Can we "generalize" results discovered from samples to similar populations?

For example, we might want to understand students' AP scores compared to the AP scores of all similar students in the state. Will understanding the sample distribution of scores tell us anything about the AP scores of all students? Also, if we implement a new way of teaching this course of study, might our methods be effective compared to all other AP student scores? In both cases, we can gain access to our own student's (sample) scores quite easily, but it is another matter to gain access to all the students' scores (i.e., population) in the state for our research questions!

Inferential statistics are methods that help make decisions about how real-world data indicate whether dynamics at the sample level are likely to be related to dynamics at the population level. That is to say, we need to start thinking about our *entire sample distribution* (perhaps our group of AP student scores) as being one possible sample of the overall population of AP student scores in the state (or some other level of population).

If we derive a sample that is unbiased, the sample values (mean and SD, for instance) should be similar to the population values. If, however, we intentionally make a change to see what will happen to our sample, we might observe that our sample values differ from population values. Or, to take another example, we might observe that another teacher has been using a "traditional" method of teaching AP, while I have used my new method, and I want to see which is more effective. In any case, what we are doing is:

1. Assuming at the outset that our sample reflects the population values from which it supposedly comes
2. Changing our sample somehow or observing different conditions between our sample and another similar sample
3. Seeing if our changed sample is now different from before or different from the other sample

In all these cases, we are comparing a sample to a population, not examining individual scores within a sample. We no longer think of our sample values individually but as *one set that could be derived from a population along with many more such sets*; our sample set of values are now seen as simply one possible set of values alongside many other possible sample sets. That is the difference between inferential and descriptive statistics. We therefore change the nature of our research question from Are our sample values normally distributed – descriptive statistics? to Do our sample values likely reflect the known (or unknown) population values from which our sample supposedly came – inferential statistics?

TERMS AND CONCEPTS

Additive rule of probability: Combining the probabilities of many mutually exclusive events by adding the separate probabilities to determine the probability of any of these events occurring.

Bayes' theorem: The notion that initial estimates of an event can be revised, made more accurate, by adding information from known subsequent information about the event.

Dependent events: Events that are tied together or related such that changing one event will have an effect on the value of another event; understanding the probability of occurrence of a single event GIVEN the fact that something else has already occurred.

Conditional probability: The likelihood that an event will take place given the fact that other events have taken place.

Empirical probability: The number of occurrences of a specific event divided by the total number of possible occurrences.

Independent events: The probability of one event happening is in no way connected to the probability of the other event happening.

Joint rule of probability: See "multiplication rule of probability."

Multiplication rule of   Multiplying the separate (independent) probabilities in
probability: order to find out the probability of them occurring
                                   together. (Also known as the "joint probability.")
Mutually exclusive: Those events that cannot be two (or more) things at once.
                                   For example, I cannot be said to own a black car if my
                                   car is green.
Probability: The realm of expectation measuring the extent to which
                                   a certain action/event is likely to occur; the field of
                                   mathematics that studies the likelihood of certain events
                                   happening out of the total number of possible events.
Prior probability: The likelihood of the occurrence of an event before it is
                                   measured.
Posterior probability: Revisions of the initial estimates of the likelihood of an
                                   event due to research or other information gathering.

DATA LAB AND EXAMPLES (WITH SOLUTIONS)

Problem 1

Using Bayes' theorem, find the conditional probability that a person has a certain
form of obsessive compulsive disorder (OCD) with an approximate 1% prevalence in
the population, given an OCD test that correctly identifies the disorder about 95% of
the time and incorrectly identifies (false positive) the disorder about 3% of the time.

Problem 2

Table 5.3 shows example data regarding the health score ratings of a small sample of
baristas in a certain metropolitan area. Use these data (with population SD) to respond
to the following questions:

TABLE 5.3   Health Score
Ratings of Baristas

Health Score Ratings
3
10
7
8
12
4
7
5
7
6

a. Using the data from Table 5.3, identify the rating scores that exclude 8% of the distribution.

b. What is the probability of obtaining a health score rating between 6 and 8?

c. What is the exact probability of obtaining a health score rating of 10?

DATA LAB: SOLUTIONS

Problem 1

Table 5.4 shows the conditional probability elements for OCD.

$$P(\textbf{OCD} \text{ given} + D) = \frac{P(+D \text{ given } \textbf{OCD}) \times P(O)}{[P(+D \text{ given } \textbf{OCD}) \times P(O)] + [P(+D \text{ given no } \textbf{OCD}) \times P(\text{no } O)]}$$

$$P(C \text{ given} + D) = \frac{0.95 \times 0.01}{[0.95 \times 0.01] + [0.03 \times 0.99]}$$

$$= \frac{0.0095}{[0.0095] + [0.0297]}$$

$$= \frac{0.0095}{0.0392}$$

$$P(C \text{ given} + D) = \frac{0.95 \times 0.01}{[0.95 \times 0.01] + [0.03 \times 0.99]} = \frac{0.0095}{[0.0095] + [0.0297]} = \frac{0.0095}{0.0392}$$

Answer: $P(C \text{ given} + D) = 0.242$

TABLE 5.4 Conditional Probability Elements for OCD

P(OCD given +D)		Probability of OCD given a positive Diagnosis	
P(O)	Prior Probability	Probability of the Occurrence of OCD in the population	1% (.01)
P(no O)		Probability of no OCD in the population	99% (.99)
P(+D given OCD)	True Positive	Probability of a positive Diagnosis given the *presence* of OCD	95% (.95)
P(+D given no OCD)	False Positive	Probability of a positive Diagnosis given the *absence* of Cancer	3% (.03)

Problem 2

  a. Using the data from Table 5.3, identify the rating scores that exclude 8% of the distribution.

Answer: 2.441 and 11.359

    Discussion: Remember that excluding 8% of the distribution means "splitting" the excluded area into both tails (i.e., 4% in each tail). Use the Z Table of Values to identify the z scores that exclude 4% in the tails (−1.75 and 1.75), and then use the formula to calculate raw scores from z scores.

$$X = Z(\text{SD}) + M$$

Mean $= 6.9$
(Population SD) $= 2.548$

  b. What is the probability of obtaining a health score rating between 6 and 8?

Answer: 0.30

    Discussion: Convert both raw scores to z score with the formula
$Z = \frac{X-M}{\text{SD}}$
Z_1 ($X = 6$) is −0.35 and Z_2 ($X = 8$) is 0.43.
Use the Z Table of Values to identify the proportion of the distribution that lies between the values of −0.35 and the mean of 13.683 and 0.43 (16.64) to get 30.323 or probability of 0.30.

  c. What is the exact probability of obtaining a health score rating of 10?

Answer: Function formula (NORM.DIST) result: 0.075
Manual calculation estimate: 0.0746

Discussion: *Manually*

- Subtract 0.5 from 10 to get a lower limit (i.e., 9.5), and add 0.5 to get an upper limit (i.e., 10.5).
- Derive z scores for these raw score values (1.02 and 1.41, respectively).
- Derive proportions under the curve using the Z Table of Values, and subtract the lower from the upper limit (42.073 − 34.614 = 7.459).
- Transform the resulting proportion (7.459%) to a probability (0.0746).

Discussion: Discussion: Using Excel NORM.DIST function (see Figure 5.14).

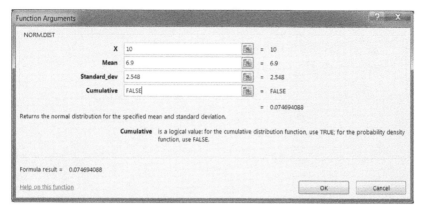

Figure 5.14   Using NORM.DIST to identify the exact probability for 10.

6

RESEARCH DESIGN AND INFERENTIAL STATISTICS

In many ways, statistics as a process finds its meaning in application to problems and questions arising from the real world. Every day, we confront social and personal issues that call for new ways of understanding and perhaps mediating those matters. Would restricting access to certain types of guns reduce violence? What is the relationship between health and wealth? Does class size really matter in explaining academic success? How can work be more satisfying and productive?

These and other questions require a way of thinking that guide problem-solving efforts toward understanding and remediation. We initiated this effort in the previous chapters dealing with how to describe data and to "see" hidden patterns that might assist our understanding. The next chapters in this book go further in two ways: (1) I discuss research design, which is the attempt to create a structure for classifying and comparing data patterns, and (2) I introduce inferential statistics as the way to understand how accessible data can help to explain unknown relationships and social realities.

RESEARCH DESIGN

Before we look in depth at inferential statistics, however, we need to cover some essential matters of research design. Statistics and research design are companion topics that need to be understood together. Sometimes, the two subjects are taught together in a single course (or courses), but more often they are taught as prerequisites for one another in college curricula. There is no best way to sequence the ideas, so I

Using Statistics in the Social and Health Sciences with SPSS® and Excel®, First Edition.
Martin Lee Abbott.
© 2017 John Wiley & Sons, Inc. Published 2017 by John Wiley & Sons, Inc.

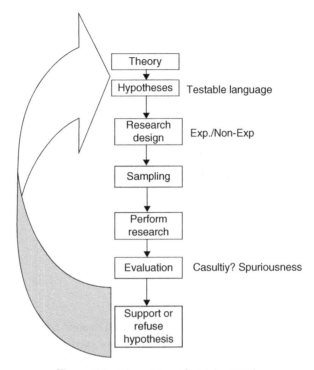

Figure 6.1   The process of social research.

simply try to introduce research design elements at the brink of discussing inferential statistics since they rely on one another.

This is a book on statistics, so we cannot hope to cover all the complexities of research design. We can only attempt to provide a research "primer." In what follows, I will outline some of the basics, but for a comprehensive understanding of research design, you need to consult further works in the field. You might start with *Understanding and Applying Research Design* (Abbott and McKinney, 2013), a book I wrote with my colleague Jennifer McKinney to explore research design in much greater depth than typically discussed in statistics textbooks.

Social and health research are fields of inquiry in which we devise standardized methods for examining available data to answer research questions. Typically, this involves collecting data from subjects or existing sources and subjecting the data to the methods of statistics to provide illumination. We may start with a research question and then figure out the best way to proceed to solve it. This procedure is research design. How can we structure our inquiry so that we can find and use data in the most defensible way to answer a research question? Figure 6.1 shows a process we might envision that will help us negotiate a research question.

Theory

As you can see, the top element in Figure 6.1 is "Theory," an abstract idea in which we state the <u>conceptual</u> nature of the relationship among our ideas of inquiry. For instance, we might state a social or health concern as a theoretical question: Does wealth result in improved health?

Hypothesis

Since a theory cannot be directly assessed (it exists on an abstract and conceptual level), we must find a way to empirically restate the theory so that it can be assessed. That is the role of the *hypothesis*, a statement that captures the nature of the theoretical question in such a way that it can be directly verified. As you can see in Figure 6.1, the hypothesis follows the statement of the theory but is written in such a way that it is "testable." In this way it will provide empirical evidence in support of, or contrary to, the theoretical question.

Let me add here that I am introducing a scientific process that underlies most all scientific attempts to understand the world. The physical sciences and social sciences alike use the methods I am describing to generate and verify knowledge. The theory testing process shown in Figure 6.1 is the heart of this process. By following the process, we can support or refute a theoretical position, but we can never "prove" it directly. If a hypothesis statement, being constructed in empirical, and therefore, limited, language, is borne out, we simply add to our confidence in the theory. There are many hypotheses that can be generated to test any one theory since the empirical world cannot completely capture the essence of the abstract conceptual world.

Here is an example of what I mean. I might generate the following hypothesis regarding the previous theoretical statement about wealth and health: "Workers with larger incomes report better health on standardized measures of health." Do you see the difference in language between theory and hypothesis? Theory is abstract; both health and wealth are recognizable concepts, but they have so much meaning that they cannot be fully understood taken singly or in relationship to one another. The hypothesis creates situations that allow the researcher to take various aspects of the concepts and describe them in ways that these limited aspects can be measured and assessed. Theory is therefore more "general," while hypotheses are more "specific."

Theory cannot be captured by a single hypothesis statement; there are simply too many empirical possibilities that can be created to "test" the theory. For example, I might suggest another hypothesis dealing with the same overall research question: "A person's combined wealth is negatively related to the number of times they visit the doctor." As you can see, this is another restatement of the theory in language that is testable. Taken together, these two hypotheses define health as a survey rating and the number of doctor visits. Both reflect the conceptual meaning of health, but even together they cannot exhaust the overall meaning of "health."

Types of Research Designs

Research designs are simply the structure within which a researcher carries out an analysis to test a theory. You can see in Figure 6.1 that the research design follows the hypothesis and enables the researcher to *situate* the hypothesis. How can we create the analysis in such a way that we can obtain data for subsequent statistical procedures that will provide evidence for assessing the theory? While there are many different possibilities, we can note three:

- Experiment
- Post facto – correlational
- Post facto – comparative

EXPERIMENT

There are two general "classes" of research designs: experimental and Non-Experimental (also known as "post facto"). Experiments are *designs in which the researcher consciously changes the values of a study variable under controlled conditions and observes the effects on an outcome variable.* Non-Experimental or post facto designs are those that involve measuring the relationships among variables using data that have already been collected.

The two examples of hypothesis I listed earlier for wealth and health are really better understood through non-Experimental designs because we cannot easily change the values of one variable to observe its effect on the other. We could change the combined wealth of individuals in a study group to see if their health improves, but this would be quite an undertaking and it would be difficult to isolate the impact of this change among many other things that are related to combined wealth (i.e., sets of friends, lifestyle habits, etc.). We might more easily change the income of a group of workers (as in the first hypothesis) to see if their health ratings change, but we would first need to overcome several ethical (e.g., do we lower the incomes of some?) and practical (e.g., are the workers randomly selected from a larger group?) matters.

A classic use of the experiment is the "randomized controlled trial" in which medications or medical treatments are tested to determine which might be considered more effective or to determine whether they may have different outcomes. Thus, a group of people are randomly selected and given different medications (or different amounts of a single medication) to determine if one is more effective for eliminating a certain medical condition. Thus, "does drug A reduce the medical condition X better than drug B?" In this example, the elements of the experiment involve changing the levels of a study variable (medication) to observe the effects on an outcome variable (medical condition X). Randomly selecting the study subjects helps to control other influences that might have different impacts on Drugs A and B.

Randomization

Experimenters use *randomization* methods to ensure comparability of experimental groups. By randomization, I mean (1) selecting subjects randomly from a larger population and (2) randomly assigning them to different conditions. The power of randomness is that it results in individual differences among subjects in the different groups that are created. If every subject has an equal chance of being chosen for an experiment and an equal chance of being assigned to a different comparison condition, then the resulting groups should be as equal as possible; there should be very little bias that would normally influence some subjects to be chosen to receive one treatment condition over another.

Control and Treatment Groups

The particular ways in which controlling all the influences other than the study variables will have a bearing on the strength and validity of the results of an experiment. The key to a powerful experimental design is limiting all influences on the outcome except for the treatment study variable. One way to do so is to create a "control group" which is typically a group similar in every way to a "treatment group" (the group targeted for change) except for the research variable of interest.

In our example, we might randomly select a study group from our study population and then randomly assign some of these to receive Drug A (treatment group: a new medicine for condition X) and others of these to receive Drug B (control group: the existing medicine for condition X). If the two groups show different effects on condition X, researchers could then point to either A or B as "causing" the changes.

Random sampling of study subjects results in all the study subjects being generally equivalent on individual attributes. Therefore, if some of these individuals show differences on condition X as a result of receiving either A or B, then the differences are attributed to the medicines (A or B) since the individuals were considered the same going into the experiment. We might say the groups are "comparable" for the experiment. Theoretically, there are no other differences present in the subjects or the design that could account for the differences to condition X. The groups are shown in Table 6.1.

As you might imagine, there are a host of potentially "confounding" conditions or ways that the two groups cannot be called comparable. Perhaps the experimenter cannot truly choose subjects randomly and/or assign them randomly to different drug conditions. If so, then there are differences being "built in" to the experiment: Was Drug A more effective than Drug B because the treatment group had more men than women? Older than younger subjects? Were there subjects of "equal" aptitudes, health histories, and personality types represented in both groups, for example?

TABLE 6.1   Experimental and Control Groups

Research Treatment Variable – Medications (A or B)		Outcome Variable
Drug A	**Treatment Group** An experimental group in which the values of the independent (or treatment) variable are changed.	Condition X
Drug B	**Control Group** An experimental group in which the treatment is not applied or administered so that the results can be compared to the treatment group	Condition X

Variables

By now, you will recognize that I have used the language of "variables" in my explanation of experimental design. Before we proceed to discuss other designs, we need to note different kinds of variables. Variables, by definition, are the quantification of concepts (like operationally defining "health" as standardized measures of health survey instruments as we discussed earlier) used in research that can take different values (i.e., vary). Thus, health is a quantified set of test scores that vary by individual subject.

Independent Variables   In research design, we often refer to certain types of variables. The "independent variable" is understood to be a variable whose measure does not relate to or depend upon other variables. Thus, in our experimental design example, "medications received" is such a variable since in our research problem; we assume that this is the influence that will lead to an impact on the outcome X. It is assumed to be a "cause" of some research action.

There are a host of problems with the independent variable designation. Typically, we refer to a variable as independent only in the context of an experiment since we are framing it as a <u>cause</u> leading to certain effects. In order for a researcher to refer to a variable as a cause, they must first ensure that there are no influences on the experiment other than changing the value of the treatment variable.

In <u>non-experimental contexts</u>, I prefer to use the designation "predictor variable" rather than independent variable since this does not evoke the language of causality. Non-experimental designs like those using survey data focus more on identifying patterns of relationship among variables rather than establishing causality. In these situations, I refer to this variable as "predictor" in that it comes first and is thought to be the influence on other variables. In like manner I use "outcome" variable for the variable that is thought to be influenced by other variables rather than <u>dependent</u> variable. As you can see predictors/outcomes correspond to independent/dependent variables but are used differently depending on the nature of the research design. A variable can be a predictor of an outcome without being assumed to be a cause.

In experimental designs, independent study variables can be "manipulated" or "non-manipulated" depending on their nature. *Manipulated independent variables* are those the experimenter consciously changes, or manipulates, in order to create the conditions for observing differential effects of treatment groups on the outcome variable. In our example, "medications" is the manipulated independent variable since the researcher could assign subjects to two different levels or conditions of this variable: Drug A or B. In this example, "medications" is manipulated (i.e., consciously changed by the researcher) by creating two groups that receive different levels of the drug.

Non-manipulated independent variables are those that cannot change or cannot be manipulated by the researcher. Typically, they are characteristics, traits, or attributes of individuals. For example, gender or age can be independent variables in a study, but they cannot be changed, only measured. <u>When these types of variables are used in a research study, the researcher cannot make causal conclusions</u>. The essence of a true experiment is to observe the effects of changing the conditions of a variable differentially for different groups and then observing the effects on the outcome. If non-manipulated variables are used, by definition the research design cannot be experimental. For example, if the researcher was interested in the effects of gender on achievement, the research design can only group the subjects by their already designated gender; no causal conclusions can be made.

Dependent Variables *Dependent variables* are those thought to be the "receivers of action" in a research study; their value depends upon (is tied to) a previously occurring variable. Where independent variables are causes, dependent variables are "effects" or results. As noted earlier, in non-experimental contexts, I like to think of these as "outcome variables" that are linked to predictors.

Quasi-Experimental Design

Experiments can be either "strongly" constructed or "weakly" constructed according to how well the experimenter can control the differences between both groups. Often, an experimenter cannot control all the conditions that lead to inequality of groups, but they still implement the study. The *quasi-experimental design* is just such a design. Here, the experimenter may be forced, because of the practicalities of the situation, to use a design that does not include all of the controls that would make it an ideal experiment. Perhaps they do not have the ability to create a control group and must rely on a similar, "comparable group" that they create, or they may be confronted with using existing groups of subjects rather than being able to create the groups of subjects randomly.

In the experimental design we discussed previously, the experimenter may not be able to randomly select subjects from some known subject "pool" and then randomly assign them to different drug conditions. Perhaps the experimenter can only assign the subjects who are available to different groups using random means. In this case, we cannot be assured that the subjects in the two groups are comparable since we could not assure complete randomness. However, we might proceed with the experiment and analyze how this potential inequality might affect our conclusions. This change on the design is shown in Table 6.2 in which the difference from the experimental design (shown in Table 6.1) is the absence of randomization and the lack of a true control group.

There are a great many variations of experimental and quasi-experimental designs. The key differences usually focus on the lack of randomization and/or true comparison groups in the latter. For a comprehensive understanding of experimental design and the attendant challenges of each variation, consult Campbell and Stanley (1963) for the definitive statement. In this authoritative discussion, the authors discuss different types of designs and how each can address problems of internal validity (whether the conditions of the experiment were present to control extraneous forces) and external validity (including generalizability).

It is probably best to think of experimental designs as being stronger or weaker rather than as specific "types" that can be employed in certain situations. Many research design books list and describe several specific (experimental and quasi-experimental) designs, noting the features that limit problems of internal and

TABLE 6.2   Quasi-Experimental Design

Research Treatment Variable – Medications (A or B)		Outcome Variable
Drug A	**Experimental Group** (Not randomly selected and/or assigned)	Condition X
Drug B	**Comparison Group** Not randomly selected and/or assigned but selected to be comparable to the experimental group)	Condition X

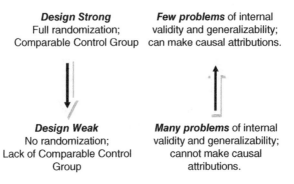

Design Strong
Full randomization;
Comparable Control Group

Few problems of internal
validity and generalizability;
can make causal attributions.

Design Weak
No randomization;
Lack of Comparable Control
Group

Many problems of internal
validity and generalizability;
cannot make causal
attributions.

Figure 6.2   The nature of experimental designs.

external validity. Figure 6.2 shows how research designs exist on a <u>continuum</u> in which they can approach "true" experimental designs on one end that limit all problems and can make causal attributions to those on the other end of the continuum that are beset with problems which limit their ability to produce meaningful experimental conclusions.

NON-EXPERIMENTAL OR POST FACTO RESEARCH DESIGNS

The hypothesis example I presented earlier ("Workers with larger incomes report better health on standardized measures of health") is more easily considered a non-experimental design; it is probably best considered a *post facto correlational* design. Here, I am simply using data that already exist (on workers' income levels and their health ratings on a standardized health measure) – hence *post facto*, which means "after the fact." I do not consciously change anything; rather I use what data I can gather *from what is already generated* to see if the two set of scores are related or correlated. This design uses the statistical process of correlation to measure the association of two sets of existing scores. (We will discuss this process at length in the correlation chapter.)

A post facto design can also *compare* conditions rather than *correlate* conditions. The *post facto – comparative* design seeks to understand *difference*. Thus, for example, I might compare two *already existing groups of workers* designated as having high or low incomes to see if they have different health measure ratings. (Or perhaps we are interested in whether one group, composed of women, has different health measure values than a group of men workers.) Statistically, the researcher can assess whether there is a <u>difference</u> between the means of the health measure values. This type of approach uses <u>methods of difference</u> like the *t* test, analysis of variance (ANOVA), and others that we will discuss in subsequent chapters. This design is post facto, since we are using data that already exist (i.e., the researcher may not have been able to randomly select and assign workers to different groups but required to use groups already operative). This design is post facto, but it is not <u>correlational</u> since we seek to assess *difference* rather than *association*.

The Nature of Research Design

I cannot hope to discuss the nuances of each type of design. However, I will introduce the different designs in the context of discussing different statistical procedures in the chapters ahead. For now, it is enough to know that there are different ways to assess theories. We devise hypotheses according to the nature of our interests and inquiry, and we thereby validate or question theories by empirical (statistical) processes.

I should mention here some important aspects of research designs that I will develop in later chapters. In brief, each design has strengths and limitations. The experiment can be a powerful way of making "causal statements" since, if only one thing changes (the main treatment) while everything else is similar between the groups being tested, we can attribute any effects or changes in outcomes to the thing that was changed. Using the first example again, if we chose and assigned subjects to different drug conditions using random means and if the only difference between the two groups was the different drug received, then the researcher could attribute any resultant differences in outcome X to the different drugs. (Of course, as we will learn, we have to take great care to control all other influences besides the treatment conditions in order to make a causal conclusion.)

<u>Post facto designs cannot lead to causal attributions</u>. Since the data are already collected, a number of different influences are already "contained in the data." In this event, any two groups we compare have differences other than the research interest (exposure to different drugs) that will intrude upon differences in test outcomes. It is a matter of controlling these influences that is the difference between an experiment and a post facto design.

Research Design Varieties

There is another dimension to research design: the variety of ways in which it is carried out to collect data. Experiments can take place in the <u>laboratory</u> or in the <u>field</u>, for example. Post facto designs can use <u>self-report instruments</u> (i.e., questionnaires) or <u>researcher observation</u> to generate outcome data. More generally, research can be <u>quantitative</u> (focusing on the statistical analysis of numerical measures for the concepts studied) or <u>qualitative</u> (focusing on the aspects of research assumed to be irreducible to numbers, like the emergent meaning of a concept among a group of people.)

Sampling

I have already alluded to the importance of sampling. By now, sampling is generally understood to be the process by which a small group of elements is chosen from a larger (population) group so that the small group chosen is representative of the larger group. Thus, for example, in my hypothesis cited earlier, sampling might involve choosing a group of subjects from a large hospital dealing with the condition X. In this way the researcher would have a number of subjects from which to create two different comparable groups rather than including everyone in the population (i.e., in this case, the hospital). The purpose is to create a representative group for study; the conclusions of the study are then thought to characterize the entire population. The sampling "step" of research thus follows the hypothesis "step" shown in Figure 6.1.

As you might imagine, the sampling process is vulnerable to problems. How do you choose the sample so that you can be assured it is representative of the entire population from which it was drawn? There is no way to be entirely certain! But, if the researcher chooses a sample randomly, where each element has an equal probability of being chosen, they can rest assured that we will have the most representative sample possible. What we are saying here is that we are using a *probability sampling process*; that is, we are using the methods of probability to arrive at a sample group in which the variability of the sample reflects the variability of the population. The chosen sample should have the same gender, age, and other characteristic mix as the population.

Sampling is more complex than I am making it out; however, at its heart, it really is a simple principle. The situation I described earlier is the *simple random sample*. There are other types of sampling that recognize the complexity of the process and the nature of a research problem. *Stratified random sampling*, for example, allows the researcher to build in *levels or categories* so that they can ensure each of the crucial components of a population is taken into account. If our population has unequal numbers of men and women, for example, we might want to sample randomly within sex categories to ensure we have a representative sample group.

What makes sampling difficult is that we often cannot control certain features of the process that would result in a representative sample. Often, we do not have the ability to use probability sampling procedures. Perhaps we are studying a phenomenon in which it is difficult or impossible to identify the population from which to sample. In such cases, we need to use whatever procedures are available. I did a study a number of years ago on street-corner preachers. It would be impossible to identify the population of street-corner preachers, so I interviewed and observed those street-corner preachers that were convenient. The *convenience sample* is obviously not representative, but it may be a researcher's only option.

Another nonrepresentative sampling process is *snowball sampling*. Often, because a study population is secretive or difficult to identify, the researcher might gain additional subject interviews from an existing interview. Then, the additional interviews might uncover other potential subjects, like a snowball gathering momentum rolling down a hill. I was forced to resort to this process when conducting a special census some years ago. The population was resistant and secretive, so I had to carefully construct an interview list through existing contacts. This and other nonprobabilistic sampling methods are available to researchers, but the limitations need to be identified in the study. Any problems in creating a representative sample will be registered in the conclusions of the research conducted.

INFERENTIAL STATISTICS

Now that I have covered some of the essentials of research design, we can return to the topic of inferential statistics. The two topics are highly intertwined. As I mentioned in Chapter 5, inferential statistics involves a shift in thinking from individual scores to sets of scores (or samples).

The main requirement for understanding inferential statistics is to learn to think abstractly. We have dealt with descriptive statistics, which, in a sense, are procedures to measure what you see. Inferential statistics looks at data on a different level of abstraction. We must learn to understand the connection between what data we see before us and the statistical world that lies outside and beyond what we see.

One Sample from Many Possible Samples

We need to begin thinking of our data as a sample that we have drawn from some larger population rather than a set of data that is a sample unto itself. Or, stated differently, we must move from measuring distributions of raw scores to measuring the probability of sample distributions belonging to certain populations.

In order to pursue the matter of whether income affects health, for example, we can use inferential statistics to help us understand whether our observed changes from a sample study likely apply to the population of all subjects. Figure 6.3 shows how this works.

When we conduct a research study, we typically select a sample that we try to ensure is representative of a population of interest. Figure 6.3 shows that this sampling process, if it is random, can result in a sample group drawn from across a population distribution. There are four samples shown in Figure 6.3 to show that most samples will be selected from the area close to the mean of the population if probabilistic methods are used. We discussed this in Chapter 5 dealing with probability and the normal curve. The greatest likelihood in sample selection is that it will come from the area massed most closely to the mean. There are probabilities that the sample can be drawn from out in the tails, but that is not as likely.

Returning to our example of the class of AP scores, we can understand the population of interest to be students in all AP classes and our sample to be the students in the one class from which we obtained AP scores. I must note the issue of generalizability here. If our population is limited to one school, then the conclusions of our study can only extend to the students from which it is drawn. In this case, this would mean that the AP scores constitute their own population. The conclusion, in this case, would be quite limited; it would only apply to the dynamics of our particular school and would

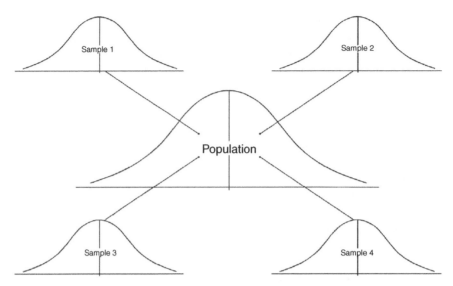

Figure 6.3   The sampling process for inferential statistics.

constitute a *case study*. If we were to conduct a national study and select a larger group of students from the national population, then our conclusions could extend to the national population.

For discussion purposes, Figure 6.3 shows that if we were to create a sample four times, our samples would fall within the large area close to the mean and not in the tails. If we were to select 1000 samples (or the scores of students in each of 1000 classes), we would likely observe the mean of most of the samples from around the population mean but several in the tails as well. That is the nature of the normal distribution.

Of course, we do not need to create four samples for our study. The figure is just to underscore the fact that when we create samples, they are likely to come from the area closer to the mean than in the tails. We assume, when we take a sample, that it represents a population by coming from the area close to the mean. Even though our sample mean will not likely be exactly the same as the population mean, nevertheless it will likely be close.

Sampling error is the difference between the sample and population means among other aspects of the distribution. Whenever we take a sample, we are not likely to create a small group with exactly the same mean and standard deviation as the overall population. This doesn't make the sample problematic or unrepresentative unless it is widely divergent from the population mean. Some error (difference between sample and population means) is expected in sampling. The extent of the error is the subject matter of inferential statistics.

Central Limit Theorem and Sampling Distributions

Here is a curious fact. Suppose we did gather 1000 samples from a large population of students. *If we used only the sample means of each sample to represent their entire*

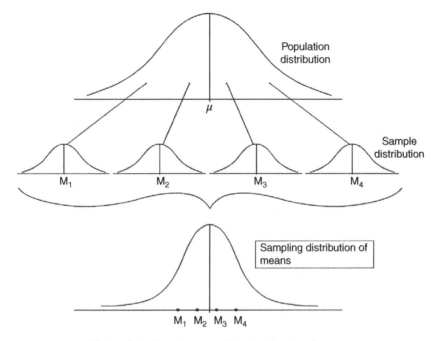

Figure 6.4 Creating a sampling distribution of means.

sample groups, we could create a new distribution just made up only of these sample means. In such a process most of the sample means in this new "sampling distribution" would lay close to the overall population mean with some spreading out into the tails. In fact, the sampling distribution of means would be normally distributed, and its mean would be equal to the population mean.

Researchers and statisticians refer to this process as resulting from the assumptions of the *central limit theorem*. This theorem states that means of repeated samples taken from a population will form a standard normal distribution (assuming a large sample size) even if the population was not normally distributed. The sampling distribution that results will have important properties to researchers conducting inferential studies.

As you can see in Figure 6.4, the four hypothetical samples are taken from the population, and their individual means make up a separate distribution called the *sampling distribution*. You can see from Figure 6.4 that the individual means, which represent their sample distributions (M_1, M_2, M_3, M_4), lay close to the population mean in the new distribution. We can say that the sampling error is smaller as we get closer to the population mean. Figure 6.4 shows this process using only four samples for illustration.

There are other important features of the sampling distribution created by using the means of repeated samples. As you can see in Figure 6.4, the following are true:

1. The sampling distribution will be normally distributed.

2. The mean of the sampling distribution will be equal to the population mean. That is, if you added up all the sample means and divided by the number of sample means, the resulting average of sample means would equal the population mean.

3. The standard deviation of the sampling distribution will be smaller than the standard deviation of the population since <u>we are only using the individual mean scores from each sample distribution to represent the entire set of sample scores</u>. Using only the mean of each sample group results in "lopping off" most of the variability of individual scores around their contributing group means with the result that the sampling distribution will have a smaller "spread."

The importance of the sampling distribution of means is that it will be normally distributed. If we take repeated random samples and make a separate distribution from just the sample means, the resulting distribution will be normally distributed <u>even if the original population is not normally distributed</u>. You can see this feature of the central limit theorem in Figure 6.5. Since it is normally distributed, you can see how a single sample mean relates to all other possible sample means. If you think of your study being one such sample, is your study mean close to the population mean? How close or far away is it?

You are probably asking yourself, "so what? What does this have to do with anything since I would only select one sample for my study?" This is the crux of inferential statistics, so let me answer this (anticipated) question.

Sampling distributions are not empirical; they provide the framework within which you can understand your sample as one of several possible samples. <u>You don't actually select multiple samples</u> for a study such as I described, so <u>the sampling</u>

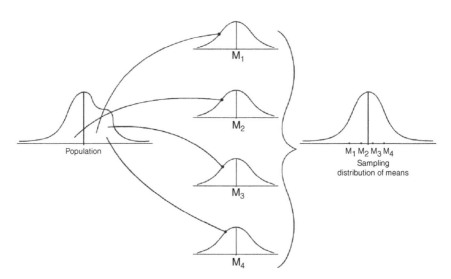

Figure 6.5   The nature of the sampling distribution.

distribution is not created; it exists to provide a benchmark that can be for comparisons of one's actual sample. But you should understand that, when you obtain the results from studying your sample, the results will reflect two things: the impact of the independent (predictor) variable on the dependent (outcome) variable *as well as the distance of the sample mean from the population mean*. If your sample is drawn randomly, it should be close to the population characteristics, and this source of "error" should be minimized. But the fact of the matter is you could select a sample from the tails of a distribution just by chance. It certainly happens; that is the nature of probability.

The important question is, how far away from the population mean can I select a sample, and still assume it is representative? This is the operative question at the center of inferential statistics and the reason we need to envision the sampling distribution. *Even though we will never actually create a sampling distribution by repeatedly sampling from a population, the known features of the sampling distribution will help us to answer the question of representativeness of values.*

The Sampling Distribution and Research

In research, you draw a sample from a population and use the sample to reflect the population characteristics. If you select the sample using probabilistic methods, it will be representative. That is, the sample mean will likely not fall far from the population mean.

Next, you "use" the sample to make a careful study. Perhaps, as a simple example, we perform an "experiment" by selecting a sample of AP students and introduce some new way of teaching the material that we think will affect an outcome measure (such as the AP exam). In this example, we would form the class (randomly if possible!) and then use the new teaching approach for a period of time before which we measured the outcome of the study (student SP test scores). Do our students have a larger or smaller test average than "normal" AP students (i.e., those not exposed to the new teaching method, assumed to be the case for the population of students)?

Since we are hypothesizing that the new teaching method is helpful to learning, we would anticipate that the average AP student test scores in our sample group would be higher than the AP test scores of the general population of students. That is, over the duration of the class, the teaching method would result in higher achievement (test scores) than in students in other AP classes. If we now compared our class achievement average to the average achievement of the population of students, it might be quite   higher.   But how much higher would it have to be for us to conclude that the new teaching method had a   *significant impact*   on student learning? This is the importance of the sampling distribution.

When we compare a sample mean to the population mean *after we change the sample in some way* (e.g., by an experimental treatment), it may no longer be close to the population mean. In effect, our treatment may have "moved the sample mean away" from the population mean a certain distance as a result of the experimental treatment. We use the sampling distribution of means to "measure" this distance. How far away from the population mean does the sample mean now fall after the treatment?

The answer to this question is found in probability theory. If we assume that we will get a sample mean close to the population mean by choosing it randomly, then we assume that a sample mean, *once changed by an experimental treatment*, will be moved further away from the population mean if the treatment is effective. If the (changed) sample mean now falls in the tail area (exclusion area) of the sampling distribution, that is tantamount to saying that it is no longer representative of the population; the sample mean falls too far away from the sample mean.

How far is too far? Statisticians and researchers have assumed that if a sample mean falls into the tails of a distribution, it is not representative; but how far into the tails? The consensus is generally the 5% exclusion area, that is, the area in the tails (both sides) that represents the extreme 5% of the area under the standard normal distribution (i.e., 2.5% on either side).

Therefore, go back to our example. If our sample students' AP test scores are substantially higher than those of the population, perhaps falling into the tails of the population distribution, we would say that the new teaching method "pushed" the sample test mean away from the population mean so far into the tails of the distribution that our students are no longer representative of the students in the population.

Figure 6.6 shows how you might visualize this. The sampling distribution is drawn (in theory) from the population of all students. After the experiment, the students' scores (as represented by the sample mean) are now ahead of the other students' scores as represented on the sampling distribution (the sample mean value is on the far right of the test score distribution of all students).

The sampling distribution thus becomes a kind of "ruler" that we can use to apply our findings. It is (theoretically) created according to the central limit theorem and therefore reflects a "perfect" distribution: a standard normal distribution. *It now stands in the place of the population as our comparison figure.* We can now see where our sample mean falls on this perfect comparison distribution. If it falls

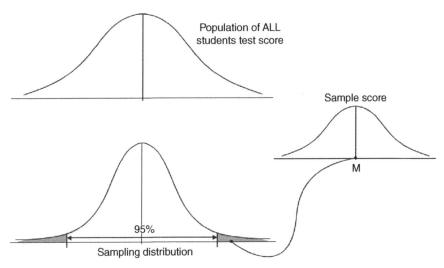

Figure 6.6 Using the sampling distribution to "locate" the sample mean.

in the tails, as it does in the example in Figure 6.6, we would say that the treatment changed the group to such an extent that it no longer is the same as the group of all other students (i.e., population); it is too far away from the population mean.

Another way of saying this is that, after the experiment, our one sample of many possible samples is now not in the area of a "normal" sample. All possible samples are represented by the sampling distribution. Our *changed* sample is now moved into the tails, and we can say it is now different from the possible samples that could be created.

Populations and Samples

Parameters refer to measures of entire populations and population distributions. This is distinguished from *statistics, which refer to measures of sample data taken from populations.* We need to distinguish these measures since inferential statistics is quite specific about the measures available for analysis. One way they are distinguished is by their symbols; population parameters are typically represented by Greek symbols.

This is a good place to review some symbols that will distinguish population measures from sample measures. Since we are now beginning to think of different levels of data, we need to be able to be precise in how we speak of both. Table 6.3 is a chart showing the symbols for population and sample sets of data.

The Standard Error of the Mean

This is a new term for a measure we have already discussed: the standard deviation of the sampling distribution of means. The designation "standard error of the means" is used because it is much shorter! Hopefully you can see why we give it this name. Both are simply ways of saying that σ_M is a standard deviation of a standard normal distribution consisting of all possible sample means.

TABLE 6.3   Population and Sample Symbols for Inferential Statistics

POPULATION AND SAMPLE SYMBOLS	
M	The mean of the sample.
SD	The standard deviation of the sample (assumes the sample is its own population)
μ	The Greek letter 'Mu' is the symbol for the population mean.
M_M	This is the symbol for the <u>mean of the sampling distribution of means</u>. You can see how this works by observing that it is a mean (M), but a mean of the sampling distribution indicated by the subscript. Thus, it is the *mean of the distribution of means*, or the 'mean of all possible means.' Since it is (theoretically) created by all possible samples, it is a parameter.
σ_X	"Sigma X" is the Standard Deviation of all the population raw scores. This differs from SD in that it does not refer to a sample, but to the entire population of individual raw scores.
σ_M	The standard deviation of the sampling distribution of means; also called the *Standard Error of the Mean*.

The standard error of the mean is a standard deviation. But recall that it is a standard deviation of a distribution that is "narrower" than the population standard deviation since we only use the mean scores from repeated sampling to make it up. You can see this by looking again at Figure 6.4.

Since the standard error of the means (σ_M) is different from the population standard deviation (σ_X), we need to be able to *estimate* its value. One way of doing this is by the following formula:

$$\sigma_M = \frac{\sigma_X}{\sqrt{N}}$$

We use this formula since it includes the sample size (N) of the sample we select as a way of helping us make the estimate. The sample size will ultimately determine the size of the σ_M since the group size is registered in the sample means that make it up. As N increases, the σ_M will decrease; you can see this from the formula. When you divide a number by a large number, the result will be a smaller number. Conceptually, however, this simply refers to the fact that larger sample sizes are better estimates and therefore the standard deviation of the sample means will likely be smaller.

Rule of thumb to remember is $\sigma_M < \sigma_X$.

"Transforming" the Sample Mean to the Sampling Distribution

Remember that "sampling error" is the distance of a sample mean from the population mean. Remember also that the sampling distribution of means is perfectly normally distributed and its mean is equal to the population mean ($M_M = \mu$). When we "fit" our *sample* mean (M) onto the sampling distribution as shown in Figure 6.6, the distance of our sample mean from M_M can be expressed as a "standard distance" by referencing it to the standard deviation of this (perfect) distribution (σ_M).

The resulting distance is therefore like a z score that is expressed in standard deviation units of the distribution of means. In effect, we are transforming a raw score mean to a standard value in the sampling distribution so that we can compare it to all possible sample means that could be taken from a population. It therefore helps us to answer the question, how good of an estimate of the population mean is our sample mean?

We "transform" the sample mean to a standardized value on the sampling distribution of means just as we did when we created a z score. Here is the formula we used when we were dealing only with single sample scores:

$$Z = \frac{X - M}{\text{SD}}$$

We can use the same formula with some changes to reflect that we are using population rather than only sample values:

$$Z = \frac{M - \mu}{\sigma_M}$$

Compare the two formulas. They look alike, because they do the same thing. The z score formula (top) is used to *transform a raw score to a standard score*. These are both at the sample distribution "level."

The bottom formula is used to *transform a sample mean to a standard score in the distribution of means*. These are measures used when we are dealing with both population and sample values.

Example

Let's take an example using our hypothetical AP scores. For the purposes of this example, assume that I selected a sample of AP students at random from all AP students in my region's universities. The following values resulted from the study:

1. The mean aggregate AP test score of the population of students: $\mu = 48.00$. (This hypothetical value represents the average AP test score for students in every university in the region.)
2. The population standard deviation (σ_X) of AP test score values $= 15.00$. (Hypothetical population value.)
3. The mean AP test score for the sample ($N = 31$): $M = 53.68$. (This example value is calculated and discussed in previous chapters.)
4. The standard deviation of AP test scores (SD) $= 20.028$. (This example value is calculated and discussed in previous chapters.) This value is not needed for this procedure since we are using the population standard deviation (μ) as our comparison.
5. The standard error of the mean (σ_M) $= 2.69$:

$$\sigma_M = \frac{\sigma_X}{\sqrt{N}} = \frac{15.00}{\sqrt{31}} = 2.69$$

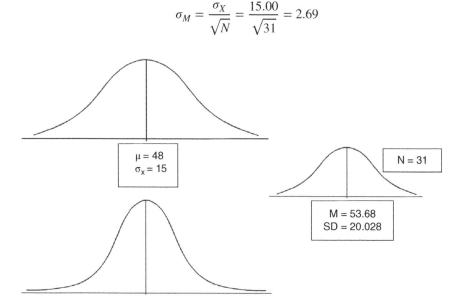

Figure 6.7   Using the sampling distribution and the standard error of the mean.

Figure 6.7 shows how these values are "placed" so you can visualize the various measures. The research question is: Is the AP test mean of our sample (of AP students) different from the AP scores from students in the region's universities? What we need to do is to see where our sample mean falls in the sampling distribution of means so that we can compare it to the population mean:

$$Z = \frac{X - M}{SD}$$

$$Z = \frac{M - \mu}{\sigma_M}$$

If we calculate the *standardized sample mean score*, Z:

$$Z = \frac{M - \mu}{\sigma_M} = \frac{53.68 - 48.00}{2.69} = 2.11$$

Findings

What does this figure of $Z = 2.11$ indicate? Consider the following findings based on our calculations:

- The resulting Z value indicates that the difference between the sample mean and the population mean, which is the top part of the formula $(M - \mu)$ is 5.68. This indicates that our sample math achievement mean lies above the population AP mean by 5.68 points on the AP test.
- When we divide this distance (5.68) by the standard error of the mean (2.69), it *transforms* the sample-population distance into a standard measure, like we did with a z score. The resulting figure $Z = 2.11$ means that our sample mean falls about 2 and 11/100 standard deviations above the population mean.
- If you recall the Z Score Table of Values, this means that our sample mean falls well into the right (positive) tail of the standard normal comparison distribution.
- Using the NORM.S.DIST function from Excel, you can calculate the area of the standard normal distribution falling below 2.11 to be 98.66%. You can locate the same value in the Z Score Table of Values, which also identifies the $Z = 2.11$ as excluding approximately 1.74%. In terms of probability, that would mean that our sample mean is extremely atypical; it is nowhere close to the population mean.
- The probability of $Z = 2.11$ falls "beyond" the exclusion area defined by the extreme 5% (or 2.5% on each side of the standard normal distribution) that researchers use to conclude that the sample mean is not typical. This exclusion value for the Z distribution is ± 1.96.
- Since our $Z = 2.11$ value fell beyond (into the tails) of the 5% exclusion area, we can conclude that the AP mean for our students is significantly above the AP scores of students in the region's universities. In fact, we can suggest that our AP sample mean is so different from the population mean that our students cannot be considered belonging to the students in the region's universities. The

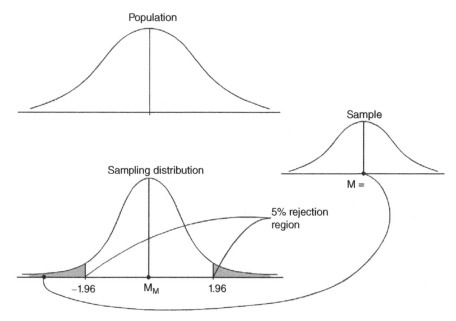

Figure 6.8 Using the sampling distribution to make a statistical decision.

implication is that our new teaching method "pushed" the sample AP scores very far away from the population mean of AP scores.

Figure 6.8 shows how this result looks using the findings from our former figure. Since a Z value of 2.11 is greater than the Z score of 1.96 that identifies the 5% exclusion area, we conclude that the sample of AP values does not represent the population of AP values.

Discussion

We need to remember that these findings probably could not be generalizable because I realistically could not choose a class made up of randomly chosen students for an AP class. This would be a difficult undertaking and points out the problems that beset research efforts. Consider the following findings:

- We discovered a finding that we <u>assumed</u> would be true, given our belief in the new teaching method. Real research might conclude the opposite: that our sample mean AP value was significantly <u>below</u> the population mean value. For example, calculate the Z value assuming that the population mean value = 59.36 (all other values remaining the same). This would result in $Z = -2.11$. The value would still not be typical since it would fall in the 5% exclusion region, but it would be on the left of the distribution, meaning that our students performed much worse than the students in the population. Researchers should be aware of this possibility. In a later chapter, I will have more to say about ways to address the potential direction of findings.

- This design would not be experimental if I used AP test scores from an existing class design since I would in that case use scores from an <u>existing</u> (and therefore not randomly chosen) group of students. To constitute an experiment, I would have had to randomly select students from across the population of regional universities and then contrive a way to invite AP student participation in the class, convince my university to pay for students to attend, assign university credit to students who finished the class, and so on.

- The results of such a study would not be definitive (or causal) since I could not control all of the extraneous influences that would impact the study. However, if done well, the study might suggest "trends" in outcomes using this new teaching method. Before I sold all of my possessions to implement the teaching method on a larger scale, I might more cautiously seek further studies that would have a bearing on my outcome.

Z TEST

Congratulations! Without being aware of it, you just performed your first inferential statistical test, the Z test. As you can see, it is not really that difficult to understand. We simply transformed a sample mean so that it could be compared to all possible sample means. By doing so, we can see how it "falls" on a standard normal distribution of values and calculate a probability for this score occurring by chance. If it falls too far into the tails (i.e., beyond the extreme 5% area), we can conclude that it is not representative of the population.

THE HYPOTHESIS TEST

What we have done is to perform a <u>hypothesis test</u>. This is the formal, logical process established to make a scientific decision. If you look at Figure 6.1, the bottom step in the process is to support or refute a hypothesis and thereby inform a theory.

If we identify the steps we used in our example, you will find that these steps form the general procedure for a hypothesis test that we will follow on all our remaining statistical tests (with some variations for each procedure). Here are the steps with our (contrived) results applied so you can see how it works:

1. The null hypothesis or (H_0): $\mu_1 = \mu$

   Researchers begin by considering a statement that can be measured and then verified or refuted. They begin with the assumption that there will be no difference between the mean of the study sample (μ_1) and the mean of the population (μ). The objective of the research process it to see if this is an accurate assumption or if our sample violates that assumption by being either too large or too small. Our null hypothesis was that a sample of AP student scores would have the same AP mean test score as that of the population consisting of AP students in regional universities.

2. The alternative hypothesis or (H_A): $\mu_1 \neq \mu$

This statement is created in order to present the finding that would negate the null hypothesis – thus the alternate finding. In our study, we proposed that a sample of students would show higher AP test score values than the population. Technically, our alternate hypothesis allows findings to be *not equal to* and thus either higher or lower than the population values. (This would help to account for negative as well as positive departures from the population mean.)

3. The critical value: ± 1.96 z values (5% exclusion area)

Recall that we need to have a benchmark to help us decide whether our actual, calculated results are considered typical or atypical. Actually, we are using this benchmark to help us decide which hypothesis (null or alternate) is more accurate. As I discussed before, for this particular situation researchers use a 5% benchmark. That is, if a calculated/transformed sample mean falls into the 5% exclusion area (the 2.5% in each tail) of a standard normal distribution, then it would be considered atypical. In probability terms, this would represent a probability of occurrence of $p < 0.05$ or $p < 0.025$, either positive or negative. Stated differently, it would be considered not likely to occur just by chance; rather some reason other than chance would create a finding this extreme.

4. The calculated value (2.11)

This is the Z test value that we calculated from the values we had available. It represents the results of the Z test formula that transformed the sample value into a standard score so that we can compare it to other possible sample outcomes.

5. Statistical decision: Reject null hypothesis?

This step asks us to compare the calculated value (step 4) to the benchmark value (step 3) in order to see which hypothesis (null or alternate) is more likely. In our study, the sample students had much higher AP test scores than those of the population students, assumed to be a result of the new teaching method. If we had simply chosen a sample of existing student scores by chance without using the new teaching method, the sample mean would likely not have been this extreme since most chance selections would be much closer to the population mean and would not reflect the changes due to the test or treatment value.

The calculated Z value "pushed" the sample AP test mean into the right tail of the distribution. Given this result, there would be an extremely small probability ($p < 0.01743$) of a Z test value this large falling into the tails simply by chance alone, and we would "reject the null hypothesis." That is, we could conclude that the null hypothesis is not supported by our findings; the alternate hypothesis is supported by our findings.

6. Interpretation

Researchers must make statistical decisions through the previous steps. However, they must *place the findings in the language of the question* so that it has meaning to the audience. We obtained an atypical finding. We would need to capture this in an interpretive discussion. We might say something like "Our sample group of students ($N = 31$) had a much higher mean AP test score (53.68) than the mean of the population of schools (48.00) as evidenced by the Z ratio (2.11, $p < 0.05$)." (Reporting the $p < 0.05$ finding simply is a general statement that the probability of our sample mean had a much smaller probability of a chance finding, that is, in the extreme 5% of the tails of the distribution.)

STATISTICAL SIGNIFICANCE

In probability terms, any finding of $p < 0.05$ is considered "statistically significant." Researchers and statisticians have a specific definition for statistical significance: it refers to the likelihood that a finding we observe in a sample is too far away from the population parameter (in this case the population mean) *by chance alone* to belong to the same population. The 5% exclusion area is typically identified to define statistical significance.

PRACTICAL SIGNIFICANCE: EFFECT SIZE

I will develop this measure much further in the following statistical procedures, but a word is in order here. Researchers and statisticians have relied extensively on statistical significance to help make statistical decisions. You can see how this language (i.e., using p values) permeates much of the research literature; it is even widespread among practitioners and those not familiar with statistical procedures.

The emphasis in statistics and research now is on *effect size*, which refers to the "impact" of a finding, regardless of its statistical p value. The two issues are related to be sure. However, effect size addresses the issue of the extent to which a difference or treatment "pushes a sample value away from a parameter". That is, how much "impact" does a research variable have to move a sample value?

Consider our example problem shown in Figure 6.8. We performed a statistical significance test with these findings and concluded that the sample mean of AP student test scores was too far into the (positive) tails of the sampling distribution to be considered a chance finding. *The effect size consideration is a completely different issue*. It does not concern itself with probability, but rather, how far away from the population mean has our sample mean been driven as result of a lower ratio? According to Figure 6.8, the sample mean has been pushed far into the right tail of the sampling distribution as a result of having a higher value than the population – a distance of about 2 and 11/100 standard deviations!

Z TEST ELEMENTS

In order to use the Z test, you must know the population parameters and the sample statistics. This is often not possible since little may be known about the population. In our example, we assumed that we had population (mean and standard deviation) information on all AP students in the population set of regional universities. We did not have data on all schools in the United States, so our definition of the population was restricted.

We will discuss similar procedures in the next chapter, but with the assumption that we do not have population information. As you will see, this makes an interesting situation since we must "estimate" the population parameters in order to use the process we learned in the Z test.

USING SPSS® AND EXCEL FOR THE Z TEST

The conditions for using the Z test are rarely met. It is not typical to know either the population mean or standard deviation. Since this is the case, SPSS® does not have a way to directly calculate values for the Z test through its drop-down menu interface.

Excel has a function that can be used, but it is not located in the "Data – Data Analysis" list of procedures. In order to initiate the Z test, you can use the "FORMULAS" menu in the main menu bar. After "FORMULAS," you will find the Z test in the list of functions available in the "Statistical" list of functions. (From the main menu, choose FORMULAS and then "More Functions" and then "Statistical.") The Z test formula is located at the end of the list.

Figure 6.9 shows the specification window that opens when you choose the Z test formula. You can see that I placed the values in the appropriate windows for the AP score example question we discussed earlier. The "Array" window identifies the AP values that we wish to consider our sample; the "X" window calls for the population mean against which we are comparing our sample mean ($M = 53.68$ in this example); "Sigma" calls for the known population standard deviation (σ_x).

When you choose "OK" the formula returns the p value under the "Formula Result =") line near the bottom left side of the menu. In this case, the result = 0.01754, which indicates the probability that the sample mean (53.68) represents the known population mean of 48.

Interpreting this result is a bit difficult at this point because we have not covered some of the relevant concepts. Here are some observations of this result:

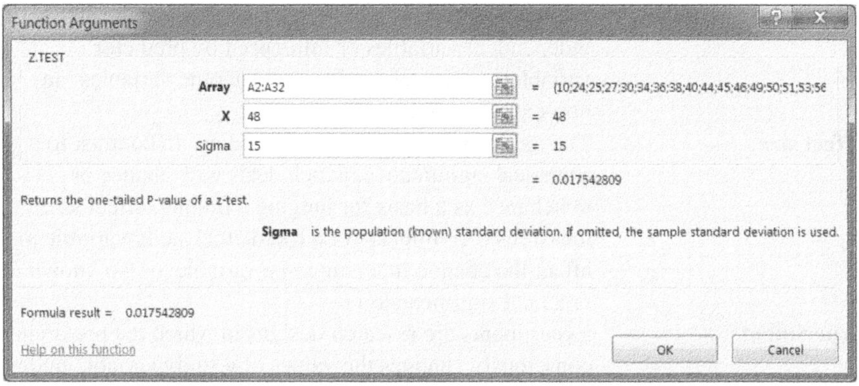

Figure 6.9 The Excel Z test formula specification menu.

- The $p = 0.01754$ value corresponds to the Z ratio (2.11) we calculated previously. If you look in the Z score table of values, the "tail" of the Z distribution contains this proportion (1.743%, or 0.01743 at $Z = 2.11$) of the distribution (equivalent to the returned value of 0.01754 accounting for rounding with raw data).
- This represents a "one-tailed" hypothesis test, which we discuss in Chapter 7. Essentially, it means that we "stack" all the exclusion area into one tail (as the Z Table of Values does by presenting proportions in the tail column) as a way of evaluating the calculated Z ratio.

TERMS AND CONCEPTS

Alternative hypothesis: The research assumption that is stated in contrast to the null hypothesis.

Case study: A study that focuses entirely on one setting rather than making inferences from one study setting to another.

Central limit theorem: The statistical notion that means of repeated samples taken from a population will form a standard normal distribution (assuming a large sample size) even if the population was not normally distributed.

Control group: An experimental group in which the treatment is not applied or administered so that the results can be compared with the "treatment group." This is a group similar in every way to a "treatment group" except for the research variable of interest.

Convenience sample: A nonprobabilistic sample selected from available elements. Usually, this method is used when the researcher has no opportunity to use random sampling methods as in studying secretive groups or groups with difficult-to-identify populations.

Dependent variables: Study variables thought to be "receivers" of the action of independent variables or influenced by predictor variables. Often referred to as "outcome variables" in non-experimental contexts.

Effect size: The meaningfulness of a study finding. In contrast to statistical significance, which deals with chance or nonchance as a basis for judging a finding, effect size measures the "impact" of a (predictor) study variable to affect the change in an outcome variable. (Also known as practical significance.)

Experiment: Experiments are research designs in which the researcher consciously changes the values of a study variable under controlled conditions and observes the effects on an outcome variable.

Hypothesis: A statement that captures the nature of the theoretical question in such a way that it can be quantified and directly verified.

Hypothesis test: The formal process of assessing whether or not a test statistic is judged to be similar to the population elements from which it was drawn or statistically different from those elements.

Independent variables: A designation in experimental research for treatment variables or those study variables that are consciously changed to observe effects on outcome variables.

Manipulated independent variables: Independent variables that the experimenter consciously changes, or manipulates, in order to create the conditions for observing differential effects on the outcome variable.

Non-Experimental designs: Those designs that involve measuring the relationships among variables using data that have already been collected. (Also known as "post facto" designs.)

Non-manipulated independent variables: Independent variables that cannot be changed by the researcher. Typically, they are characteristics, traits, or attributes of individuals.

Null hypothesis: The assumption in an hypothesis test that there is no difference between the study population yielding a particular sample statistic and the population from which the sample supposedly came.

Parameters: Characteristics or measures of entire populations.

Post facto research: These study designs are those that involve measuring the relationships among variables using data that have already been collected. The focus of the study may be to determine differences among study variables ("post facto – comparative") or correlations ("post facto – correlational"). (Also known as Non-Experimental designs.)

Practical significance: See Effect size.

Predictor variables: Study variables that are considered prior to and influential upon other study variables. In experiments, these are typically called independent variables; in post facto research, they are simply the alleged variable of influence upon an outcome variable.

Probability sampling: The process of using probability methods in sampling to ensure that the sample elements are representative of the elements in the population.

Quantification: Operationally defining a concept by expressing it numerically. In this chapter we quantified "health" as a standardized measures of a health survey instruments.

Qualitative research: Focusing on the aspects of research assumed to be irreducible to numbers, like the emergent meaning of a concept among a group of people.

Quantitative research:	Focusing on the statistical analysis of numerical measures for the concepts studied.
Quasi-experimental design:	Experimental designs in which there are elements missing or extraneous influences cannot be controlled sufficient to ensure that the researcher can make causal conclusions. Ordinarily in program evaluation, this takes the form of working with "intact groups" or groups that already exist, or more generally, the inability to ensure full randomization in designing the experiment.
Research design:	Fields of inquiry in which standardized methods for examining available data are applied to answer research questions.
Randomization:	Procedure in which the study elements (i.e., sample) are chosen and assigned on the basis of equal chance or probability. These methods ensure comparability of experimental groups by (1) randomly <u>selecting</u> subjects randomly from a larger population and (2) randomly <u>assigning</u> them to different conditions.
Sampling:	The process of selecting elements from a population.
Sampling distribution:	The distribution formed from repeatedly drawn means from a population.
Sampling error:	The difference between the sample mean in a study and the mean of the population from which the sample was drawn.
Simple random sample:	A sampling process in which each element chosen from a population has an equal chance of being selected.
Snowball sampling:	A method of (nonprobabilistic) sampling in which available sample elements are identified from previous sample elements. Oftentimes, in studying secretive or difficult groups, additional contacts can be identified as the researcher proceeds with interviews, for example.
Standard error of the mean:	The standard deviation of the sampling distribution of means.
Statistical significance:	This designation is stated differently for different statistical procedures. Essentially, it refers to the likelihood that study results are not obtained by chance or happenstance, but reflect an underlying pattern in its population.
Statistics:	Characteristics or measures of samples.
Stratified random sampling:	A sampling process that recognizes inherent levels or strata in the population that can be sampled by probabilistic means.
Theory:	An abstract idea or statement that links the conceptual relationships within an inquiry.

Treatment group: An experimental group in which the values of the independent (or treatment) variable have been changed.

Variables: Concepts that have been quantified and used in research. In contrast to "constants" that cannot take different values, variables consist of elements that can vary or change.

Z test: The statistical test of the likelihood that a sample mean comes from a population with known parameters.

DATA LAB AND EXAMPLES (WITH SOLUTIONS)

Problem 1

According to a CDC report at nonfederal short-stay hospitals, the average length of stay averages about 4.8 days. The population standard deviation is unclear for the population of these facilities, but we can use the hypothetical value of 2.00 for this lab problem. A researcher proposes to compare a small sample of regionally "distinct" hospitals with this overall population information, even though the researcher's description of the sample is hazy.

Here are the researcher's data:

1. The mean population number of hospital days spent: $\mu = 4.8$.

2. The population standard deviation (σ_X) of hospital stays is 2.00 (hypothetical value).

3. The mean length of stay for the sample set of regionally distinct hospitals ($N = 30$): $M = 5.60$.

4. The standard deviation of stays at the sample hospitals (SD) = 2.80. (Remember this value is not needed for this procedure since we are using the population standard deviation (μ) as our comparison.)

Using this information, perform a Z test to determine whether the length of stay among patients at the sample of regionally distinct hospitals is representative of the length of stay among patients the population of nonfederal short-stay hospitals.

Respond to the following questions:

1. What is the standard error of the mean?

2. What is the calculated Z test ratio?

3. Perform the hypothesis test.

4. Interpret the analyses.

5. Discuss effect size.

Problem 2

Discuss the research design discussed in Problem 1: type, strength, and generalizability.

Problem 3

A national medical preparation test yielded a mean test score of 25.2 with a standard deviation of 6.4. A sample of 40 students selected from colleges deemphasizing the social sciences took the test with the following results: mean test score of 23.1. How well did the sample students perform compared to the national results?

DATA LAB: SOLUTIONS

Problem 1

1. What is the standard error of the mean?
   Answer: The standard error of the mean is 0.365. This is the standard deviation of the sampling distribution of means:

   $$\sigma_M = \frac{\sigma_X}{\sqrt{N}} = \frac{2.00}{\sqrt{30}} = 0.365$$

2. What is the calculated Z test ratio?
   Answer: The Z test ratio is 2.19. This represents the number of standard deviations that the sample mean is removed from the population mean in the sampling distribution of means:

   $$Z = \frac{M - \mu}{\sigma_M} = \frac{5.60 - 4.8}{0.365} = 2.19$$

3. Perform the hypothesis test.
   Answer: The hypothesis test follows the same steps we used in our earlier example:
   The null hypothesis (H_0): $\mu_1 = \mu$
   Our null hypothesis was that a sample of regionally distinct hospitals will have the same length of stay as the population of nonfederal short-stay hospitals.
   The alternative hypothesis (H_A): $\mu_1 \neq \mu$
   The sample of regionally distinct hospitals will not have the same length of stay as the population of nonfederal short-stay hospitals.
   The critical value: ± 1.96 z values (5% exclusion area)
   Remember if a calculated Z ratio falls into the 5% exclusion area (the 2.5% in each tail) of a standard normal distribution, then it would be considered unlikely to occur by chance.

The calculated Z ratio $= 2.19$
The calculated Z value falls into the right side of the distribution in the 5% exclusion area.

Statistical decision: reject null hypothesis
The calculated Z value fell into the 5% exclusion region indicating that the probability of the sample length of stay being this large by chance is less than 0.05 ($p < 0.05$). (Using NORM.S.DIST this Z value excludes 1.426% of the rejection area on the right side of the distribution; therefore, it is "beyond" the 2.5% rejection region used to establish significance or $p < 0.05$.) Since we reject the null hypothesis, we assume the sample hospitals are different from population of hospitals.

4. Interpret the analysis.
   Answer: *Interpretation*
   On the basis of a Z test ($Z = 2.19$, $p < 0.05$), there are statistically significant differences between a sample of regionally distinct hospitals ($N = 30$) and the population of nonfederal short-stay hospitals in terms of the length of stay. The regionally distinct hospitals report significantly longer hospital stays ($M = 5.60$ days) than the population ($M = 4.80$ days).

5. Discuss effect size.
   Answer: We rejected the null hypothesis with a Z value of 2.19, suggesting that the mean of the regional hospitals was more than two standard deviations beyond the mean of the population hospitals.

Problem 2

Discuss the research design: type, strength, and generalizability.

Answer:

- Non-experimental design since the independent/predictor variable was not changed. The stay rate for the sample of regionally distinct hospitals was already determined to be 5.60.
- Post facto – comparative since the object is to compare the results of the sample to a (known) population; are there differences between the length of stay between sample and population? (Yes.)
- The problem states that the researcher's descriptions were "hazy" indicating no information about whether the sample of hospitals were drawn by random means or using any standard protocol. Also, the researcher would need to define exactly what is meant by "regionally distinct" (e.g., those from warm climates? Those practicing alternative procedures? Specializing in certain diseases?).
- Generalizability would be limited due to lack of randomization and lack of specificity about the nature of the sample. At most, the researcher could conclude that this group ($N = 30$) of hospitals differs from the population.

Problem 3

<u>Answer:</u>

- $Z = -2.075$
- Reject the null hypothesis, $p < 0.05$.
- The students not prepared in the social sciences performed significantly worse than the national group.

7

THE *T* TEST FOR SINGLE SAMPLES

A number of years ago, my colleagues and I conducted a series of analyses on a low-income housing area in a large western city in the United States. We wanted to explore the effects of gang activity in the community on residents' ratings of their neighborhood and if a new policing model would help to improve their ratings. As I presented in Chapter 3, we compiled the Quality Index (which we called the Quality of Life (QL) Index in Chapter 3) as a way to help us understand the residents' perceptions of health services, recreational opportunities, air quality, community involvement, fear of crime, and related measures. Ratings from the measure resulted in values between 8 and 53, with 56 representing the highest rating of one's neighborhood.

Table 3.4 shows resident ratings of the quality of their neighborhoods from the survey. As a researcher, it was important to understand the residents' perceptions, but it is also important to compare these to existing national data to further understand the findings from one city. We will use the single sample *T* test with a sample of these data to address the comparability of the survey data from similar national rankings.

How would one proceed to compare the ratings from this study to those of the national level without information about the population for which to compare to the sample? This problem is one that can be addressed using inferential statistics and the "single sample *T* test."

Using Statistics in the Social and Health Sciences with SPSS® and Excel®, First Edition.
Martin Lee Abbott.
© 2017 John Wiley & Sons, Inc. Published 2017 by John Wiley & Sons, Inc.

INTRODUCTION

This chapter deals with the "full jump" to inferential statistics, so it is usually the material that you will need to review carefully before (and after) a class you may have in statistics. In the class I teach, I designate this content in my syllabus as "headache day" so that students are aware of the changes in thinking that are required. I designed Chapter 6 as the transition to this chapter, so really there shouldn't be too great a leap.

A number of years ago, one of my graduate students (and elementary school teacher) who took my accelerated course during the summer looked increasingly dour during this and subsequent chapters on inferential statistics. I asked the student one day before class began if all was well. The student replied, "Every day I go home after this class and drink a pint of gin!" After I pleaded for the student not to take this route to understand statistics and as we began to discuss the topic, the student appeared livelier and engaged with the topics. I am happy to report that the student received an "A" grade in the class and, as far as I know, does not drink a pint of gin a day!

I use this example for students who feel at this point in the class that the material is overwhelming. As my student learned, the material is not unknowable; it simply takes a different way of looking at it to see the direction we are taking in inferential statistics.

Z VERSUS *T*: MAKING ACCOMMODATIONS

Up to now, we have dealt with population values (parameters) that are <u>known</u> to the researcher. As I mentioned in Chapter 6, this is fairly rare. If you do have access to parameter values, you can use the *Z* test to help you make a statistical decision about whether your sample values are likely to be taken from that known population.

If the researcher does not have access to population values in their research, this chapter will show how to estimate the population values in order to use them in the statistical decision-making process. This will seem a little strange at first, since we will use sample values to help estimate the population values, but we are going to make use of our sampling distribution as well. In addition, we will learn to make small "adjustments" based on the sample size as a way to better understand the population values.

As we have discussed, the *Z* distribution consists of the known areas in the standard normal distribution. We learned in Chapter 6 that we could use the features of this distribution to help us understand whether a sample value could likely come from a distribution with <u>known</u> population parameters (*Z* test). Now we turn to a related distribution, the <u>*T* distribution</u>, to determine whether a sample value could likely come from a distribution with *unknown population parameters*. This is typically the situation a researcher encounters in real-life problem solving since the knowledge of parameters is unlikely in most situations.

The *T* test for a single sample is a statistical procedure similar to the *Z* test but with some limitations:

1. <u>Population parameters are unknown</u>. Typically, the population mean may be known as a general estimate based on similar research or on the basis of some

other reason. However, the standard deviation (SD) of the population is not known. Therefore, a *T* test uses estimates of population parameters based on sample values.

2. <u>Sample size is small</u>. Sample size is very important in statistics since it is used as a denominator in many calculations. Large sample sizes typically result in better estimates of population means. According to the central limit theorem, repeated large samples will more closely approximate a normal distribution. But how large is large? Researchers and statisticians vary on that score. Typically, a sample size of 30 is considered large for statistical procedures by many researchers. Other researchers suggest higher values. I often use $N = 40$ as an operational definition for "large" samples. As you will see, there is probably no best answer to this question, however.

RESEARCH DESIGN

Does community policing affect ratings of neighborhood satisfaction? This is one of the questions my researchers and I asked during the aforementioned neighborhood quality study. We wanted to see whether a community policing model would affect residents' fear of crime and other attitudes toward the neighborhood. Community policing allows police officers to have more face-to-face contact among a community by walking around rather than simply using squad car patrols.

We discussed research design in Chapter 6; I mentioned then that I would discuss various designs in more detail in subsequent chapters. The design appropriate for the subject of this chapter on *T* test is a very simple one. We will determine whether a sample group mean is likely to come from a population for which we have no knowledge of the parameters.

Experiment

If a researcher administered some treatment or manipulated some research (independent) variable with a random selection of subjects, they might create a (weak) experimental design. For example, I might have taken a (randomly selected) group of residents in the housing complex and assessed their satisfaction with the neighborhood (the dependent variable) after changing the policing model to community policing. I would then have a set of data that indicated the residents' attitudes.

As you can see, this design would be quite weak because there is really nothing to serve as a comparison: There is no control group to compare neighborhood ratings nor is there a "pretest" or assessment of the neighborhood satisfaction ratings before implementing community policing. The researcher would be left with a measure of resident attitudes but could not really attribute the attitudes to community policing; there would be nothing to indicate change from some previous set of attitudes.

Campbell and Stanley (1963) refer to this "experimental" design as the "one-shot case study" since the design does not have the requisite parts of a true experimental design. Figure 7.1 shows the diagram for this kind of design. There is only one group, the sample of residents' neighborhood satisfaction ratings; there is no comparison or

Research Treatment Variable: Community Policing		Outcome Variable
Random Sample??	Experimental Group: Residents	Neighborhood Satisfaction ratings
	(No Control/Comparison Group)	-------

Figure 7.1   The "one-shot case study."

control group. There is no "pretest" of the technology test to compare to the outcome test ("posttest"). Also, we have no information about whether or how the subjects would be identified for the study (random sampling or not).

You can see that the problems with this experimental design would lead to questionable conclusions. The research treatment (community policing) might be effective, but it would be difficult to disentangle the experimental effects from the effects of the uncontrolled influences. No causal conclusions could be made on the basis of data from this design.

Post Facto: Comparative Design

Another approach to a study of this nature is to use existing data that could be compared to some measure of national attitudes of neighborhood satisfaction. This would be a different study because there would be no attempt to measure changes on neighborhood ratings as a result of policing model. Moreover, there would be problems with this design as well since the measure I might have used may be dissimilar from the one(s) reported in national studies, my sample of residents may not be characteristic of the national sample of residents, and so on. Because of these issues, I could not use causal language with any of my findings. That is, I could not say any differences in resident satisfaction measures between sample and population would be due to any change in policing policy. I could only compare national and sample attitudes to see if there were differences apart from policing model.

My study data measured the resident's perceptions of the neighborhood before the full implementation of community policing. Therefore, I would not use these data as experimentally related to community policing. I could only determine, using the single sample, that there may be significant differences between my sample of residents and those of the population.

Generally stated, the single sample *T* test compares data from a sample group drawn from a larger population from which little or no population data are available. The researcher in this instance must compare the sample data to estimated population values (mean and SD) to determine whether or not the sample is likely to come from this population.

The post facto design does not allow causal conclusions since the requirements for a true experimental design (i.e., randomness, control group, control of extraneous variables) would not be met. Most researchers argue that a one-shot experimental design would be no better than a comparative post facto design.

The post facto design is not the strongest for many reasons. As I am using it here, the design does not include any measure of the influence of policing; the focus changes to whether or not sample and population neighborhood ratings are similar. The design can still provide meaningful data depending on the research question.

PARAMETER ESTIMATION

In the post facto design like the one I am discussing, the researcher is faced with making as strong a conclusion about the research question as possible with the available data. The first task, however, is to understand what data are available and how they can be used to make a strong conclusion.

Figure 7.2 shows the population, sample, and sampling distribution drawings that I presented in earlier chapters. As you can see, a research study will be able to provide sample information and perhaps have available some estimates of the population mean, but otherwise, there will be no additional information for the researcher.

In this event, the researcher must *estimate the key parameters* in order to carry out a study like the Z test where we compare sample to population comparisons. The most important parameter to estimate is the population SD (σ_X). Without a notion of the variability of the population, we cannot make an accurate estimate of the overall likelihood of the sample mean representing the population mean.

Estimating the Population SD

The method for estimating σ_X is fairly straightforward. In fact, it follows a common-sense logic. If you want to know what the population variance looks like, what is the best guess? The best guess is probably the variance and SD of the sample. Obviously, it may not be a perfect representation, but *the sample variance is the best estimate of the population variance and SD*.

The method statisticians have devised to create a more likely estimate than the sample SD is to adjust the sample value. The principle is that if you divide by a smaller number, the resultant calculation will be larger.

Estimating the population SD from the sample follows the same principle. If we *adjust* the SD formula for the sample by subtracting a value of "1" in the denominator, it will provide a *larger* estimate of the population SD. A larger estimate is more likely to "capture" the true population SD in the absence of the actual population SD. Figure 7.3 shows this process. The actual SD becomes "s_x" when corrected by the formula. When corrected, it becomes a more accurate estimate of the population SD, σ_X.

The left-hand formula later (SD) calculates the SD for a group of scores that constitute its own population. I discussed this formula in Chapter 3 in the context of identifying a difference in the way both Excel and SPSS® calculate SD. In fact, I

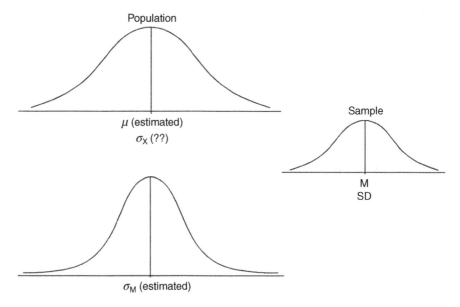

Figure 7.2   Using the sampling distribution with estimated population values.

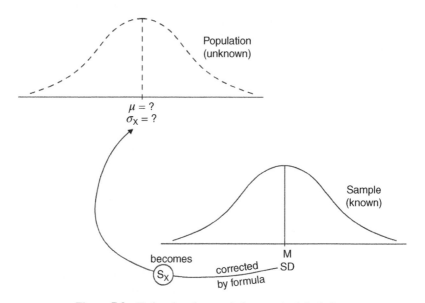

Figure 7.3   Estimating the population standard deviation.

labeled this the "population SD." This is the calculation for simply describing a set of data without making reference to a greater population from which the set of scores may have been derived. We simply consider the set of scores its own population.

Now that we are considering inferential statistics, we can modify this formula a bit to be a better estimate of the population SD on the basis of a sample value. The right-hand formula in the following "adjusts" the SD formula by subtracting 1 from the denominator in the last row of the formula ($N - 1$). Doing this makes the denominator smaller, and therefore it results in a larger estimated SD result. The reason for doing this is that we are estimating a population value from a sample value, and this adjustment "casts a wider net" to capture the true population SD, especially if we do not know what the population SD value is. By making the adjustment, we transform the population SD into the estimated population SD (s_x) which we described as the inferential SD.

$$SD = \sqrt{\frac{\Sigma X^2 - \frac{(\Sigma X)^2}{N}}{N}}; \quad s_x = \sqrt{\frac{\Sigma X^2 - \frac{(\Sigma X)^2}{N}}{N - 1}}$$

If you recall, I distinguished this population SD with the "inferential SD" that is reported by Excel and SPSS. Although I did not introduce the formula, I wanted to ensure that you understood the difference between the population SD and the inferential SD. Review the discussion in Chapter 3 to make sure you understand the difference.

New Symbol s_x: The Estimated SD of the Population

The second formula earlier for the value of "s_x" represents the "adjusted" formula for estimating a population SD from a sample SD. Many statisticians and researchers use s_x or simply "s" as the symbol for the *estimated SD of the population*. You can see the only difference between the formulas is the denominator: "N" in the SD formula and "$N - 1$" in the s_x formula. We are estimating one parameter, the population SD. As a way to be more likely of capturing the true population SD, we subtract a value of 1 from the divisor and therefore show a larger result.

Review the "Computation Method" section in Chapter 3 showing the calculation of the population SD for the AP scores. The formulas in the following show that the population SD is 20.028:

$$SD = \sqrt{\frac{101,754 - \frac{(1664)^2}{31}}{31}}; \quad SD_{(Population)} = 20.028$$

The formula as follows adjusts this calculation by removing 1 from the overall denominator, yielding the estimated population SD (s_x) of 20.359. The s_x value is reported by both Excel and SPSS:

$$SD = \sqrt{\frac{101,754 - \frac{(1664)^2}{31}}{30}}; \quad SD_{(Inferential)} \text{ or } s_x = 20.359$$

Biased versus Unbiased Estimates

Statisticians refer to the population SD (which is based on the sample) as a "biased estimator" since it does not necessarily provide a true picture of an unknown population SD. Since the sample mean is likely different than the population mean and since the sample mean is used in the calculation of the population SD, it will not provide a true representation of s_x. The estimated SD of the population s_x is therefore an unbiased estimate when it is adjusted as we discussed.

New Symbol s_m: The Estimated SD of the Sampling Distribution of Means (or Simply, "Standard Error of the Mean")

As in the Z test, we need to make use of the sampling distribution since it is a more perfect comparison distribution for our sample mean. This is especially the case because we have incomplete information about the population (especially the population SD). Therefore, *the sampling distribution stands in the place of the population as the standard of comparison for the sample*. Since it is theoretically a standard normal distribution, we can transform our sample mean into a value among other values on the sampling distribution to see how the sample mean compares to the population mean. The sampling distribution is the proxy for the population.

TABLE 7.1   Population and Sample Symbols for Inferential Statistics

POPULATION AND SAMPLE SYMBOLS	
M	The mean of the sample.
SD	The standard deviation of the sample (assumes the sample is its own population)
μ	The Greek letter 'Mu' is the symbol for the population mean.
M_M	This is the symbol for the mean of the sampling distribution. You can see how this works by observing that it is a mean (M), but a mean of the sampling distribution indicated by the subscript. Thus, it is the *mean of the distribution of means*, or the 'mean of the means.' Since it is (theoretically) created by all possible samples, it is a parameter.
σ_X	"Sigma X" is the Standard Deviation of all the population raw scores. This differs from SD in that it does not refer to a sample, but to the entire population of scores.
σ_M	The standard deviation of the sampling distribution of means; also called the *Standard Error of the Mean*.
s_x	The estimated standard deviation of the population. The subscript x identifies this estimated value as belonging to the population of all scores.
s_m	The estimated standard error of the mean. The subscript m identifies this estimated value as belonging to the sampling distribution of means. It is the estimated standard deviation of all possible sample means (theoretically) taken from the population.

Since we are making use of the sampling distribution, we need to have the values of the mean and SD for that distribution:

- The mean of the sampling distribution of means (M_M) is equal to the population mean (μ) according to the central limit theorem (see Chapter 6).
- Since the SD of the sampling distribution is smaller than the population SD (also according to the central limit theorem), we must calculate the (estimated) SD of the sampling distribution of means (or estimate the standard error of the mean) using the same procedure as in the Z test.
- The following formula calculates the estimated SD of the sampling distribution, which has a new symbol to identify it, s_m:

$$s_m = \frac{s_X}{\sqrt{N}}$$

This new symbol indicates that it is estimated (by using the lower case "s" instead of "σ") and that it belongs to the sampling distribution (since the subscript is an "m" rather than an "x"). Thus, we add two additional symbols to our earlier list shown in Table 6.3. Table 7.1 reproduces the earlier symbols and adds the two new symbols.

THE *T* TEST

When values are generated for the sampling distribution of means, the researcher can use these values to perform the T Test. Like the Z test, this procedure allows the researcher to compare a sample mean to a standard normal distribution (the sampling distribution) to see how close or far away the sample mean is from a(n) (unknown) population. The sampling distribution "stands in the place" of the population for this comparison since we can more accurately determine its values.

In order to perform a T test, we use a formula very similar to the Z test. The numerator, the difference between sample mean and population mean, is the same as in the Z test except that with the T test, we are using an estimated μ:

$$t = \frac{M - \mu}{s_m} \quad \text{where} \quad s_m = \frac{s_x}{\sqrt{N}}$$

As you can see, the T test formula parallels the Z test formula:

$$t = \frac{M - \mu}{s_m} \qquad Z = \frac{M - \mu}{\sigma_M}$$

Figure 7.4 shows the elements for creating a T Test. As you can see, a researcher can populate these elements with the calculated values of the study. In Figure 7.4, the sampling distribution is shown directly below the population so that it is apparent that the mean of the sampling distribution is equal to the mean of the population. The T Test allows the researcher to transform the mean value of the sample onto the value axis of the sampling distribution and, knowing the SD of this distribution (sM), can

POPULATION   SAMPLE

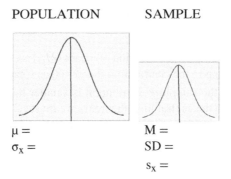

$\mu =$ $M =$
$\sigma_x =$ $SD =$
                      $s_x =$

SAMPLING DISTRIBUTION

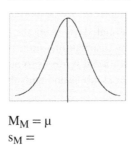

$M_M = \mu$
$s_M =$

Figure 7.4   The *T* Test elements used to compare a sample mean to all possible means from a population.

determine how many SD it falls from the population mean. The *T* value is therefore expressed in SD units.

Degrees of Freedom

Degrees of freedom (df) are important elements in statistics. Essentially, they represent *the restrictions on the values when we are estimating a population parameter*. Technically, df identify how many values are free to vary when making the parameter estimate. Another way of looking at this concept is that, when we estimate parameters, we must adjust the values so it is a better estimate. In the *T* Test, we are estimating one parameter, the SD of the population. Therefore, the adjusted formula substituted $N - 1$ for N in the bottom denominator. Estimating one parameter therefore results in an adjustment of one. The *T* Test for single samples therefore assumes that the sample size "*N*" needs to be adjusted by subtracting 1 resulting in df $= N - 1$.

Figure 7.5 shows an example table of data with three columns. The first column lists raw score values, with the next column "$X - M$" showing the deviation scores in which the mean is subtracted from each raw score. These are the "deviation amounts" that I discussed in Chapter 3 (see Figure 3.7). The last column shows the squared deviation values "$(X - M)^2$" used to calculate the SD.

DF Example	X - M	(X-M)2
3.7	0.5	0.25
3.7	0.49	0.24
3.6	0.43	0.18
3.5	0.33	0.11
3.5	0.3	0.09
3.5	0.3	0.09
3.4	0.21	0.05
3.4	0.17	0.03
3.4	0.17	0.03
3.3	0.13	0.02
3.2	0.03	0
3.2	0.02	0
3.2	−0.04	0
3.1	−0.1	0.01
3.1	−0.11	0.01
3.1	−0.13	0.02
3.1	−0.14	0.02
3.1	−0.15	0.02
3.0	−0.16	0.03
3.0	−0.17	0.03
3.0	−0.17	0.03
3.0	−0.18	0.03
3.0	−0.18	0.03
3.0	−0.18	0.03
3.0	−0.21	0.04
2.9	−0.27	0.07
2.9	−0.33	0.11
2.7	−0.55	0.31
3.2	**0**	1.88

Figure 7.5   Understanding the concept of degrees of freedom.

Recall that the deviation scores when added together equal 0 for the reasons we discussed in Chapter 3. Here is the curious fact: When we use these values to estimate a parameter, we may be using a mean value that varies slightly from an unknown population mean. Therefore, the values in the "$X - M$" column can change slightly, but one must be "fixed" to ensure the deviations still add to 0. Look at the $X - M$ values in Figure 7.5; in order for the sum of the values to equal 0, the last value ("−0.55") must take this specific value. If the other values change, one value must take a specific value in order to ensure the outcome of 0.

This example is just to show that *estimating parameters places restrictions on our data*. In the case of the *T* test with one sample, only one value cannot vary. Thus we can calculate df to be $N - 1$. This represents the sample size minus one value.

Each statistical procedure that we encounter will have a different way of calculating df since each will be estimating different parameters. We will make note of df as we discuss the hypothesis tests.

THE *T* TEST: A RESEARCH EXAMPLE

Returning to the research question I posed in the discussion of this chapter "Do policing models affect resident perceptions of the community?," we can explore how to calculate the *T* Test (as we did with the *Z* test in Chapter 6) but this time using adjusted values. In many cases, a researcher is forced to use a different statistical test (than the *Z* test) when it is apparent that they have no information about some population values.

Let us assume that I as a researcher obtained community attitude data AFTER a community instituted community policing and I knew what the population mean was likely to be prior to installing community policing. We can assess whether the sample of community values taken after the change are statistically different from the population by using the *T* Test.

The hypothesis for the research question before is: "Did community policing change residents' perceptions of the community?" Thus, we are asking whether our (known) sample mean is representative of a(n) (assumed) population mean but without knowing the value of the population SD. (In many cases such as this example, researchers may have an approximated value for the population mean but almost never have the population SD value.)

The outcome variable is residents' perceptions of the community (using QL data) that I described in Chapter 3. For this example I will use a sample of the QL data but will suggest a <u>hypothetical population mean</u> to illustrate this *T* test procedure.[1] The sample group consists of 10 residents' QL Index values.

Obviously, this "study" is for illustration, so we cannot hope to make generalizable conclusions. If it were an actual study, it would be post facto, and we could not make causal attributions about policing since the policing model would already have been implemented, there would be no control or comparative group, and extraneous influences would not be adequately controlled.

---

[1] Because this is hypothetical data used for illustration, no conclusions should be made about the substance of the data (i.e., community policing and resident perceptions).

TABLE 7.2   Quality of Life (Hypothetical) Sample Data

Resident Perception of Neighborhood (Quality of Life)
8
11
16
22
26
19
31
36
25
28

Table 7.2 shows the QL sample data. Remember, I am creating a hypothetical sample of data (from actual study values) in order to illustrate the *T* test process.

With the values shown in Table 7.2, we can calculate the *T* Test using the formula I presented previously:

$$t = \frac{M - \mu}{s_m} \quad \text{where} \quad s_m = \frac{s_x}{\sqrt{N}}$$

Sample and Population Means ($M - \mu$)

For the purposes of this research example, assume that the population mean (μ) is 15.8. That is, the entire population of residents[2] indicates a mean rating of 15.8 on the perception of their neighborhoods according to the QL Index. We can calculate the mean QL rating from the sample ($N = 10$) of residents in this particular neighborhood to be 22.2. Therefore, the sample residents rated the neighborhood quality higher than the population (22.2 vs. 15.8, respectively). The question is, how big does this discrepancy have to be before we conclude that a sample value this large could not be a random sample drawn from a population with a mean of 15.8?

$$(M - \mu) = 6.4$$

The Estimated Population SD (s_x) and Estimated Standard Error of the Mean (s_M)

In order to answer this question, we must use the *T* test, which is very similar to the *Z* test except that with the *T* test, we do not know the value of the population SD (σ_X). Using the aforementioned process for estimating the population SD (resulting in s_x), we can add information that will be helpful in assessing the difference in population–sample means by creating a standard measure of the distance.

---

[2]The "population" in this case needs to be defined. If this were an actual study, the description of the population would be crucial in determining the generalizability of the findings, among other concerns.

QL Data Summary	
Mean	22.2
Standard Error	2.79
Median	23.5
Mode	#N/A
Standard Deviation	8.82
Sample Variance	77.73
Kurtosis	−0.67
Skewness	−0.19
Range	28
Minimum	8
Maximum	36
Sum	222
Count	10

Figure 7.6 Excel descriptive statistics for QL.

Review the process in Chapter 3 for calculating the population SD and s_x using Excel and SPSS. Remember, Excel and SPSS both provide s_x as the default calculation. Figure 7.6 shows the descriptive summary for the QL variable from Excel. The reported SD (s_x) is 8.82. The population SD from Excel[3] is 8.36 (use the "STDEVP" function). The discrepancy between the actual SD and s_x is not large; however the larger s_x value provides a better estimate of the population SD, which is not known in this study.

Both Figures 7.6 and 7.7 (dark shaded values) also report the estimated standard error of the mean (or s_M, the estimated SD of the sampling distribution of means). By calculation,

$$s_m = \frac{s_x}{\sqrt{N}} = \frac{8.82}{3.16} = 2.79$$

$$S_x = 8.82$$

$$S_M = 2.79$$

Figure 7.7, the SPSS output, yields the same value for SD (s_x) as reported in Excel (8.817 or 8.82 rounded). Note that the estimated standard error of the mean shows the same value in both Excel and SPSS as indicated by the dark highlighted values. (Also in both reports, the sample group appears to be normally distributed as indicated by skewness and kurtosis figures.)

---

[3]Remember, as we have used it, the "population SD" refers to the sample values taken together as the entire set of values. We will use this to estimate the standard deviation of the population, which is not known in this example or other studies like it.

Descriptive Statistics

	N	Minimum	Maximum	Mean		Std. Deviation	Skewness		Kurtosis	
	Statistic	Statistic	Statistic	Statistic	Std. Error	Statistic	Statistic	Std. Error	Statistic	Std. Error
QLIndex	10	8	36	22.20	2.788	8.817	−.194	.687	−.668	1.334
Valid N (listwise)	10									

Figure 7.7   SPSS® descriptive statistics for QL.

Calculating the *T* Ratio Value

With the values thus determined, we can use the *T* Test formula to calculate a value for the *T* ratio, which allows a test of the hypothesis of whether or not the "sample" mean of QL values is likely to come from a population of QL values with an assumed mean (μ) and no known SD (σ_x). If the sample mean is determined to be close to the population mean on the sampling distribution, we would conclude that the sample was likely the same as any other sample of QL values that could have been drawn from the population.

However, if the sample mean is determined by the *T* Test to be statistically <u>different</u> from the population mean (i.e., the transformed sample mean falls into the exclusion region of the comparison distribution), then we could conclude that the sample is different from the population; one possible reason for which might be that changing to community policing could have affected resident's perceptions of the community.

A researcher would use the "*T* Test of a single sample" in this study. It is a <u>*T* test rather than a *Z* test</u> because we (1) do not have population values, especially σ_x, and (2) we are using a small sample from which to make population estimates. We will use the same procedure that we used with the *Z* test, except now we must use the estimated parameter s_x that is an adjusted value based on the sample SD:

$$t = \frac{M - \mu}{s_m}$$
$$t = \frac{22.2 - 15.8}{2.79}$$
$$= \frac{6.4}{2.79}$$
$$= 2.29$$
$$t = 2.29$$

Therefore, our sample mean of 22.2 is transformed into a *T* ratio of 2.29. This value indicates that the sample mean value lies over 2 and one-fourth SD above the population mean when transformed to a standard normal distribution using the *T* test formula.

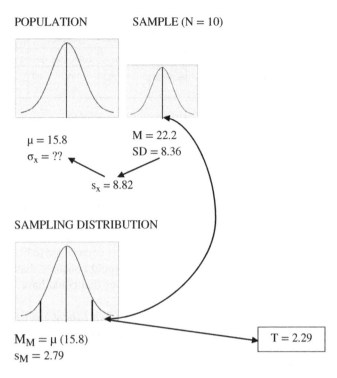

Figure 7.8 Transforming the sample mean value to a value on the sampling distribution.

Figure 7.8 shows how to visualize these values:

- The mean of the sampling distribution (M_M) is equal to the (assumed) population mean (μ).
- The sample SD estimates the (unknown) SD of the population σ_x to be the estimated value $s_x = 8.82$.
- The estimated standard error of the mean (s_M) is calculated from s_x to be 2.79.
- The resulting *T* ratio of 2.29 falls on the axis of the sampling distribution at a distance of 2.29 SD from the mean. This is indicated by the arrows showing the sample mean being "transformed" to the sampling distribution at a value well to the right of the curve and in an exclusion region (which we discuss later).

INTERPRETING THE RESULTS OF THE *T* TEST FOR A SINGLE MEAN

As with the *Z* test, the researcher must determine whether or not it is likely that a sample mean derived from the raw data represents a population mean from which it is supposedly drawn. In order to make this determination, the researcher uses the hypothesis testing process we reviewed in Chapter 6. In this process, the researcher determined the exclusion regions of the comparison distribution to see whether a calculated Z ratio could be considered significantly different.

We must use the *T* Test in our research example rather than the Z Test because we do not know the population values (and we have a small sample size). The steps in the hypothesis test are the same, however. I will review those steps later for this example, but it is first important to discuss the adaptations that we need to make to determine an accurate exclusion region for the comparison distribution of this example and those like it.

THE *T* DISTRIBUTION

Before we proceed to a hypothesis test, we need to discuss the *T* distribution. It is essentially the same as the Z distribution in terms of being a standard normal distribution. That is, it is normally distributed with known proportions between the mean and each SD.

Because the *T* distribution is typically based on small sample sizes, however (along with estimated parameters), the *T* distribution "varies" by sample size. Figure 7.9 shows how different sample sizes affect the T distribution. As you can see, the larger the sample size, the more the *T* distribution looks like the Z distribution with the large "hump" in the middle with smaller tails on both sides. The smaller the *T* distribution, the fewer the comparison values that make it up, with the result that it appears flatter as the sample sizes decrease.

The result of these dynamics of size is that the *T* distribution is often thought of as a *series of distributions that are linked to the size of the sample to be compared.* Since the shape of the curve alters drastically with smaller sample sizes, the exclusion/rejection region for a hypothesis test changes as well. *It takes a higher calculated T ratio to reject the null hypothesis the smaller the sample size.* This is because the 5% exclusion area "moves" away from the mean with smaller sample sizes due to the changing shape of the distribution.

The rejection values for the 5% exclusion area get smaller and smaller as the sample sizes increase. With very large numbers in the sample, the *T* distribution is indistinguishable from the Z distribution (the top curve in Figure 7.9).

Using df with the *T* Distribution

Because the *T* Test is used with small sample sizes and because it involves estimated values, the exclusion region for hypothesis tests using the *T* ratio must involve an adjustment to the Z table of Values we described in Chapter 4. The df provide this adjustment so that the researcher can establish an exclusion region tailored to their research study.

In our example, $N = 10$; therefore, df $= 9$ (since df $= N - 1$). In order for us to reject the null hypothesis at the 5% exclusion region, we would need the *T* ratio to be at least 2.262 (positive or negative). You will find the exclusion regions described in the statistical tables in Appendix C. In this case, for the single sample *T* Test, the researcher would use Table B that lists the exclusion values for the *T* distribution.

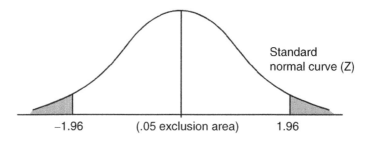

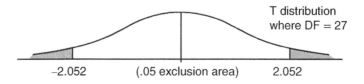

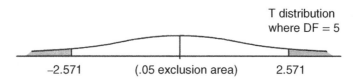

Figure 7.9   The nature of the *T* distribution.

Use the "df" column to locate the df of a particular study (in this example, df = 9) and follow the row to the values in the columns that describe a series of possible exclusion percentages (in this case, the 5% exclusion region).

THE HYPOTHESIS TEST FOR THE SINGLE SAMPLE *T* TEST

Recall that our hypothesis asked, "do policing models affect resident perceptions of the community?" In order to assess this hypothesis, we can proceed to the hypothesis test as we did with the *Z* test using the same procedural steps:

1. **The null hypothesis** or (H_0): $\mu_1 = \mu$
     Do the QL values of a sample of residents differ from the population of residents' QL values after community policy was instituted?
2. **The alternative hypothesis** or (H_A): $\mu_1 \neq \mu$
     The sample QL values do not represent the population of residents' QL values.

3. **The critical value**: T table values of $= (\pm)$ 2.262 (5% exclusion area)

   If the calculated T ratio value exceeds this value from the statistical table (either positively or negatively), we reject the null hypothesis. In such a case, our sample value being so high would be considered not likely to occur just by chance; rather some reason other than chance would create such a difference from the population QL value. The researcher could ASSUME that the reason for the difference might be the effect of community policing, but this could not be determined with this research design.

4. **The calculated value** (T ratio $= 2.29$)

   This is the t ratio value that we calculated earlier. It represents the results of the T test formula that transformed the sample mean value into a standard score on the T distribution so that we can compare it to other possible sample outcomes.

5. **Statistical decision: reject null hypothesis**?

   We reject the null hypothesis since our calculated value ($t = 2.29$) exceeds the t table value (df $= 9$) for the 5% exclusion area of 2.262 (either positively or negatively). In our study, the sample residents' QL scores were significantly different from the QL scores of the population of residents.

6. **Interpretation**

   The QL scores of residents ($M = 22.2, N = 10$) were significantly higher than those of the population of residents ($\mu = 15.8$) in an urban area that implemented community policing. The T test ratio ($T = 2.29$) exceeded the tabled value of T (df $= 9$) at ± 2.262 indicating a statistically significant difference between sample and population QL scores. The researcher might suggest from these findings that <u>one possible reason</u> for the difference might be the effect of community policing, but this conclusion would not be determined with a study using this research design.

TYPE I AND TYPE II ERRORS

As I have continually noted, statistics deals with uncertainty. You can begin to get a better picture of this through our discussion of inferential statistics. The hypothesis test attempts to establish *the extent to which it is likely* that a certain sample mean reflects a population mean, not the absolute certainty.

This being the case, statisticians and researchers often can make mistakes in their conclusions from hypothesis tests. These errors can be presented in two "groups."

Type I (Alpha) Errors (α)

The type I error is mistakenly rejecting the null hypothesis when it should be accepted. That is, we might reject the null hypothesis, as we did in our QL–community policing study, concluding that a sample mean this high, vis-à-vis an assumed population mean of a certain value, could not have happened by chance. That is, some reason other than chance resulted in the difference between sample and population QL values: perhaps the introduction of community policing. However, it is possible that our sample mean was one of the few in the exclusion area just by chance rather than a mean that reflected a different population.

Remember, in essence the statistical test compares <u>one</u> sample mean to the theoretical collection of <u>all</u> possible mean values that make up the sampling distribution. It is possible, though not likely, that our observed sample mean just happened to be one of the samples that was located in the exclusion region just by chance. After all, there are 5% of sample mean values located in the exclusion region that we are using as a comparison; those that by chance fall in the tails of the distribution (i.e., the 5% exclusion area).

We rejected the null hypothesis, but perhaps there really is no difference between sample and population mean QL values. Perhaps our "sample" group of residents was just a chance finding. So, even though we rejected the null hypothesis on the basis of the size of the *T* ratio, it perhaps was one of the small likelihood samples that just happened.

The 5% exclusion area that statisticians and researchers use for hypothesis tests is somewhat arbitrary. No matter what the exclusion area set, however, there is the small possibility that the sample mean comes from beyond the limit of the exclusion area <u>by chance alone</u> and not due to anything connected to the research study. Figure 7.10 shows this possible error using the results from the aforementioned *T* test.

As you can see in Figure 7.10, the *T* ratio of 2.29 (the calculated value of the sample mean translated into a value on the sampling distribution of means) landed "beyond" the exclusion values of ± 2.262 (i.e., the value was in the tails of the distribution), so we rejected the null hypothesis. This result may be because (1) there really was a significant difference between sample and population QL values or (2) this *T* ratio was one that could have been obtained just by chance, without any differences between sample and population having to do with community policing or other influences. The sample of QL values may have chosen with 10 people who just happened to

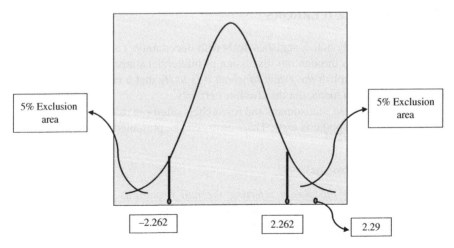

Figure 7.10   The *T* test exclusion areas.

have a larger mean than the population. Therefore, our decision about the sample not representing the population, or being different than the population, may be in error. It may be more an issue of <u>chance</u> than the <u>meaningfulness</u> of the research treatment/variable.

When we use the designation "$p < 0.05$" in announcing our statistical decision (from the hypothesis test), we are saying that the probability (p) is less than 0.05, or 5 chances in 100; we would obtain a test value (T ratio in this example) that large <u>by chance alone</u>. Therefore, we reject the null hypothesis. However, note that our test result may be one of those chance findings that happen to be in the "0.05" area of the distribution. The upshot of all this is that we must understand that our alpha (type I) error is 0.05. Whatever exclusion area we announce (5%, 1%, etc.) defines our alpha error.

The type I error is mistakenly rejecting the null hypothesis when it should be accepted. If we got the result we did, but it was really only due to the chance of selecting a sample of 10 people who differed from the population for any number of reason, we commit a type I error.

Type II (Beta) Errors (β)

Beta errors are quite interesting for many reasons. We will examine several of these in the chapters ahead. For now, however, we will define the type II (beta) error as *not rejecting the null hypothesis when it should be rejected*.

In some ways, this is the opposite of the alpha error. Just as there is the possibility that we could reject the null hypothesis due to chance alone, rather than for some substantive reason, we could also *not* reject a null hypothesis when we really should have.

<u>Some possible reasons for type II errors are as follows:</u>

<u>Sample selection</u>: Perhaps our sample was taken by chance from residents who initially had a <u>lower</u> QL mean than the population, and whatever research influence was involved "moved" it toward the right side <u>but not far enough</u> to fall in the right-hand rejection region. That is, perhaps the influences acting on the sample group had to "work harder" to move the sample mean value toward the rejection region.

In the example before, this might be the case if we had chosen a sample group with a mean QL much lower than the population that resulted in a calculated T ratio value of 22.0 instead of 22.2. In that event, we would have calculated a T value of 2.222, which would not have exceeded the 2.262 value defining the exclusion region. Therefore, we would not have been able to reject the null hypothesis even though there was a powerful influence in the study that resulted in a large change among the sample. In this analysis, the substantive reason for the movement of the T ratio was real, but because of a sample that started so far below the mean, it did not reach the exclusion region.

<u>Small sample size</u>: Other reasons why a research finding may not be able to reject the null hypothesis despite being a meaningful finding include a <u>small sample size</u>. As we discussed earlier, if we had an N of 15 in the study rather than 10, we would only have needed a T ratio of ± 2.145 to reject the

null hypothesis rather than ±2.262. Therefore, by increasing the sample size of a study, whatever substantive reasons for affecting a sample mean would have an easier time concluding a significant finding. Studies with smaller sample sizes would therefore have a more difficult time, even if the substantive reasons for changes were the same.

Rejection region: A further reason for a potential type II error is that a study may have an exclusion region smaller than the one defined by the 5% level. Suppose a researcher wanted to lessen the possibility of a chance finding and chose a 1% exclusion region, thereby making it more difficult to achieve a significant result but being more confident that such a result was not by chance. We discussed the 5% exclusion for the *Z* distribution as ±1.96. If we chose a 1% exclusion region, this would identify values of ±2.58 (use the *Z* Table of Values to determine this number). In our example using the *T* distribution with df = 9, the 1% exclusion value would be ±3.250. Under these circumstances, making it more difficult to reject the null hypothesis also might result in a substantive finding not being able to be achieved simply due to the exclusion region boundaries.

Areas of Comparison Distributions

Figure 7.11 shows the type II error among other considerations. The example is a general one, using the *Z* distribution, but it applies to other distributions as well. As you can see in Figure 7.11, the mean of a sample group (shown in cross-hatching) was calculated to be very close to the rejection region of 1.96 (the 5% rejection region for the *Z* distribution) but not beyond the limit. The sample mean in this case, although it may have moved quite a distance from its initial state, would not result in a rejection of the null hypothesis.

Look in Figure 7.11 at the distance between the population mean and the sample mean (shown by a two-sided arrow). This shows some substantive research effect "moving" the sample mean away (to the right) from the population mean some distance. The horizontally hatched region of the sample distribution is the area that lies above the rejection region in the comparison distribution. Any sample mean test value

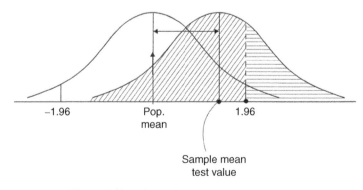

Figure 7.11   Visualizing beta and nonbeta areas.

that would fall in this region would result in the null hypothesis being rejected and therefore would be a "correct" decision.

The possibility of the beta error would lie in the diagonally hatched region of the test distribution. This is the region that would not result in a rejection of the null hypothesis since this is the area that falls below the rejection region of 1.96. As you can see, our sample test value fell just below the rejection region and therefore in the beta error section representing a possible type II error.

The beta error can be measured like the alpha error. The diagonally hatched region would represent the proportion of beta (β), while the horizontally hatched section of the test distribution represents the non beta area ($1 - \beta$).

EFFECT SIZE

Effect size is a very important concept in statistics as I have mentioned in past chapters. It refers to the *strength or impact of a finding*. Although related to statistical significance, it refers to the distance a research variable or treatment "moves" a sample test mean away from a population mean. That is, irrespective of a hypothesis test finding, how far away from the population mean did the substantive influences in a study "push" the sample mean away?

Figure 7.11 shows the effect size by the double-sided arrow separating the population and sample means. In our previous example, the sample QL mean value was higher than the population average due to some substantive influence like (possibly) community policing, even though the figures in Figure 7.11 show that the test mean did not exceed the exclusion value.

Here are some things to note regarding effect size:

1. It measures the impact of the research treatment/variable to move a sample test mean away from a population mean.
2. It is a separate consideration from statistical significance. Even though these are related concepts, effect size addresses the extent of the sample mean being moved away from the population, while statistical significance refers to whether this is a chance finding.
3. Statistical tests indicate effect size measurements even though the null hypothesis may not be rejected.

EFFECT SIZE FOR THE SINGLE SAMPLE *T* TEST

Each statistical test procedure we will discuss in this book has an effect size measurement. For the single sample *t* test, the effect size formula is

$$d = \frac{M - \mu}{s_x}$$

This formula is derived from Cohen's *d*, the classic formula for transforming the distance between two means (in the single sample *t* test, this is the distance of the sample mean from the population mean) into SD units by dividing the $M - \mu$ distance by the SD (s_x). Substituting our values from the QL research example,

$$d = \frac{M - \mu}{s_x} = \frac{22.2 - 15.8}{8.82} = 0.726$$

Therefore, the effect size of the research study is 0.726. This represents the difference in the population and sample mean <u>in SD units</u>. Several values are suggested for interpreting the magnitude of effect size, like the following from Cohen (1988):

0.20: small effect
0.50: medium effect
0.80: large effect

In this study, the effect size of 0.73 is "medium" but close to "large." The population and sample means were nearly three-fourths of a SD apart. Whether this distance is considered to be statistically significant as determined by a hypothesis test (which it was), it shows how far the sample mean was pushed away from the population mean by the substantive forces in the research study.

Another Measurement of the (Cohen's *d*) Effect Size

You may notice that the effect size calculation d is similar to the T ratio. However, the T ratio transforms the $M - \mu$ distance into SD units of the sampling distribution (s_m), whereas the effect size uses the estimated SD of the population (s_x). Since these are similar measures, we can use another calculation to achieve similar results (Cohen, 1988):

$$d = \frac{t}{\sqrt{N}} = \frac{2.29}{\sqrt{10}} = 0.724$$

The chief difference between these methods is that the second formula is more sensitive to sample size.

POWER, EFFECT SIZE, AND BETA

There are relationships between type II error, effect size, and power. Power represents *the ability of a statistical analysis to detect a "true" finding*. The larger the power, the greater the probability of rejecting the null hypothesis when it should be rejected. As we discussed earlier, type II (beta) error is the probability of not rejecting the null hypothesis when it should have been rejected. Power and beta are complementary: Power is therefore defined as $(1 - \beta)$.

Look again at Figure 7.11 which shows all these measures.

- Beta (β) is the area of the sample distribution diagonally hatched and represents sample test mean values that do not reject the null hypothesis.

- Power $(1 - \beta)$ is represented by the area horizontally hatched. Sample test means that fall in this section will reject the null hypothesis correctly; this represents the power of the relationship among the test variables.
- Effect size is represented by the double-sided arrow, the distance the sample test value moves away from the population mean and measured in SD units.

Power tables exist in which the researcher can determine the sample size and magnitude of Cohen's d to achieve certain "levels" of power (Cohen, 1988).

ONE- AND TWO-TAILED TESTS

Up to now, we have assumed that when researchers create a rejection region, or exclusion area of the comparison distribution for the hypothesis test, that they will split the exclusion area into both tails. Figure 7.12 shows the two-tailed test in which the rejection region is split into the two tails of the distribution. (The figure shows the Z distribution since it is easier to understand as an example.) The top figure shows the 5% exclusion area. As you can see, the 5% must be split in half so that both tails will have half the rejection region. Thus, $2.50\% + 2.50\% = 5\%$.

Figure 7.12 also shows the 1% exclusion area in which the 1% is split into both tails of the distribution (1/2% or 0.5% are located in each tail).

Two-Tailed Tests

The "default" hypothesis test used by researchers is the two-tailed test since it allows for the possibility that a research finding may be changed in either direction, positive

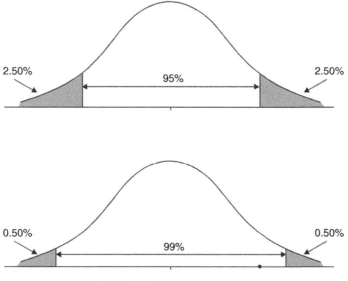

Figure 7.12   The two-tailed test.

or negative. If you recall, I mentioned before that exclusion area of 5% for the *Z* distribution consists of the *Z* values of ± 1.96. The 1% exclusion area in the *Z* distribution split into two tails would result in the exclusion values of ± 2.58.

As we discussed previously, the exclusion values change when using the *T* distribution since the sample values are often smaller. In the example we discussed in this chapter, our *T* ratio of 2.29 was large enough to reject the null hypothesis since the exclusion value was ± 2.262. If we had wanted to use the more stringent 1% exclusion area for the *T* distribution (with df $= 9$), the exclusion values would have been ± 3.250. The exclusion values for the *T* distribution must be evaluated differently for each statistical test since the sample sizes can vary.

One-Tailed Tests

Researchers can also establish <u>one-tailed</u> tests by "stacking" the entire rejection region in one tail or the other but not both. Figure 7.13 compares the one- and two-tailed 5% exclusion areas for the *Z* distribution. The top figure shows the two-tailed test with the 5% split into both tails; the exclusion value is ± 1.96. The bottom figure shows a one-tailed test with all 5% loaded into one tail. In this case, the exclusion value is 1.65. (If we had loaded the 5% in the left side of the distribution, the exclusion value would have been -1.65.)

Table 7.3 shows the exclusion values for the *Z* distribution for both the one- and two-tailed tests. As you can see, it matters a great deal which to choose for a research problem.

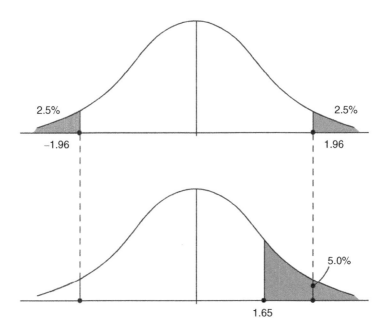

Figure 7.13   One- and two-tailed exclusion values.

TABLE 7.3   Exclusion Values for the Z Distribution

	One Tail Test	Two Tail Test
5% Exclusion Area	1.65 (either pos. *or* neg.)	+/- 1.96
1% Exclusion Area	2.33 (either pos. *or* neg.)	+/- 2.58

TABLE 7.4   Exclusion Values for *T* Distribution (df = 9)

	One Tail Test	Two Tail Test
5% Exclusion Area	1.833 (either pos. *or* neg.)	+/- 2.262
1% Exclusion Area	2.821 (either pos. *or* neg.)	+/- 3.250

To provide a sense of how the exclusion values differ for the *T* distribution, Table 7.4 shows the values for df = 9, the sample size we used in the QL example. Recall that our test value (*t* ratio) was 2.29. We rejected the null hypothesis using a two-tailed test and could have rejected the null more easily with a one-tailed test. However, we could not have rejected the null hypothesis at the 1% exclusion region using either a one- or a two-tailed test.

Choosing a One- or Two-Tailed Test

It is up to the researcher to choose which type of exclusion value to include in the hypothesis test. There is no absolute rule about which should be used. However, the researcher should be ready to defend their choice. The 5% exclusion area of a two-tailed test is considered a standard for researchers. However, researchers exploring potential relationships among variables may choose a much lower exclusion region.

One potentially thorny issue in using a one-tailed test is which tail to identify as the exclusion area. The logical sequence of the hypothesis test requires researchers to choose, before they calculate the t ratio, whether they will use a one- or two-tailed test. So, you should use some criteria for deciding which tail to use, if you decide on a one-tailed test.

One criterion is the expectation, based on the research literature, or other research findings, that the study finding will tend toward one direction or the other. For example, if you have noted in the literature that student technology skills almost always eclipse teacher's skills, you might use the right tail as the exclusion area if you are comparing teachers and students on a technology learning task.

Another criterion is to think about the nature of the sample. If you are working with a sample group that is "extreme" on some measure (e.g., introducing a new method for teaching AP subjects among students without limited chemistry exposure), you might anticipate that the students' scores would <u>increase</u> if the new instructional method is designed to integrate chemistry concepts in a novel way. This is somewhat intuitive. Among a group of students with no chemistry background, for example, there would only be one way to go, up!

Therefore, the nature of the group would determine the likely increase of scores rather than anything special about a new teaching method. In this case, the researcher could capitalize on the "regression to the mean effect." A group's scores will generally increase upon retesting if they are low to begin with or if the group is extreme on some measure. On the other hand, if the group's measure is high initially, retesting runs the risk of lowering the scores. Likewise, assuming a positive result may be met with failure.

In some sense, it is a gamble as to whether you use a one- or two-tailed test. It is easier to reject the null hypothesis with a one-tailed test, but it is also riskier if there is a reasonable possibility that the direction of your findings will tend to the opposite side from what you expect.

A Note about Power

We discussed power earlier, but I wanted to note here that there are ways a researcher can increase the power of a finding. The following are some of the factors I have discussed or hinted at thus far that might increase power:

1. <u>Using a one-tailed test</u>, depending on the nature of the research question.
2. Using a <u>lower exclusion value</u> (5% vs. 1%).
3. <u>Increasing the sample size</u> since this will generally lower the size of the standard error with the result of increasing the test ratio
4. <u>Considering the nature of the sample</u>

We will add to this list as we proceed. For now, remember that the researcher is in the driver's seat of their research. Use appropriate methods, pay attention to power and effect size, and be systematic in obtaining the most accurate results with the appropriate statistical procedures.

POINT AND INTERVAL ESTIMATES

In conducting the analysis of a *T* test of a single mean, we transformed a sample mean to see where it would fall on the sampling distribution of means. This resulted in a decision about whether the sample mean likely came from the population. To researchers, the *T* test procedure is called a "point estimate." The object of the procedure is to create one point in the sampling distribution of means so that we can compare it to the population mean. In order to do this, we had to have some idea of the population mean. Ordinarily, the population mean is not known, so the researcher must posit a value, based on past research or other criterion. This value is more than a guess; however it still is likely not exactly equal to an unknown population value.

Another way to proceed with a research study is to estimate the population mean within a certain range of values. This is known as a "confidence interval." *This interval is the range of values that will likely contain the true population mean within a certain percentage of certainty.* We often use the same benchmark of probability as we do for a point estimate to create the range of values: $p = 0.05$. Thus, we speak of the 0.95 confidence interval to mean the range of values within which the true population mean will fall with 95% certainty. We might also choose a more "certain" range of values by using a benchmark of $p = 0.01$. I will show how this works.

Calculating the Interval Estimate of the Population Mean

What would this interval of values look like? How can it be created? The short answer is that we will use the "inclusion area" to create the range of values, rather than the exclusion area that we used in the *T* test before. This procedure allows the researcher to identify what the population mean is likely to be the majority of the time when it is estimated from the sample values. Therefore, this procedure differs from the point estimate.

Point estimate: What is the value of the sample mean when it is transformed to fit the sampling distribution so that it can be compared to all possible sample means?

Confidence interval: Since we do not know a population mean value, what would an estimate of the population mean be 95% of the time using sample values for the estimate?

Look at Figure 7.12 again. I used this figure to discuss the two-tailed test. However, the figure also illustrates the inclusion area that will "capture" the true population mean. The top figure shows a 0.95 inclusion area (indicated by the double-sided arrow), and the bottom shows a 0.99 inclusion area. These areas conform to the 0.95 confidence interval ($\text{CI}_{0.95}$) and the 0.99 confidence interval ($\text{CI}_{0.99}$), respectively.

A statistical formula is used to identify the limits of this interval, that is, the specific values on the sampling distribution of means that bracket the inclusion area. These values represent the confidence interval. The formula is not new to you. If you recall, you learned in Chapter 5 to transform a z score into a raw score as follows:

$$X = Z(\text{SD}) + M$$

We can use this formula to create the confidence intervals by adapting it to the *T* distribution, since we are dealing with unknown population parameters. The adapted formula is

$$\text{Confidence interval} = \pm t(s_M) + M$$

As you can see, the Z value is replaced by $\pm t$ and SD is replaced by s_m in the formula. Beyond these changes in symbols that represent the difference between the Z distribution and the T distribution, the formula is the same. Examining each element of the formula:

- $\pm t$ is the exclusion value of the T ratio, <u>determined by the T table of values</u> that recognizes the appropriate df value. For example, in our research question before, the (two-tailed) T value at df $= 9$ was ± 2.262.
- s_m is the estimated standard error of the mean. In our example, $s_m = 2.79$.
- M, the sample mean in our example, was 22.2.

Substituting these values into the formula will yield the CI. In this example, we can use $CI_{0.95}$ since that is the assumption used to create the appropriate t value from the table (i.e., the 5% exclusion – 95% inclusion area).

$$CI_{0.95} = \pm 2.262(2.79) + 22.2$$

You will notice that the t value from the T table is both a positive and a negative number since we are using it in a two-tailed procedure; we want to identify values on the left and right of the sample mean that will <u>bracket</u> the population mean estimate. Therefore, we need to calculate the confidence interval twice: once with T as a negative value and once as a positive value:

$$CI_{0.95} = -2.262(2.79) + 22.2$$
$$CI_{0.95}(\text{left bracket value}) = 15.89$$
$$CI_{0.95} = +2.262(2.79) + 22.2$$
$$CI_{0.95}(\text{right bracket value}) = 28.51$$

Figure 7.14 shows these values. The T table values capture the 95% inclusion area. Below these brackets are the calculated values that define the $CI_{0.95}$ interval. We can summarize by stating that with a 95% certainty, the true population mean will fall between 15.89 and 28.51.

We can in like fashion calculate the 0.99 confidence intervals as follows:

$$CI_{0.95} = -3.250(2.79) + 22.2$$
$$CI_{0.95}(\text{left bracket value}) = 13.13$$
$$CI_{0.95} = +3.250(2.79) + 22.2$$
$$CI_{0.95}(\text{right bracket value}) = 31.27$$

This is quite a different process than the point estimate, but the procedures are created to answer different questions:

- *Point estimate*: Is the sample mean of 22.2 likely to be from a population with an assumed mean of 15.8 (from our example)?
- *Confidence interval*: Based on the sample values, what is the population mean likely to be? The true population mean is likely to range between 15.89 and 28.51 with a 95% certainty.

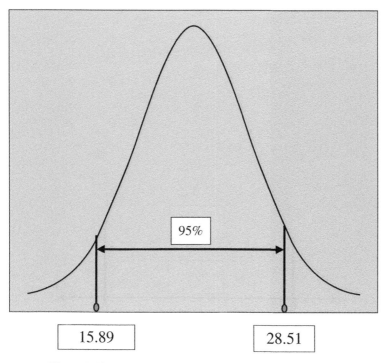

Figure 7.14 Confidence interval values for the QL example.

The Value of Confidence Intervals

As you will see, confidence intervals are quite important in statistics. We have learned how to create brackets that will contain a population parameter. That is, we have estimated a population parameter within a certain probability level.

Confidence limits can be placed around any parameter estimate. We will learn to create CIs with each procedure we discuss.

You may notice that you can create a 95% or a 99% CI. Both CIs are created in the same fashion; the difference being the tabled T value that defines the inclusion/exclusion area. The value of the $CI_{0.99}$ is that it is *more likely to contain the true population estimate*, since it will create a wider interval of values. However, in doing so it will be *less precise*. Look at our two examples:

$$CI_{0.95} \quad \text{Interval values}: \quad 15.89 \dots 28.51$$

$$CI_{0.99} \quad \text{Interval values}: \quad 13.13 \dots 31.27$$

Figure 7.15 compares the $CI_{0.95}$ and $CI_{0.99}$ for our example. As you can see, the $CI_{0.99}$ interval is wider and therefore more likely to contain the actual population mean. However, the width of the interval makes it a *less precise* estimate than the $CI_{0.95}$.

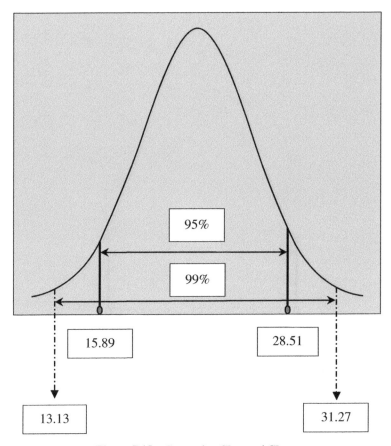

Figure 7.15   Comparing $CI_{0.95}$ and $CI_{0.99}$.

USING SPSS® AND EXCEL WITH THE SINGLE SAMPLE *T* TEST

We can use both SPSS and Excel to evaluate a single sample *T* test, although SPSS is more straightforward. Both provide the same results.

SPSS® and the Single Sample *T* test

SPSS provides a very easy way to perform this test with a drop-down menu. As you can see in Figure 7.16, you can access the "One-Sample *T* Test … " menu through the Analyze menu on the main screen and then choosing "Compare Means." When you choose the one sample t test, you are presented with the menu in Figure 7.17.

This menu allows you to specify which dependent (outcome) variable you are testing by specifying the appropriate variable in the "Test Variable(s):" window using the arrow button. Include the assumed population mean value in the "Test Value" window near the bottom of the menu. As you can see in Figure 7.17, I included the

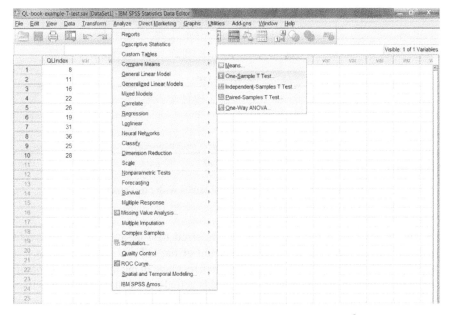

Figure 7.16 Selecting the single sample *t* test in SPSS®.

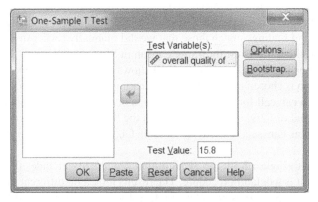

Figure 7.17 Specifying the single sample *T* test in SPSS®.

value 15.8 since this was the value I assumed the population mean to be in our QL research question.

Figure 7.18 shows the SPSS output tables including descriptive statistics and *t* test results. The top panel provides the descriptive statistics on QL values, including mean (22.2) and estimated population SD (8.817) values. It also provides the s_m value (2.79).

The bottom panel shows the calculated t ratio (2.295) and the df (9) values. The significance reported (0.047) is the *actual probability value* of values occurring

One-Sample Statistics

	N	Mean	Std. Deviation	Std. Error Mean
overall quality of life index	10	22.20	8.817	2.788

One-Sample Test

	Test Value = 15.8					
					95% Confidence Interval of the Difference	
	t	df	Sig. (2-tailed)	Mean Difference	Lower	Upper
overall quality of life index	2.295	9	.047	6.400	.09	12.71

Figure 7.18 The SPSS® output tables with *t* test results.

"beyond" this result. Up to now, we have referred to a table of values to create numerical values that exclude a certain portion of the tails for our hypothesis test (i.e., 0.05, 0.01). SPSS provides the exclusion percentage in the tail *from the point of the calculated t ratio* (2.295 in this case). If this actual probability value is less than (i.e., smaller) the tabled exclusion value of 0.05, the *t* test is considered a significant finding since the test value would fall into the exclusion area.

In our QL research example, we can reject the null hypothesis since our test value (2.295) fell at the probability point that excluded 0.047 of the distribution in the tail. In order to reject the null hypothesis and therefore have a probability of occurrence that falls in the exclusion area, the Sig. number reported must be smaller than 0.05. These values and findings match those that we did manually earlier in the chapter.

When I specified the *T* test for a single mean in SPSS (see Figure 7.18), I had the option of requesting CI values. Figure 7.19 shows the menu that appears when the "Option" button is chosen in the *T* Test specification window (shown in Figure 7.17). Notice that you can call for CI values other than 0.95, which is the default value. To choose a CI level of 0.99, simply include it in the "Confidence Interval Percentage" window. As you can see, I used the default $CI_{0.95}$ values in running the *T* test procedure.

If you refer to Figure 7.18, the SPSS output file already includes the confidence intervals since it is a default procedure. The results look a bit different than those we discussed since SPSS shows confidence interval values placed around the *assumed population mean*. This is the way to view the output values:

Assumed population mean ("Test Value") = 15.8

$+0.09 = 15.89$ Lower limit

$+12.71 = 28.51$ Upper limit

These values correspond to the values we calculated manually previously. You can check the $CI_{0.99}$ values in the same way as before. Simply change the default 0.95 in the "One-Sample *T* Test: Options" window to 0.99, and SPSS returns the following values for the lower and upper interval: Lower $= -2.66$ and upper $= 15.46$. Using the

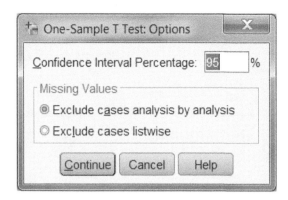

Figure 7.19   The SPSS® output tables with *t* test results.

same process as before, you can confirm the $CI_{0.99}$ values. The values are the same as our manually calculated CI values, accounting for slight differences due to rounding:

$$\text{Assumed population mean ("Test Value")} = 15.8$$

$$-2.66 = 13.14 \quad \text{Lower limit}$$

$$+15.46 = 31.27 \quad \text{Upper limit}$$

Excel and the Single Sample *T* test

The Excel program makes you work a bit harder than SPSS, but you can use it effectively to conduct a single sample *T* test. The "Data – Data Analysis" submenus do not include the single sample *T* test. However, the descriptive analysis that you performed on the **QL study** (see Figure 7.6) provides all the information you need to conduct the analysis.

If you recall, here are the relevant information taken from the descriptive analysis:

$$\text{Mean} = 22.2$$

$$\text{Standard deviation } (s_x) = 8.82$$

$$\text{(estimated) Standard error } (s_m) = 2.79$$

$$\text{Count}(N) = 10$$

You can simply substitute the values earlier in the *t* test formula. The only thing you need to remember is the assumed population mean (15.8):

$$t = \frac{M - \mu}{s_m} = \frac{22.2 - 15.8}{2.79} = 2.294$$

As you can see, your calculation of *t* using Excel's descriptive summary is the same as our own calculation and that derived from SPSS.

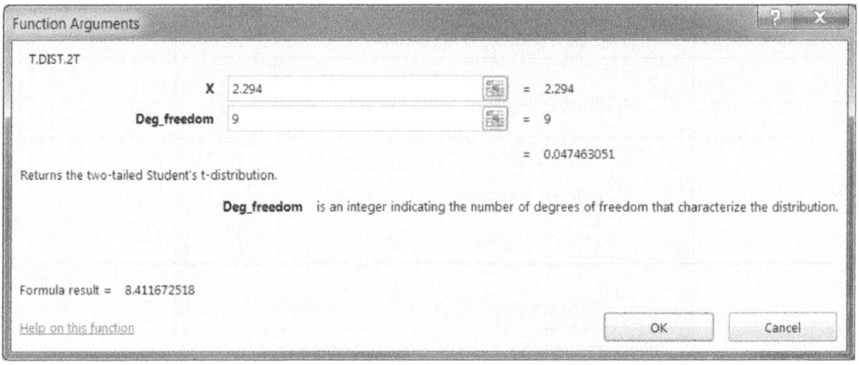

Figure 7.20   The T.DIST.2T function in Excel.

The next step in the hypothesis test is to determine whether the calculated *t* ratio (2.294) is "extreme enough" to reject the null hypothesis. You could proceed as you did in the manual calculation by comparing the t ratio to the tabled value of *t* (± 2.262). This comparison would lead you to be able to reject the null hypothesis since 2.294 exceeds the exclusion value of 2.262.

You may access the *T* table in Excel through the use of the "T.DIST.2T" function.[4] This function is available by choosing the Statistical Functions from the Formulas menu on the main page. (Review the material in Appendix B dealing with the Excel functions.) When you choose T.DIST.2T, the window in Figure 7.20 appears.

As you can see, I entered the relevant information in the T.DIST function windows. The "X" window is the place to enter the calculated *T* ratio (2.294). Excel compares this value to *T* table values using df (9) and tail (2) information.

When this information is entered, you can select "OK" to paste the resulting value to your spreadsheet. However, note that the result ("0.047463051") is returned in the middle of the function screen. Like SPSS, this value is the actual probability of values greater than the sample mean occurring on the comparison distribution. If the value is beyond (smaller than) the 0.05 level (the standard exclusion area used by researchers), then you would reject the null hypothesis. The values returned by Excel match those returned by SPSS (see Figure 7.18).

You must calculate the CI values manually as we did before since Excel does not provide this information for the single sample *t* test. You need to have access to a *T* distribution table for this calculation since you need the 0.05 (or 0.01) exclusion values to calculate the estimated population mean interval. Since Excel (T.DIST.2T) returns the actual probability of a result, you cannot use this for the CI. (The Excel function "CONFIDENCE.T" calculates confidence intervals, but it requires a known population SD, so it wouldn't be completely reliable for the single sample *T* test.)

---

[4]Excel also has functions for one-tailed left (T.DIST) and right (T.DIST.RT) hypothesis tests as well.

TERMS AND CONCEPTS

Biased estimator: A sample measure that does not provide an accurate measure of the population characteristic.

Confidence interval: Creating a range of values that will likely contain the true population value within a certain level of certainty.

Degrees of freedom: The restrictions on the sample values when estimating a population parameter.

Effect size: The strength or impact of a finding, typically the amount of distance the test value is "pushed" away from the population value.

Estimated standard deviation of the population: Determining a value for the standard deviation of the population when it is not known by "adjusting" the sample SD value.

Estimated standard deviation of the sampling distribution of means: Determining a value for the standard deviation of the sampling distribution of means through the use of the estimated standard deviation of the population (also called the "standard error of the mean").

One-tailed tests: Locating the exclusion area in one tail of the comparison distribution (either to the right or to the left).

Point estimate: Transforming a sample value (e.g., sample mean) to a comparison distribution to determine whether it is statistically different from a population value (e.g., population mean).

Power: The ability of a statistical analysis to detect a "true" finding.

Standard error of the mean: See "estimated standard deviation of the sampling distribution of means."

T distribution: A series of distribution curves like the Z distribution but adjusted for different sample sizes. Used to assess the statistical significance of hypothesis tests.

Two-tailed tests: Locating the exclusion area in both tails of the comparison distribution.

Type I (alpha) error: The type I error is mistakenly rejecting the null hypothesis when it should be accepted.

Type II (beta) error: Not rejecting the null hypothesis when it should be rejected.

DATA LAB AND EXAMPLES (WITH SOLUTIONS)

Problem 1

The following values represent Job Satisfaction Scores (JSS) for a sample of baristas from Southern California. Compare these scores with baristas from Seattle who are assumed to show a JSS mean of 50. (JSS maximum score = 60, with higher scores representing higher satisfaction.) Is the Southern California sample of baristas more satisfied with their work than those in Seattle? Perform the appropriate hypothesis test and provide an interpretation of your results. How would you describe the impact of these findings?

JSS scores of Southern California baristas: 48,42,55,35,50,47,45,45,39,42

Problem 2

The following are scores on a parasite identification test among students in an introductory epidemiology class: 25,19,18,17,15,12,9,6.

Estimate the population mean from these scores. What is the population mean likely to be at the $CI_{0.95}$ level?

Problem 3

The sample group of observations[5] in Table 7.5 consists of observations of math classrooms in grades $K - 8$th across several schools. The study variable (i.e., outcome variable) is an overall measure of the extent to which Powerful Teaching and Learning was present during a classroom observation in year four of a study.

TABLE 7.5   The STAR
Classroom Observation
Protocol™ Data

Overall
4
3
3
2
2
3
4
2
3
3
3
3
4
2
2
4
2
3

[5]This problem uses STAR Classroom Observation Protocol™ data provided by The BERC Group, Inc. The data are measures of the extent to which Powerful Teaching and Learning™ is present during a classroom observation. The BERC Group, Inc., has performed thousands of classroom observations of all grade levels and subject areas.

The study variable "Overall" scored observations of teachers in the following categories:

Score	Category
1	Not at all
2	Very little
3	Somewhat
4	Very much

The purpose of this lab is to respond to the following research question: "Do $K-8$ math classrooms demonstrate different levels of Powerful Teaching and Learning than the population of all classrooms observed?" The population of classrooms of all grades and subjects is assumed to have an Overall average of 2.45.

1. Calculate the single sample t test manually and perform the hypothesis test.

2. Calculate the effect size and $CI_{0.95}$.

3. Perform the single sample t test through Excel and SPSS.

4. Provide a summary of your findings.

DATA LAB: SOLUTIONS

Problem 1

- $M = 44.8$.
- $S_x = 5.692$.
- $S_M = 1.80$.
- T ratio $= -2.889$.
- Rejection region (df 9): ± 2.262 (two-tailed test, 0.05 level).
- Reject the null hypothesis, $p < 0.05$.
- The Southern California baristas show lower values on the JSS measure, which suggests they are less happy with their work than Seattle baristas.
- Effect size: $d = 0.91$, large effect.

Problem 2

- $M = 15.13$
- $S_x = 6.034$
- $S_M = 2.133$
- Table T value (0.05, df 7) $= \pm 2.365$

$$CI_{0.95} = -2.365(2.133) + 15.13$$

$$CI_{0.95}(\text{left bracket value}) = 10.09$$

$$\text{CI}_{0.95} = 2.365(2.133) + 15.13$$

$$\text{CI}_{0.95}(\text{right bracket value}) = 20.17$$

Problem 3

1. Calculate the single sample *t* test manually and perform the hypothesis test.

$$s_x = \sqrt{\frac{\Sigma X^2 - \frac{(\Sigma X)^2}{N}}{N-1}} = \sqrt{\frac{160 - \frac{2704}{18}}{17}} = 0.758$$

$$s_m = \frac{s_x}{\sqrt{N}} = 0.179$$

$$t = \frac{M - \mu}{s_m} = \frac{2.89 - 2.45}{0.179} = 2.458$$

- $H_0: \mu_1 = \mu$. (There is no difference between the Overall mean of the sample of $K-8$ math classrooms and the classrooms in the study population.)
- $H_A: \mu_1 \neq \mu$. (The sample group Overall mean is not the same as all classrooms in the study population.)
- The critical value: The two-tailed *T* table value $(t_{0.05,\ 17\ df}) = 2.110$.
- Calculated $t = 2.458$.
- Statistical decision: Reject the null hypothesis since the calculated value of the t ratio (2.458) exceeds the exclusion value on the distribution (2.110).
- Interpretation: The single sample *t* test revealed that the sample group of $K-8$ math classrooms showed higher average observed Powerful Teaching and Learning scores than the population of classrooms observed at all grade levels and in all subject areas.

2. Calculate the effect size and $\text{CI}_{0.95}$.

$$d = \frac{t}{\sqrt{N}} = \frac{2.458}{4.24} = 0.58 \quad \text{(medium effect)}$$

Confidence interval $= \pm t(s_M) + M \qquad (t_{0.05,17df}) = 2.110$

Lower interval value $= -2.110\,(0.179) + 2.89 = 2.512$

Upper interval value $= +2.110\,(0.179) + 2.89 = 3.268$

$\text{CI}_{0.95}$ consists of an interval of 2.512–3.268 for the population *from which this sample came*. Notice that this interval does not contain the assumed population mean (2.45). <u>Since we rejected the null hypothesis</u>, we concluded that our *sample mean was so different that it must have come from a population mean much higher than the general population with an assumed Overall mean of 2.45.*

3. Perform the single sample *t* test through Excel and SPSS. Figure 7.21 shows the Excel descriptive statistics output for Overall. The calculated values needed for the single sample *t* test are shaded.

Overall	
Mean	2.889
Standard Error	0.179
Median	3.000
Mode	3.000
Standard Deviation	0.758
Sample Variance	0.575
Kurtosis	−1.118
Skewness	0.195
Range	2.000
Minimum	2.000
Maximum	4.000
Sum	52
Count	18

Figure 7.21   The Excel descriptive data for the sample group Overall scores.

Using the shaded mean and s_m values from Figure 7.21, the calculated t ratio is the same as our manual calculation under #1 earlier:

$$t = \frac{2.89 - 2.45}{0.179} = 2.458$$

Using the Excel T.DIST.2T function, the calculated value is $p = 0.025$. Since this value is lower (i.e., more extreme) than the 5% exclusion value, we can reject the null hypothesis. The hypothesis test results in #1 previously are verified.

The SPSS single sample *t* test results are shown in Figure 7.22. As you can see, the *t* ratio (2.455) is the same as those calculated manually and through Excel (slight differences due to rounding).

Other relevant findings from the SPSS output in Figure 7.22 are the following:

o The significance (0.025) like that reported by Excel is the actual probability of a finding at least this extreme; that is, the *t* ratio (2.455) falls into the exclusion area at the point where only 0.025 probability of a sample value are more extreme. Thus, since this value of 0.025 is smaller (more extreme) than the 0.05 exclusion area, we can reject the null hypothesis.

o The confidence interval values are the same as those we calculated manually under #1 before:

One-Sample Statistics

	N	Mean	Std. Deviation	Std. Error Mean
Overall	18	2.89	.758	.179

One-Sample Test

	Test Value = 2.45				95% Confidence Interval of the Difference	
	t	df	Sig. (2-tailed)	Mean Difference	Lower	Upper
Overall	2.455	17	.025	.439	.06	.82

Figure 7.22   The SPSS® results of the single sample *t* test.

Assumed population mean ("Test Value") = 2.45

$$+0.06 = 2.51 \quad \text{Lower limit}$$

$$+0.82 = 3.27 \quad \text{Upper limit}$$

4. Provide a summary of your findings. A single sample t test of a randomly chosen group ($N = 18$) of $K - 8$ math classrooms revealed significant differences in their overall Powerful Teaching and Learning scores from the population of observed classrooms in all grades and subjects with an assumed mean of 2.45 ($T = 2.46$, $p < 0.025$). The $K - 8$ math classrooms demonstrated higher average Overall scores than the population. This study revealed a medium effect size ($d = 0.58$) indicating a meaningful sample mean score difference from the population of classrooms.

8

INDEPENDENT SAMPLE *T* TEST

You have arrived at an important benchmark in the book. By now, you have gained an understanding of descriptive statistics, and you are working your way toward an understanding of sampling distributions and how they are helpful in making statistical decisions. I have discussed two inferential tests: the *Z* test and the single sample *T* test.

In the chapters ahead, you will build upon your understanding of inferential statistics. This chapter extends what we learned in Chapter 7 about the *T* test. As you will see, there is a logical process of extending the single sample *T* test to the two-sample (independent) *T* test.

A LOT OF "*T*s"

In the previous chapters, we discussed several "*t*" statistics and measures:

- Single sample *T* ratio
- Two-tailed *T* table of values
- One-tailed *T* table of values

To these we add yet another *T*, the two-sample *T* test for independent samples, or simply the independent *T* Test. This is a "workhorse" test in statistics because it is so versatile and straightforward. The reason it is so common is that it allows the researcher to perform a very basic function in statistics and common practice, *compare*. The nature of statistics is comparison as you learned from the inferential process of comparing sample measures to population measures.

Perhaps you have heard an advertisement like the following: "New Drug X (fill in whatever drug comes to mind) is 25% better!" The immediate question that should

Using Statistics in the Social and Health Sciences with SPSS® and Excel®, First Edition.
Martin Lee Abbott.
© 2017 John Wiley & Sons, Inc. Published 2017 by John Wiley & Sons, Inc.

spring to mind is, "compared to what?" Old Drug X? A vomit bag? Other brands of the drug? In order to find out whether the claim has merit, <u>you must compare it to something else</u> to see if there is a difference.

In Chapter 7, you used a sample mean to estimate a population mean. In essence, you compared a sample value to an (assumed) population value. We will extend this comparison to include a second sample group through the independent sample *T* test. This statistical procedure assesses whether two samples, chosen independently, are likely to be similar or sufficiently different from one another that we would conclude that they do not even belong to the same population.

RESEARCH DESIGN

As you encounter new statistical procedures, I want to draw us back to the examination of research design. It is important to understand *how a statistical procedure should be used* rather than simply how to calculate it.

If you recall, I distinguished experiment from post facto designs in Chapter 6. One of the key differences was whether the researcher manipulated the independent variable (experiment) or simply measured what data already exists (post facto). The independent *T* test can be used with either design.

EXPERIMENTAL DESIGNS AND THE INDEPENDENT *T* TEST

Figure 8.1 shows the diagram for an experimental design in which there are two groups: experimental group and control group. As you can see, the treatment variable is manipulated by assigning one group (experimental) one level of a treatment and the other group (control) a different level (or no treatment at all). The dependent (outcome) variable is tested after the independent variable has been changed to see if there is a difference between the outcome measures of the two groups. *If there is a difference, the researcher attributes the change to the presence or action of the independent variable (i.e., makes a causal attribution), depending on the control of extraneous influences.*

The researcher may only make causal attributions if there is randomization in which subjects are chosen and assigned to groups randomly. If randomization is

Research Treatment Variable (Independent or Predictor)			Dependent Variable (Outcome)
Random Selection and Assignment?	Pre-Test Scores	Experimental Group	Outcome Test Scores (Post-Test Scores)
Random Selection and Assignment?	Pre-Test Scores	Control Group	Outcome Test Scores (Post-Test Scores)

Figure 8.1 The research design with randomness and two comparison groups.

present, then the assumption is that both groups (experimental and control) are equal at the outset. Then, if they are different on the dependent variable measure after the experiment is over, the differences must be because of the treatment that was introduced to change the experimental group and not the control group.

Under these conditions, the researcher compares the outcome measures of both groups when the experiment is over to see if there is a difference. The independent T test is the statistical procedure to use in this case since the researcher compares two sample groups. Formally stated, this is a test of the difference between two sample groups to see if they belong to the same population after the experimental manipulation. It is assumed that they belong to the same population at the <u>beginning</u> (before the independent variable is manipulated).

DEPENDENT SAMPLE DESIGNS

In research designs like those shown in Figure 8.1, the researcher compares the (post-test) outcome measures of both groups. Note that this statistical test uses *independent samples*. This means that choosing subjects for one group has nothing to do with choosing subjects for the other group. Thus, if I randomly selected Bob and assigned him randomly to group 1, it has nothing to do with the fact that I chose Sally and assigned her randomly to group 2. This is an important assumption since it assures the researcher there are no "built-in linkages" between subjects. The power of randomization results in the comparability of the two groups in this way.

Dependent samples consist of groups of subjects that have some structured linkage, like using the same people twice in a study. For example, the researcher might use pre-test scores from Bob and Sally and *compare them with their own post-test scores*. Using dependent samples affects the ability of the randomness process to create comparable samples; in such cases, the researcher is assessing *individual* change (before to after measures) in the context of the experiment that is assessing *group* change.

Figure 8.2 shows how <u>dependent samples</u> might be used in an experimental context. Extending the example shown in Table 6.1, the researcher might create a "pre–post" design in which subjects take a pre-test measure, become exposed to some experimental condition, and then take a post-test measure. This would mean that the pre-test group would be very specifically related to the post-test group (since they would be the <u>same</u> people) and therefore not independent.

Research Treatment Variable (Independent or Predictor)			Dependent Variable (Outcome)
Random Selection and Assignment?	Fear of Hospitals (Pre-Test measure scores)	In-patient video on hospital procedures, organization, and personnel (Experimental Treatment)	Fear of Hospitals (Post-Test measure scores from the same subjects)

Figure 8.2 Using dependent sample measures in experimental designs.

Research Treatment Variable (Independent or Predictor)			Dependent Variable (Outcome)
Matched group of M/W with a range of anxiety	Fear of Hospitals (Pre-Test Scores)	In-Patient Video (Experimental Group)	Fear of Hospitals (Post-Test Scoresfrom different but <u>matched</u> subjects)
Matched group of M/W with a range of anxiety	Pre-Test Scores	Control Group	Outcome Test Scores (Post-Test Scoresfrom different but <u>matched</u> subjects)

Figure 8.3   Using matched groups in experimental designs.

A different dependent sample design uses *matched samples*, a situation in which the <u>researcher purposely chooses and assigns subjects to comparison groups</u> based on similar characteristics relevant to the study rather than choosing and assigning randomly. For example, the researcher might be concerned about gender and/or general anxiety and the effects of these characteristics on fear of hospitals. The researcher might therefore purposely assign equal numbers of men and women, and subjects who were equally anxious, to the two study groups. As you can see in Figure 8.3, the randomness criterion in the first column is replaced by "matching" to indicate that the design uses two groups of different subjects (not the same people twice), but two groups of subjects who are *structurally linked by the decision to purposely "build in" some group similarity.*

BETWEEN AND WITHIN RESEARCH DESIGNS

Research designs differ as to whether they measure independent samples, dependent samples, or both. The design in Figure 8.1 illustrates all three processes. *Between-group designs are those in which the researcher seeks to ascertain whether the <u>groups</u> demonstrate unequal outcome measures.* That is, are there differences *between* the groups' post-test scores? In Figure 8.1, this would be comparing the post-test scores for the experimental group versus the control group. It is represented by the "vertical" distance in the "Outcome" measure column.

Within-group designs are those in which the researcher seeks to ascertain whether <u>subjects</u> in a group change over time. In Figure 8.1 the within group design would be the change from a group of subjects' pre-test scores to their post-test scores. This would be represented by the "horizontal" difference of a group; that is, are the scores *within* a specific group different after the treatment than they were at the beginning?

Mixed designs are those in which both within- and between-group measures can be taken. The design in Figure 8.1 is one such design. The vertical comparison of post-test scores is between groups, and the horizontal comparison of pre-test to post-test difference is within subjects.

USING DIFFERENT *T* TESTS

Depending on the nature of the design, an experiment may call for different *T* test procedures. With independent samples, the researcher might use an independent *T* test by comparing the post-test measures between two treatment groups. This procedure is the focus of this chapter.

If the researcher used dependent samples, they would need to use another kind of *T* test called a *dependent sample T test*. Other names for this test are repeated measures *T* test, within-subject *T* test, and paired sample *T* test. Both Excel and SPSS® refer to these as paired sample *T* tests. Chapter 15 discusses these procedures.

Pre-test or No Pre-test

Experimental research designs differ in terms of whether they include a *pre-test* of the dependent variable measure. A pre-test is simply administering the dependent variable measure before the experiment begins to insure that the two groups are in fact equal. Some experimental designs that include full randomization do not use a pre-test since the researchers assume that randomization results in equal groups; therefore, there is no need for a pre-test. In fact, under these conditions, eliminating a pre-test might eliminate potential problems since research subjects can often be affected by receiving a test of the outcome measure before the study. (This is known as *pre-test sensitivity*.)

Example of Experiment

When I was an undergraduate student, I performed an experiment on the effects of noise on human learning. I randomly selected students and randomly assigned them to either a high- or low-noise condition (by using a white noise generator with different decibel levels). Then, I gave the students in both groups the same learning task and compared their performance. The learning task (the outcome measure) was simple word recognition. Figure 8.4 shows the research design specification for this experiment.

Research Treatment Variable (Noise)			Dependent Variable (Word Recognition)
Random Selection and Assignment	No Pre-Test	Experimental Group (High noise level)	Outcome Test Scores (# of recognized words)
Random Selection and Assignment	No Pre-Test	Control Group (Low noise level)	Outcome Test Scores (# of recognized words)

Figure 8.4 Example of experimental research design using *T* test with two groups.

Note some features of the experiment shown in Figure 8.4:

- I randomly selected students and then randomly assigned them to the two treatment groups.
- I did not use a "control group" (the "absence of the treatment") but rather a second level or condition of the treatment variable to yield two treatment groups.
- I did not pre-test the subjects on word recognition before exposing them to different experimental treatment conditions because the subjects were randomized.
- I administered the word recognition test (outcome measure) to both groups after exposing the subjects to different experimental treatment conditions.

I randomly selected and assigned students, which allowed me to assume they were equal on all important dimensions (to the experiment). I exposed the two groups to different conditions, which I hypothesized would have differential effects on their learning task. Thus, if I had observed that one group learned differently (either better or worse) than the other group, I could attribute this difference to their exposure to the different conditions (high or low noise). If their learning was quite different, I could conclude, statistically, that the groups were now so different that they could no longer be thought to be from the same population of students I started with. That is the process I used for testing the hypothesis of difference. Specifically, I used the *T* test with independent samples to detect differences between post-test scores.

I will discuss this experiment in subsequent chapters as well. The short answer as to whether or not I observed statistical differences between the high- and low-noise outcome measure is no. This did not necessarily mean that noise does not affect learning; it just gave me a way to look at the problem differently. As you will see, this example shows several features of the theory testing process as well as the *T* test procedure.

Post Facto Designs

In Chapter 6, I discussed the post facto design as one in which the researcher compares group performance on an outcome measure after experimental treatments or study procedures have already taken place. These designs can be correlational or comparative depending on how the researcher relates one set of scores to the other (i.e., using correlation or difference methods, respectively).

A post facto design compares conditions with one another. Thus, for example, rather than perform an experiment to detect the impact of noise on human learning, I might ask a sample of students to indicate (1) how loud their music is when they study and (2) their GPA. Then, I could separate the students into two groups on the basis of (high and low) study noise and compare their GPA measures to detect possible differences between the two types of studiers.

In this design, therefore, I would not manipulate the noise measure; I would simply create groups on the basis of already existing differences in noise conditions. Notice that by articulating the design thus, "noise" is operationally defined as "loudness of

Studying under high noise	Studying under low noise
GPA scores	GPA scores
GPA scores	GPA scores
.	.
.	.
Mean GPA$_{High}$	Mean GPA$_{Low}$

Figure 8.5   The post facto comparison for independent *t* test.

music." If the outcome measure (GPAs) was different between the groups, I would conclude that noise would *possibly* be a contributing factor to GPA. I could not speak causally about noise since many other aspects of studying may have affected GPA (and most decidedly would!).

Figure 8.5 shows how the post facto design might appear using my noise research question. I would simply use an independent *T* test to compare the GPA measures for high- and low-noise studiers.

This same design could use dependent samples if I deliberately "stack" the two samples to be the same on some issue. For example, I might equate the numbers of women and men students and equivalent numbers of freshmen, sophomores, juniors, and seniors in both noise groups. If I did this, I would be *matching* the groups and therefore creating dependent samples. Under these circumstances, I would need to use the dependent sample *T* test.

INDEPENDENT *T* TEST: THE PROCEDURE

In the independent *T* test, the researcher takes a pair of samples to see whether these can be said to be from a single population. The experimental and post facto designs that we discussed earlier both would yield sample data for two sample groups. Figure 8.6 shows how the two-sample process works.

The chief concern with this test is the difference in the means of the two samples. If the samples are chosen randomly, by chance the means will both be close to the actual population mean (the value of which is unknown). By chance alone, the difference between the means should be fairly small.

If we chose two sample groups (or, in an experiment, we randomly chose a group and randomly assigned them to two groups), we would therefore expect the group means to be similar. In research, we start with this assumption but observe whether the two sample means are still equal after an experimental treatment or whether the group means are different when we compare different conditions of the research variable.

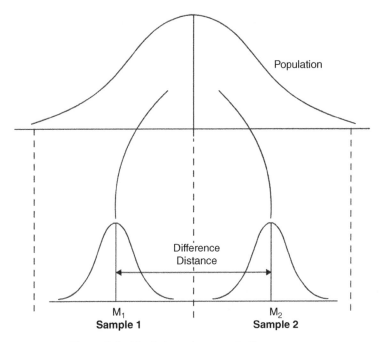

Figure 8.6   The independent sample *T* test process.

Using the post facto example earlier (see Figure 8.5), my reasoning would be the following:

- I have two groups of students, some who study under high noise and some who study under low noise.
- I assume the groups of students were equivalent before they developed their habits of studying under different amounts of noise.
- My task is to determine whether, now that they have developed their habits of study, they are still equivalent or different on a word recognition task; if I reject the null hypothesis, that will indicate they no longer belong to the same population of students.
- If they are different now, then I can say that the different (study music loudness) noise may have affected their ability to recognize words. However, there were surely other influences that led them to develop their study habits, so I cannot say the different word recognition ability is caused only by the study music loudness.

But how large does this difference have to be before it could be said that a difference so large could not be explained by chance and therefore the two groups do not represent a single population? That is the nature of the *T* test process that we examined with the single sample *T* test in Chapter 7.

CREATING THE SAMPLING DISTRIBUTION OF DIFFERENCES

In Chapter 7, you learned that in order to decide whether a (single) sample mean came from a(n) (assumed) population, you had to use the sampling distribution of means as a standard of comparison. Since you will now ask a similar question with two sample groups, you need to think about a sampling distribution created not by repeated sampling of a single group, but created by sampling *pairs of groups*.

The *sampling distribution of differences* is the sampling distribution that you use as a standard of comparison in the independent *T* test. It is called the sampling distribution of differences since it focuses on the *differences between the means of pairs of sample groups*. Figure 8.7 shows the process used to create the sampling distribution of differences (remember this is not something the researcher does, but it is simply to show the conceptual steps for creating the sampling distribution of differences).

Figure 8.7 shows pairs of samples being randomly selected from a population. The sampling distribution is made up of *all possible pairs of sample means*; Figure 8.7 simply shows four such pairs as an example of how it works. When all possible pairs of samples are taken from a population, a distribution can be created on the basis of the *differences between the means of the pairs* (designated in the figure by the lines titled "*D*"). Figure 8.8 represents the process of creating the "*D*" values (differences between pairs of sample means) that form the sampling distribution of differences.

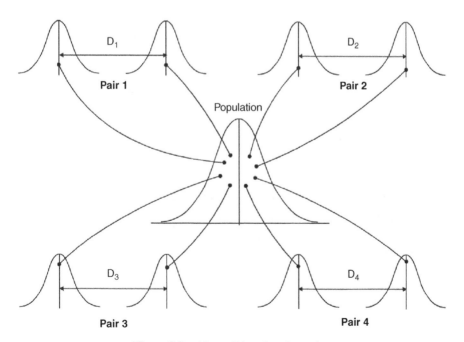

Figure 8.7 All possible pairs of samples.

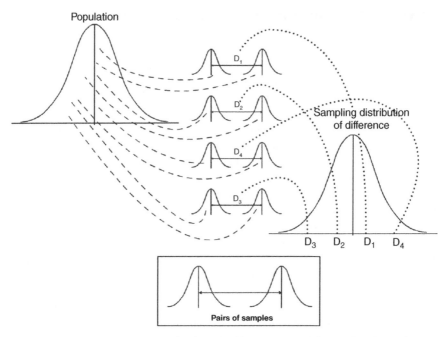

Figure 8.8   The sampling distribution of differences created from pairs of samples.

THE NATURE OF THE SAMPLING DISTRIBUTION OF DIFFERENCES

In Figure 8.8, the sampling distribution of differences is created by differences between all possible pairs of sample means. This sampling distribution of differences will now serve as the standard of comparison to see whether a pair of sample means a researcher randomly selects could be said to be representative of a research population. In effect, *how does the difference between the sample means compare to all possible sample mean differences?*

The Mean and Standard Deviation of the Sampling Distribution of Differences

The mean of the sampling distribution of differences ($\mu_{m_1 - m_2}$) should be equal to 0, since if we select pairs of groups randomly, they will by chance come from both sides of the distribution; the positive and negative values of the means, when added, would cancel one another out resulting in a total of 0.

Because all pairs of samples are hypothetically taken to create the sampling distribution, *this distribution should be normally distributed.* Therefore, if a researcher observes that a pair of samples in their study results in a difference in means that is significantly removed from 0 on the sampling distribution of differences, the researcher can conclude that the research samples cannot be said to come from the same population.

In order to transform the difference in sample means from our research study to a point on the sampling distribution of differences, we need to be able to specify the standard deviation of this sampling distribution of differences. The standard deviation of the sampling distribution of differences is known as the standard error of difference and symbolized by (s_D). The small "s" identifies this as an estimated standard deviation, and the subscript "D" identifies it as belonging to the distribution of differences. The shorthand designation for s_D is the *estimated standard error of difference.*

Technically, s_D is the *estimate of a parameter.* If you can imagine it, the standard deviation of all possible mean differences that forms the sampling distribution of differences is symbolized by $\sigma_{m_1-m_2}$. Since we could never calculate this, we must *estimate* this population parameter which is our estimated value of s_D.

We can now introduce these new symbols to the list I compiled in Table 7.1. Table 8.1 shows the entire list of symbols including the two new entries. Figure 8.9 shows the placement of the symbols that are relevant to the distribution of differences.

TABLE 8.1   New Entries to the List of Population and Sample Symbols

POPULATION AND SAMPLE SYMBOLS	
M	The mean of the sample.
SD	The standard deviation of the sample (assumes the sample is its own population)
μ	The Greek letter 'Mu' is the symbol for the population mean.
M_M	This is the symbol for the mean of the sampling distribution. You can see how this works by observing that it is a mean (M), but a mean of the sampling distribution indicated by the subscript. Thus, it is the *mean of the distribution of means*, or the 'mean of the means.' Since it is (theoretically) created by all possible samples, it is a parameter.
σ_X	"Sigma X" is the Standard Deviation of all the population raw scores. This differs from SD in that it does not refer to a sample, but to the entire population of scores.
σ_M	The standard deviation of the sampling distribution of means; also called the *Standard Error of the Mean.*
s_x	The estimated standard deviation of the population. The subscript x identifies this estimated value as belonging to the population of all scores.
s_m	The estimated standard error of the mean. The subscript m identifies this estimated value as belonging to the sampling distribution of (single) means.
$\mu_{m_1-m_2}$	The mean of the sampling distribution of differences; a parameter. This value is 0 since if all possible samples are taken, half of the means will be negative and half will be positive, resulting in a 0 value when the means are subtracted.
$\sigma_{m_1-m_2}.$	The population standard deviation of all mean differences; a parameter.
s_D	The estimated standard deviation of the sampling distribution of differences. Also known as the estimated standard error of difference.

CALCULATING THE ESTIMATED STANDARD ERROR OF DIFFERENCE WITH EQUAL SAMPLE SIZE

Figure 8.9 shows the <u>conceptual</u> method for understanding and calculating s_D. As you can see, in order to create the estimated standard error of difference, we must *combine the information from two separate samples*. Each sample standard deviation is important to the overall estimate, so we must "pool" the sample standard deviations to create a single sampling distribution standard deviation. Technically, we *pool the variances* from the two research samples to obtain s_D.

The pooled variance is a way of weighting the sample variances (with dfs) to ensure a better estimate. This is simply the *average of the variances from which we can derive s_D as long as the sample sizes are equal*. Because sample sizes (n_1 and n_2) are so critical in estimating variance, the formula for this process requires equal sample sizes. (If sample sizes are unequal, we would need to estimate s_D with a different formula since estimates of the population variance based on the samples, s^2, will not be equally weighted.)

The following is the formula for calculating s_D <u>*when there are equal sample sizes*</u>. Notice the sequence of calculations necessary to calculate s_D. You must calculate the estimated standard deviation (s_x) from each sample; then you must use s_x to calculate s_m for each sample. This is the same process we used in the single sample *T* test. We are simply performing the calculation twice since there are two samples involved.

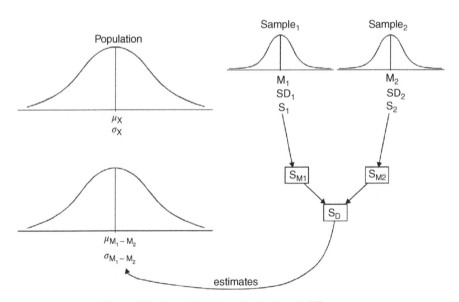

Figure 8.9   Symbols in the distribution of differences.

Finally, the separate s_m values are <u>pooled</u> to create s_D. This is the point at which you combine the sample values to create the standard error of difference[1]:

$$s_D = \sqrt{s_{m_1}^2 + s_{m_2}^2} \quad \text{where} \quad s_{m_1} = \frac{s_1}{\sqrt{n_1}} \quad \text{and} \quad s_{m_2} = \frac{s_2}{\sqrt{n_2}}$$

The Degrees of Freedom for the Independent T Test

With two samples, the researcher combines the degrees of freedom as well as the variation measure. In the independent T test with two samples, the degrees of freedom is thus equal to

$$(\text{df}_1 = n_1 - 1) + (\text{df}_2 = n_2 - 1) = n_1 + n_2 - 2$$

USING UNEQUAL SAMPLE SIZES

Unequal sample sizes present the researcher with the problem I mentioned previously. Since you need to pool the estimated population variances, unequal sample sizes will affect the overall estimate according to the magnitude of the differences. An *average* places the estimated value directly in the middle of both sample estimates. However, when one sample is larger, the pooled "average" is influenced more greatly by the value with the bigger sample size.

To account for the different "weights" presented by different sample sizes, researchers use a different formula for s_D. This formula looks quite complex, but it makes conceptual sense if you look carefully. The formula uses elements that you have learned before. Here is the formula:

$$s_D = \sqrt{\left(\frac{(\text{SS}_1) + (\text{SS}_2)}{(\text{df})} \right) \left(\frac{1}{n_1} + \frac{1}{n_2} \right)}$$

Derivation of the Formula for Unequal Sample Sizes

If you recall from Chapter 3, I used the sum of squares (SS) value to calculate a global measure of variation for a set of values. The following is the formula for that procedure:

$$SD = \sqrt{\frac{\Sigma X^2 - \frac{(\Sigma X)^2}{N}}{N}}$$

---

[1]Notice that the formula for s_D combines the estimated *variances* from both samples but produces the standard error of difference which is a standard deviation measure.

The <u>SS</u> part of that equation is the overall numerator, without the square root sign:

$$SS = \sum X^2 - \frac{\left(\sum X\right)^2}{N}$$

When the SS is divided by the sample size, it is a calculation for population variance (or the total variance of a set of scores as its own population):

$$\text{Variance} = \frac{SS}{N} \quad \text{or} \quad \text{Variance} = \frac{\sum X^2 - \frac{\left(\sum X\right)^2}{N}}{N}$$

Under the square root sign, this became the (total) standard deviation:

$$SD = \sqrt{\frac{SS}{N}} \quad \text{or} \quad SD = \sqrt{\frac{\sum X^2 - \frac{\left(\sum X\right)^2}{N}}{N}}$$

I used these calculations to <u>estimate</u> the population standard deviation (s_x) by dividing the values by the <u>degrees of freedom</u>. In the case of a single sample, the df $= n - 1$. (See Chapter 7 to review the formula and calculation for s_x.) Looking again at the previous formula using the pooled estimate of variance for calculating s_D with unequal sample size, you will see these primary elements:

$$s_D = \sqrt{\left(\frac{(SS_1) + (SS_2)}{(df)}\right)\left(\frac{1}{n_1} + \frac{1}{n_2}\right)}$$

Here are some observations about the nature of this equation. If you take the formula apart:

The first part (left half)
   As you can see in the *first part* of the equation under the radical sign above, we are simply combining SS_1 and SS_2 values (the SS values from both samples) and dividing this sum by the <u>combined</u> degrees of freedom for both samples. *The result is the pooled variance and is shown in the following as (Pooled)* σ_X^2. Taking the <u>square root of the pooled variance yields the</u> *pooled standard deviation* which is useful when we calculate effect size in the following. It is shown in the following as (Pooled) σ_X:

$$(\text{Pooled}) \ \sigma_X^2 = \frac{(SS_1) + (SS_2)}{(df)} \qquad (\text{Pooled}) \ \sigma_X = \sqrt{\frac{(SS_1 + SS_2)}{df}}$$

The second part (right half)

The right half of the equation for s_D under the radical is tantamount to dividing the left half by the combined sizes of samples to yield s_D from the pooled variance. Remember what the estimated standard error of difference (s_D) represents. It is the *estimated standard deviation of the sampling distribution of difference* (or estimated standard error of difference). Whether s_D is calculated from samples that have equal sample sizes or unequal sample sizes, the s_D measure is valuable since it allows the researcher the ability to *transform* the difference in sample means $(m_1 - m_2)$ to a point on the sampling distribution. This enables the researcher to compare this point with all possible sample differences to determine if the resultant point (difference between samples) is too large to be obtained by chance.

THE INDEPENDENT *T* RATIO

What I described previously are the elements used to calculate the independent *T* test. It is an extension of the single sample *T* test in that we are simply adding a second sample value. Once you calculate s_D, you can calculate the overall *T* ratio:

$$t = \frac{(M_1 - M_2) - \mu_{M_1 - M_2}}{s_D} \quad \text{or} \quad t = \frac{(M_1 - M_2) - 0}{s_D} \quad \text{since} \quad \mu_{m_1 - m_2} = 0$$

$$\text{df} = N_1 + N_2 - 2$$

Compare this formula with the single sample *T* ratio we discussed in Chapter 10:

$$t = \frac{M - \mu}{s_m}, \quad \text{df} = N_1 - 1$$

As you can see:

- The independent *T* test adds a second sample mean value and uses a calculated standard error of difference (s_D) that incorporates the second sample (according to whether the sample size is equal or unequal).
- The population of all paired sample differences $(\mu_{m_1 - m_2})$ is subtracted from the difference in sample means $(M_1 - M_2)$. Note that the population of all paired sample differences $(\mu_{M_1 - M_2})$ is equal to 0, since the population would have equal amounts of negative and positive paired differences.
- The distance of the sample mean difference from the population value is transformed to standard deviation units on the sampling distribution when it is divided by s_D.
- This value (the independent *t* ratio) indicates that it is likely not a chance finding if it exceeds the tabled probability value for the exclusion.

INDEPENDENT T TEST EXAMPLE

I will demonstrate the independent T test with a hypothetical example. Critique the research design after you perform the hypothesis test.

The Setting

Patients at a research hospital were randomly chosen to evaluate the effectiveness of an information session on reducing fear of colonoscopies. Patients were randomly assigned to two conditions: (1) upon admittance a medical practitioner spent about one-half hour with the patient reviewing the myths of the colonoscopy procedure (i.e., it will hurt, embarrassment, cleanliness of the instrument, etc.), or (2) patients spent the same amount of time reading general literature about the procedure in a quiet room.

Immediately before the procedure, the patients were given a hospital survey measuring their fear level of the procedure. The Fear of Procedure (FOP) survey resulted in fear index scores between 0 (no fear) and 30 (complete fear).

The Research Data

Table 8.2 presents the data I will use for this example. As you can see, there were 14 patients randomly assigned to two conditions.

The research question is: Do the different sessions differ in FOP scores?

HYPOTHESIS TEST ELEMENTS FOR THE EXAMPLE

The Null Hypothesis

The null hypothesis for the independent sample T test is similar to that for the single sample T test:

$$H_0 : \quad \mu_1 = \mu_2$$

TABLE 8.2 Procedure Information and Fear of Procedure Scores

Practitioner Session	Reading Session
21	20
9	28
12	15
9	11
11	16
9	18
7	14

Technically, the null hypothesis states that the population from which group 1 came is the same as the population from which group 2 came. This is a formal way of stating that the sample group means are equal.

The Alternative Hypothesis

The alternative hypothesis is that the populations from which the samples came are not equal:

$$H_A : \quad \mu_1 \neq \mu_2$$

The Critical Value of Comparison

For this test, you use the T table as you did for the single sample T test. Despite the fact that the overall sample is 14, the group sample sizes (7 and 7) warrant the use of the T table. Further, we have no knowledge of the parameter values.

Remember that the degrees of freedom must be identified so we can specify the exclusion value for the T table of values. For the independent sample T test

$$df = n_1 + n_2 - 2$$
$$df = 7 + 7 - 2 = 12$$

Note: For the remainder of the text, I will use the protocol of identifying the overall group size with the capital "N" and the size of individual samples with lower case "n." This is an important distinction to keep in mind as we proceed through this and subsequent statistical procedures.

Referring to the T table with $df = 12$, you will find that the comparison value for the two-tailed T test at the 0.05 exclusion level is 2.179, which identifies the 5% exclusion area on the comparison distribution. If the calculated T ratio exceeds this number, you would reject the null hypothesis and conclude that the two sample means are different from one another. Note that the comparison value is identified for a two-tailed test. Therefore, if the calculated t ratio exceeds this value either positively or negatively, you would reject the null hypothesis. The comparison value is identified; thus $t_{(0.05,12)} = \pm 2.179$.

The Calculated T Ratio

Table 8.3 shows the data with calculations for most of the elements of the T test. Go over the process and the results for a better grasp of the procedure.

Recall the formula for the independent samples T ratio using the s_D formula for equal cell sizes.

Using these formulas and the data from Tables 8.2 and 8.3, calculate the t ratio:

$$s_D = \sqrt{s_{m_1}^2 + s_{m_2}^2} \quad \text{where} \quad s_{m_1} = \frac{s_1}{\sqrt{n_1}} \quad \text{and} \quad s_{m_2} = \frac{s_2}{\sqrt{n_2}}$$

TABLE 8.3   Minutes Pacing for Low and High Perceived Stress Assessments

	Practitioner		Reading	
	X_L	X_L^2	X_H	X_H^2
	21	441	20	400
	9	81	28	784
	12	144	15	225
	9	81	11	121
	11	121	16	256
	9	81	18	324
	7	49	14	196
Mean	11.14		17.43	
Σ	78		122	
ΣX^2		998		2306
$(\Sigma X)^2$	6084		14884	
s_x	4.634		5.473	
s_m	1.752		2.069	
s_D		2.711		

$$2.711 = \sqrt{3.07 + 4.281} \quad \text{where } 1.752 = \frac{4.634}{\sqrt{7}} \quad \text{and} \quad 2.069 = \frac{5.473}{\sqrt{7}}$$

$$t = \frac{(M_1 - M_2) - \mu_{M_1 - M_2}}{s_D}$$

$$= \frac{(11.14 - 17.43) - 0}{2.711}$$

$$= -2.320$$

The calculated t ratio for the independent sample T test (with df $= 12$) is -2.320. This value represents the transformed difference in the sample group means of a value in standard deviation units on the sampling distribution of differences. It shows where the two-sample group difference in means fall on the comparison distribution so we can decide if it is either a chance difference or if the difference is too large by chance to be considered a common population.

Statistical Decision

Since the calculated t ratio (-2.320) exceeded the exclusion value (± 2.179), you would reject the null hypothesis. The t ratio represents the point on the sampling

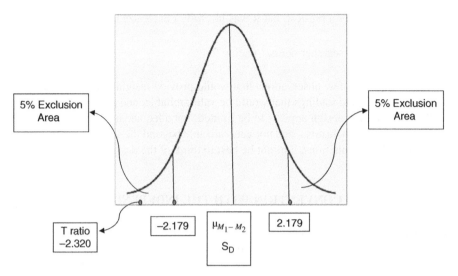

Figure 8.10   The statistical decision for the FOP example question.

distribution of difference where the difference between the Practitioner and Reading measures of the FOP scores of the study samples would be placed. Since this value lies beyond the rejection region, you would conclude that it is likely not a chance finding. Thus, you would conclude that the difference in FOP scores between Practitioner and Reading groups came from different populations. Figure 8.10 shows how these values compare.

Interpretation

The independent sample T test revealed that patients in the Practitioner group had lower mean FOP values ($M = 11.14$) than patients in a Reading group ($M = 17.43$). The T ratio of -2.319 is statistically significant ($p < 0.05$), indicating that the difference in group means is not likely due to chance.

Research Design of the Example

This is a form of an experiment but has features that detract from a true experiment, which could yield causal conclusions:

- No information is given about the "pool" of patients; was it large, randomly chosen, a convenience sample, etc.?
- The study group was randomly <u>assigned,</u> so there was an attempt to include as much randomization as possible, but the overall study cannot be said to be randomized.
- There was no FOP measure taken before the session (Practitioner or Reading) – thus no pre-test. If this had been a fully randomized study, there would

be less need for a pre-test, but it was not fully randomized, and it was a small sample.

- How did the researcher define "pacing?"

These are only a few observations that would provide insights into the adequacy of the design to yield findings that would be valid, reliable, and generalizable. Generally speaking, the design appears to be limited, not adequate as an experiment for providing causal conclusions, and not generalizable beyond the subjects in the study. Because of these limitations, it might be best to think of the design as post facto.

BEFORE–AFTER CONVENTION WITH THE INDEPENDENT *T* TEST

Which group to consider group 1 or group 2 in an independent sample *T* test is an important consideration. As you can see from the formula, the researcher can consider *either group* to be group 1 or group 2. *Depending on how they are entered into the formula, the sign of the t ratio will differ.*

If we had considered Reading to be group 1 and Practitioner to be group 2 in the previous example, the resultant *t* ratio would have been $T = 2.320$ instead of $T = -2.320$. This would not have altered the finding (rejection of the null hypothesis) unless we had specified a one-tailed test in the positive exclusion region, but it might have affected the wording of the interpretation.

This example points out that you need to use caution in specifying group identification. This is as much an issue for experimental studies as well as post facto studies since the researcher can assign the treatment group as either group 1 or group 2.

Let me suggest a convention for this dilemma. When you are dealing with a research design that uses "before" and "after," you can think of the "before" as what you are measuring the "after" against. By convention, *subtract the "before" score from the "after"* so that you can show the change "leftover" once the before score is subtracted out. This convention would yield the following conceptual design (the general experimental pattern):

$$t = \frac{\text{After} - \text{before}}{\text{StError}}$$

If you subtract out the before from the after scores, you will just have the increment leftover that is due to your program or whatever you designed to move the sample data "away" from the population data. Thus, for example, if you are dealing with a program that reduces stress and you posit that a treatment program will result in lower stress scores after the program is completed, then using the previous formula revision should show negative values if your research hypothesis is accurate. If a research hypothesis suggests that higher scores should result from training designed to increase management potential, then using the aforementioned should yield positive values if the research hypothesis is accurate.

This convention is perhaps less clear with post facto designs since the researcher may not be aware which direction the results may tend. The key issue is *being aware of the nature of the data and how the signs should fall if your alternate (research) hypothesis is true.* In the post facto example cited earlier, the researcher may have been aware from previous observation or research literature that patients experience greater fear if they are isolated during pre-surgery rather than being in the position of being able to discuss specific fears with practitioners. In this case, the researcher might have placed the Reading group as group 1 and the Practitioner group as group 2 so that the probable lesser fear scores of the Practitioner group would be subtracted out of the likely higher fear of group 1. This would likely yield an *increment of difference as a positive value* assuming the alternative hypothesis is accurate.

There are exceptions to this process. It is up to you as the researcher to make sure that you understand which value you place first in the formula and how that decision will affect your conclusions. One obvious exception is if your research hypothesis is not true or if in fact it is the opposite of what you expect!!

CONFIDENCE INTERVALS FOR THE INDEPENDENT *T* TEST

Remember that the *T* test cited earlier is a <u>point estimate</u>. We transformed the group mean difference to a point on the sampling distribution in order to see if it fell into the exclusion area (which it did). However, if you were interested in <u>estimating the population value</u>, you would use the confidence interval (CI) procedure I discussed in Chapter 7 with a couple of changes to the formula.

The following formula is for the single sample (refer to Chapter 7 for a complete analysis of the formula):

$$CI_{0.95} = \pm t(s_M) + M$$

The independent sample *T* test formula is almost identical, but includes some changes:

$$CI_{0.95} = (\text{table value of } \pm t)(s_D) + (M_1 - M_2)$$

As you can see, the tabled value of *T* is the same. The changes are due to using a <u>different sampling distribution</u> with consequent changes in the standard error (s_D rather than s_M) and due to having two sample means rather than a single mean (thus using $M_1 - M_2$ rather than M).

Using the data available from the previous analyses,

$$CI_{0.95} = -2.179(2.711) + (11.14 - 17.43)$$

$$CI_{0.95}(\text{lower or left bracket value}) = -12.197$$

$$CI_{0.95} = 2.179(2.711) + (11.14 - 17.43)$$

$$CI_{0.95}(\text{upper or right bracket value}) = -0.383$$

CI with the sampling distribution of difference are placed in reference to a value of "0" since the population mean of all differences ($\mu_{M_1-M_2}$) is 0. Therefore, in the previous example, we can conclude that the true <u>population mean difference value</u> from which we derived the <u>sample group difference</u> is between -12.197 and -0.383.

Notice that the CI does not include 0, the population mean of differences. This indicates that the difference in sample means is likely significantly different since "their" reference population is different from the true population mean of differences.

EFFECT SIZE

Effect size is very important and has a number of calculations depending on how it is used. In what follows I will discuss two primary calculations: the Cohens (d) method of difference and the eta squared method. Cohen's d is valuable because it demonstrates the magnitude of the difference in means. The eta squared method expresses the importance of the main factor of a study (i.e., the primary influence of the predictor/independent variable) in explaining the overall variance of the outcome variable. I will discuss this second method for other statistical procedures that follow in this book.

Cohen's d Method

You can use this method to calculate effect size in a way similar to the calculation for the single sample T test. As you recall, you calculated *Cohen's d* for the single sample T test according to the following formula:

$$d = \frac{t}{\sqrt{N}}$$

Since you add another sample group for the independent T test, you need to adjust the formula. Cohen (1988) lists this (adjusted) calculation as follows:

$$d = \frac{M_1 - M_2}{\sigma}$$

Cohen noted that the denominator (σ) is the <u>population standard deviation</u>. He further specified that for the formula, the researcher could use the standard deviation for *either group since they are assumed to be equal.* (Another approach is to use σ for the *entire set of scores* as the denominator.) Since you learned to create the pooled variance and the pooled standard deviation as the combined estimate of the population standard deviation, you could use this as the denominator:

$$d = \frac{M_1 - M_2}{(\text{Pooled})\sigma_X}$$

Using this adjusted formula, we find the following:

$$d = \frac{11.14 - 17.43}{5.07}$$

Therefore, $d = -1.24$ (the negative sign indicates direction of the finding, not magnitude).

You can use the same criteria for judging the magnitude of the effect size (d) that you did in Chapter 10: 0.20, small; 0.50, medium; and 0.80, large. In this example the effect size is judged to have a large effect.

An alternate method (Cohen, 1988) that does not include the <u>pooled standard deviation</u> is

$$d = t\sqrt{\frac{n_1 + n_2}{(n_1)(n_2)}} = -2.319\sqrt{\frac{7+7}{49}}$$

This alternate formula provides essentially the same value of $d = -1.24$. In both cases, the effect size is judged large. In terms of the research problem, this indicates that the predictor variable "information condition" had an impact on the FOP scores such that the difference between Practitioner and Reading groups "moved" the FOP measures about 1.24 standard deviation units apart (based on the population standard deviation).[2]

The Eta Squared Method

Another method for calculating effect size for the independent T is "eta square," symbolized by "η^2" and calculated by the following formula:

$$\eta^2 = \frac{T^2}{T^2 + df}$$

Also by Cohen (1988), this effect size calculation describes the impact of a predictor variable on an outcome differently from the d formula. Eta square creates a value that expresses the amount of variation in the outcome attributed to the predictor variable. Thus, in the previous example

$$\begin{aligned}
\eta^2 &= \frac{T^2}{T^2 + df} \\
&= \frac{(-2.319)^2}{(-2.319)^2 + 12} \\
&= 0.31
\end{aligned}$$

In this example, knowing the information group assignment (predictor variable) explains 31% of the variation among FOP scores (outcome variable). There are a lot of reasons why fear occurs; information is only one possible determinant. If the "variability space" of fear is 100%, then the information group assignment explains 31% of fear, leaving 69% of fear yet to be explained.

Cohen's (1988) guidelines for interpreting explained variance are as follows:

- 0.01 – small
- 0.06 – medium
- 0.14 – large

---

[2]Note that in the explanation, I emphasize the magnitude of the finding, not the direction.

These may not appear to very large numbers, but as we will see with subsequent procedures, explaining 1%, 6%, and 14% of the variance in an outcome will be a most substantive outcome.

THE ASSUMPTIONS FOR THE INDEPENDENT *T* TEST

All statistical tests require that the researcher first assess whether the conditions are appropriate for using a specific procedure. *Using the correct statistical procedure for a given research problem ensures a greater likelihood of not committing type I and type II errors.* This is a general statement that applies to all statistical procedures, not just the independent *T* test.

Many statistical tests, including the *T* test, are called "robust," since they can be relied upon to deliver valid results even if some of the assumptions are not perfectly met. However, the researcher should always assess the assumptions prior to using a statistical procedure.

Here are the requirements for the independent *T* test:

1. The samples are independent of one another.
2. Dependent variable is interval level.
3. Sample populations are normally distributed.
4. Both populations have equal variance (this is also known as the "test of homogeneity" since we are assessing "sameness").

Assumptions 1 and 2: Independence and Interval Level

The researcher can assess the first two of these assumptions easily. Whether or not the samples are independent of one another is connected to the method and purpose of the research. As we discussed earlier, the cases for both of our sample groups must not be connected to one another. That is, the membership of one group must not rely on the membership of another. (We will discuss the "dependent sample *T* test" in a later chapter.) The researcher likewise can assess whether or not the outcome variable is <u>interval</u> level.

Assumption 3: Normal Distribution of Sample Groups

The third assumption requires a bit more investigation. Whether the samples are <u>normally distributed</u> call for the researcher to use the descriptive statistical procedures I discussed in Chapters 2 and 3. Are skewness and kurtosis values "in bounds"? Does the graphical "evidence" match the numerical assessment of skewness, kurtosis, and so on? These procedures should be assessed before the researcher proceeds to the independent *T* test. The caveat is to remember that <u>checking for normal distribution should be done for the outcome measure in groups of the independent variable.</u>

I introduce you to another procedure in the following text for assessing the normality of sample groups. The Explore procedure in SPSS provides several results for checking whether the data meet the assumptions of normality (Assumption 3) and equal variance (Assumption 4).

Assumption 4: Equal Variance

The fourth assumption requires a separate statistical test. The descriptive statistical summary produced to check the third assumption will reveal the values for variance and standard deviation. However, the researcher cannot conclude they are equal or unequal simply by looking at them!

SPSS® EXPLORE FOR CHECKING THE NORMAL DISTRIBUTION ASSUMPTION

The Explore procedure in SPSS provides a great deal of information for checking both assumptions of normality and equal variance. I introduce it here because with this (independent T test) and subsequent procedures, there are more than one group to compare. The Explore procedure can also be used with a single group however.

Figure 8.11 shows the SPSS menus that provide results for checking assumptions (Explore). As you can see, I specified "Explore" from the "Analyze – Descriptive Statistics" menus. Choosing Explore results in the further specification window shown in Figure 8.12.

Figure 8.12 shows the Explore window allowing the researcher to identify the variables used in the study. As you can see, I listed the FOP scores as the dependent or outcome variable and group (Practitioner or Reading) as the predictor variable.[3]

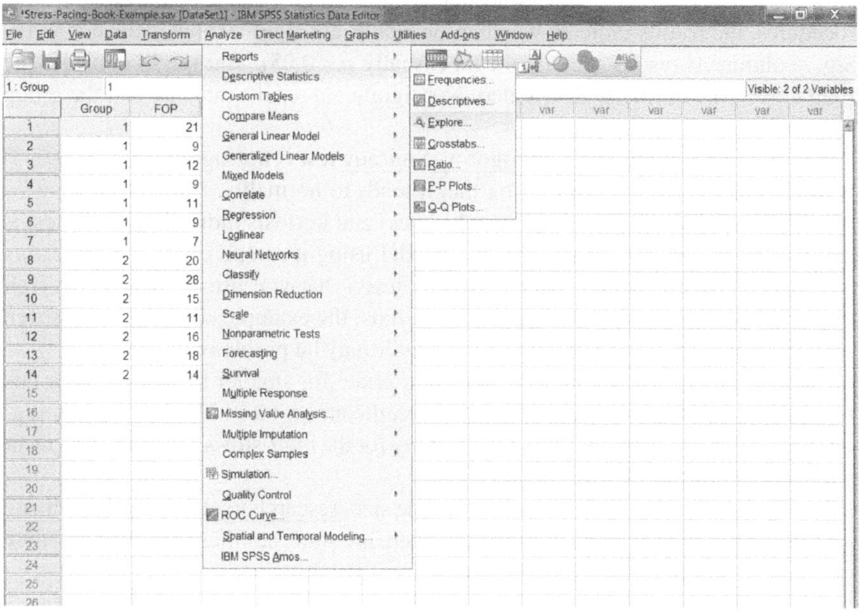

Figure 8.11   Accessing the SPSS® Explore procedure.

[3] SPSS® and other statistical programs identify the independent (or predictor) variable as a <u>factor</u>. I discuss this in subsequent chapters.

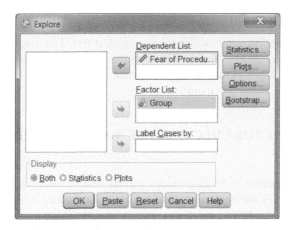

Figure 8.12   Specifying the variables to check the normality assumption.

The output derived from this procedure is shown in Figure 8.13. As you can see in the two panels below (for Practitioner and Reading groups), it appears that the Practitioner group shows a possibly skewed and leptokurtic distribution, while the Reading group appears to be normally distributed by these values.

The second panel of the output ("Tests of Normality") in Figure 8.13 shows two statistical tests designed to assess normality. In both of these specialized statistical procedures, the results indicate whether the results are significant as indicated in the "Sig." column. If results are significant (usually $p < 0.05$), you might consider the group to NOT be normally distributed. Nonsignificant results indicate that the group IS normally distributed.

In the example study, the Kolmogorov–Smirnov test is not significant ($p < 0.093$) for the Practitioner group, indicating that it tends to normality. It therefore shows a different result than that derived from skewness and kurtosis indications. This test is sensitive to sample size, so you might consider using it as one of several indicators (skewness and kurtosis and other normality tests) that you use to make an overall determination of normality. In this example study, the example study has only seven cases per group, so relying on any one indicator may be problematic.

The Shapiro–Wilk test may be more appropriate for smaller samples, and in this case it shows the Practitioner group to be significant ($p < 0.017$). Therefore, it suggests a violation of the assumption of normality for the high-stress group in agreement with the skewness and kurtosis assessment.

I would suggest that with this small sample size, researchers use caution with any one test for normality. In the present case, there are some conflicting results, but they may be the result of conservative assumptions of the tests.

Descriptives

Group				Statistic	Std. Error
Fear of Procedure	Practitioner Session	Mean		11.14	1.752
		95% Confidence Interval for Mean	Lower Bound	6.86	
			Upper Bound	15.43	
		5% Trimmed Mean		10.83	
		Median		9.00	
		Variance		21.476	
		Std. Deviation		4.634	
		Minimum		7	
		Maximum		21	
		Range		14	
		Interquartile Range		3	
		Skewness		2.011	.794
		Kurtosis		4.515	1.587
	Reading Session	Mean		17.43	2.069
		95% Confidence Interval for Mean	Lower Bound	12.37	
			Upper Bound	22.49	
		5% Trimmed Mean		17.20	
		Median		16.00	
		Variance		29.952	
		Std. Deviation		5.473	
		Minimum		11	
		Maximum		28	
		Range		17	
		Interquartile Range		6	
		Skewness		1.246	.794
		Kurtosis		2.100	1.587

Tests of Normality

		Kolmogorov-Smirnov[a]			Shapiro-Wilk		
Group		Statistic	df	Sig.	Statistic	df	Sig.
Fear of Procedure	Practitioner Session	.284	7	.093	.763	7	.017
	Reading Session	.176	7	.200*	.917	7	.443

*. This is a lower bound of the true significance.

a. Lilliefors Significance Correction

Figure 8.13   Explore output for assessing normal distribution of sample groups.

EXCEL PROCEDURES FOR CHECKING THE EQUAL VARIANCE ASSUMPTION

Excel provides a way to assess the equality of variances in the two samples used in a research study. The "F-Test Two-Sample for Variances" is available through the "Data – Data Analysis" series of menus. Figure 8.14 shows the submenu called out from the Data Analysis menu.

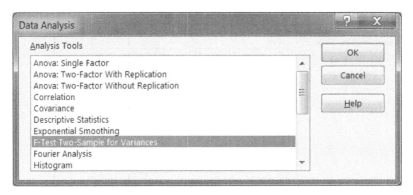

Figure 8.14   The Excel equal variance test menu.

	Practitioner	Reading
Mean	11.14	17.43
Variance	21.48	29.95
Observations	7	7
df	6	6
F	0.72	
P(F<=f) one-tail	0.35	
F Critical one-tail	0.23	

Figure 8.15   The Excel output for the two-sample variance test.

When you choose this option, you must specify the range of values for groups 1 and 2. When you run the procedure, an output sheet with the results of the test appear in a separate sheet, as shown by Figure 8.15. As you can see, the output includes some descriptive analyses in for each group in addition to the *F* test results.

I will discuss the *F* test in much greater detail in later chapters. But for now, think of the *F* test as a way to compare <u>variances</u> rather than <u>means</u>. I compared sample means in Chapter 7 (single sample) and in this chapter (two sample means) using the sampling distribution of means. The *F* distribution is a *sampling distribution of variances*. So, when you are interested in <u>whether the variances of two sample groups are equal</u>, you compare their differences to the <u>sampling distribution of variances</u>. The following is the formula used to create the *F* ratio to test whether it exceeds chance expectation:

$$F = \frac{s^2_{\text{Group 1}}}{s^2_{\text{Group 2}}} = \frac{21.476}{29.952} = 0.717$$

You can compare the results of the analysis ($F = 0.717$) with the value in the Excel output result in Figure 8.15. If you look at the formula, it simply compares the variances to see if one is <u>substantially greater or lesser</u> than the other. If both are

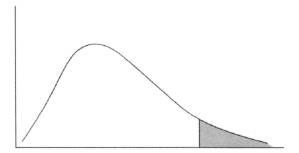

Figure 8.16   The F distribution and exclusion area.

relatively equal (or comparable), the result would be $F = 1$. To the extent the F ratio departs from 1, the less likely the group comparisons are equal. But how different do the variances have to be before we judge them not equal? We use the same logic as we did with the T tests. If the test value (the transformed score applied to the sampling distribution) exceeds the exclusion value, you conclude it is too extreme to be a chance finding. (Thus, you are performing a sort of "mini hypothesis test"!)

F Distribution

The F distribution looks different than the sampling distribution of means since you are sampling all possible <u>variances</u>. Figure 8.16 shows how this sampling distribution of variances appears.

The F distribution appears to be a normal distribution that has skewed to the right. This is because <u>variances are never negative values</u>. As you can see, all values tend to the right (positive) with the majority of observations near the left (smallest) side of the distribution. When you perform a hypothesis test for equal variance, the calculated F ratio values can fall to the left or the right side of the distribution, depending on which variance (i.e., for group 1 or group 2) has the greatest value.

Use "Right" Side Critical Values

You could place either group in the numerator or denominator in the formula; it depends on which group you identify as group 1. However, please note that "left" side values for this F test are difficult to determine, so the best rule of thumb is *place the largest variance in the numerator and the smallest variance in the denominator* since you are only trying to determine the <u>proportion</u> of the two variances. Excel will calculate both exclusion regions however.

In our example, Practitioner variance (21.476) is smallest, so you would expect the F ratios to tend toward the left exclusion area. You do not need a separate F table of values to identify the exclusion area since Excel reports the exact probability of a finding. F tables of values are common in statistics, so you may check statistical authorities (like Cohen et al. (2003)).

However, using our "right side" rule would produce the following result for the right exclusion region:

$$F = \frac{s^2_{\text{Group 1}}}{s^2_{\text{Group 2}}} = \frac{29.952}{21.476} = 1.39$$

If any research group (i.e., group 1 in this formula) has the greater value, the resulting proportion will likely tend toward the right side, in which case the right exclusion value is checked for an excessive value. If group 1 is smallest, then the left exclusion area is the one that will determine excessive calculated *F* ratios.

Figure 8.15 also reports two additional values. These are the values you use to assess equality of variances. From Figure 8.15, the following outcome indicates the likelihood of a chance finding:

$$P(F <= f) \text{ one-tailed} = 0.348$$

$$F \text{ critical one-tailed} = 0.233$$

You can interpret this result for the "left" exclusion region since sample one (Practitioner) was considered group one:

- There is a 0.348 probability that the calculated *F* ratio (0.717) could be considered a chance finding using a one-tailed table of probability. Therefore, the *F* ratio does not fall into the exclusion region and can be considered a chance finding.
- The value on the *F* distribution that identifies the one-tailed exclusion region (to the left) is 0.233. In order for the two group variances to be considered significantly different, the *F* ratio would need to be less than 0.233.

Taking both of these findings into account, you would conclude that the two group variances, while different, are nevertheless in the range of chance expectation. Since the calculated *F* ratio does not exceed the critical value that defines the exclusion area, you can conclude that the variances are statistically equivalent.

What Outcome Meets the Assumption for Equality of Variances?

Much of the time, researchers use this *F* test to determine whether sample groups are equivalent so that they might proceed with the overall statistical test. If this test indicates that the two sample groups are not equivalent, the *T* test (or whichever procedure is used) results would be conflicted. For example, if the two sample groups in this study were determined to be significantly different, then the overall rejection of the null hypothesis might reflect (i) the difference between Practitioner and Reader FOP values and (ii) the lack of group equivalence, indicating that the different subjects in the groups led to the result.

SPSS® PROCEDURE FOR CHECKING THE EQUAL VARIANCE ASSUMPTION

SPSS also has a procedure for testing the equality of variances. It is known as "Levene's test" and is reported through the Explore menu (see Figure 8.11). Choosing Explore reveals two further dialog boxes that allow you to specify the procedure. The first of these shown in Figure 8.17 shows the box in which you can specify the variables of interest. (It is the menu shown in Figure 8.12.)

As you can see, I entered the "Fear of Procedure" variable as the <u>outcome variable</u> ("Dependent List:") since that is the variable I want to check for equal variances *according to information groups.* The procedure assesses whether the Practitioner FOP values have an equivalent variance to the Reading FOP values. I also chose "Both" in the "Display" box so that the output would include visual (plots) as well as numerical (statistics) output.

Figure 8.18 shows the further specification of the Explore procedure which I accessed by choosing the "Plots … " button on the Explore menu in the top right-hand boxes (see Figure 8.17). Choosing Plots results in a further specification of the Explore procedure in which I can ask for several additional criteria to be applied. I will not explain all of these here, but I would only point out the choices for "Spread vs Level with Levene Test" in the bottom of the panel.

As you can see, there are several choices for how to manage the data to be analyzed for equality of variance. Since you are only interested in a "global" measure of equality, we can choose "Untransformed" which tests the data values "as is" or as raw data. If you were interested in "transforming" group values that may include outliers or extreme scores, you could choose "Transformed" in this panel to see how

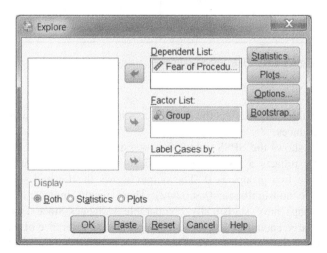

Figure 8.17   Specifying the variables of interest for equality of variances.

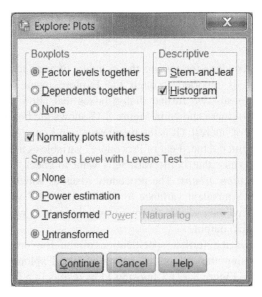

Figure 8.18   Specifying Levene's test for equality of variances.

Test of Homogeneity of Variance

		Levene Statistic	df1	df2	Sig.
Fear of Procedure	Based on Mean	.228	1	12	.642
	Based on Median	.203	1	12	.660
	Based on Median and with adjusted df	.203	1	11.960	.660
	Based on trimmed mean	.245	1	12	.629

Figure 8.19   The SPSS® output assessing equality of variance.

changing the values might affect the outcome. As it is, you are only interested in the equality of variances.

Figure 8.19 shows the SPSS output for assessing the equality of variance. The Levene statistic reflects a test of the hypothesis that the difference between the variances of the two groups is 0. The output shows the Levene statistic (based on mean) to be nonsignificant ($p < 0.642$). These results indicate that low- and high-stress groups have statistically comparable variances since Levene's value (0.228) is not large enough to reject the assumption of 0 difference of variances and therefore fall into the exclusion area. These results indicate that the group variances are equivalent.

The Homogeneity of Variance Assumption for the Independent *T* Test

Both Excel and SPSS concluded that the group variances were equal. Therefore, you can consider the fourth assumption to be met. Had the equality of variance test (*F* test) or Levene's test indicated that the group variances were not equal, you would need to discuss further whether you could proceed with the *T* test.

As I mentioned, the *T* test is robust and will provide valid results even with slightly different variances. However, with large differences, you might need to transform the values or use a different statistical procedure. Note here, however, that Levene's test is sensitive and may be overly conservative. You might use both the Excel and SPSS procedures to confirm the decision to proceed with the *T* test.

A Rule of Thumb

A simple rule of thumb might be helpful as well as these more formal procedures. If the *F* ratio we calculate according to the formula above is 2 or less, you can generally consider the variances to be equal for the purposes of using the independent *T* test. You only need a global indication of homogeneity of variance to proceed.

USING SPSS® AND EXCEL WITH THE INDEPENDENT *T* TEST

When the researcher is assured that the data meet the assumptions for the independent *T* test, they can proceed using Excel and SPSS which are both very straightforward procedures. Each provides the calculation for the *T* ratio and the pertinent information for hypothesis tests. The outputs for both preclude the necessity for using the *T* table of values.

Both Excel and SPSS provide separate *T* tests depending on whether the group variances are equal. Therefore, even if the homogeneity of variance or Levene's tests show unequal variance, the researcher can rely on the separate formulas in Excel and SPSS to provide a meaningful *T* test result.

SPSS® PROCEDURES FOR THE INDEPENDENT *T* TEST

SPSS provides a straightforward way of conducting the independent sample *T* test. You can use the "Analyze" menu to access several *T* test options that provide the output you need to conduct a research analysis. SPSS provides CI output routinely, which is an advantage over using the Excel procedure. SPSS is also limited, however, in that it does not provide results for Cohen's *d* effect size measure. However, this is a simple manual calculation, so the researcher can provide this critical information.

Figure 8.20 shows the Analyze menus for accessing the independent sample *T* test. As you can see, the "Compare Means" submenu provides the option for the independent *T* test.

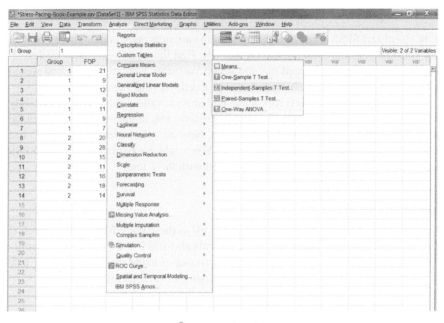

Figure 8.20 The SPSS® menus for the independent sample *T* test.

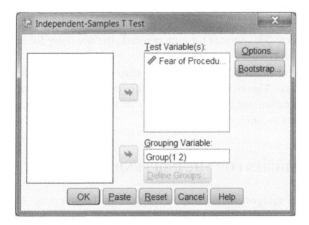

Figure 8.21 The Independent-Samples *T* Test callout window for specifying the analysis.

In Chapter 9, I discussed the single sample *T* test, which is the choice immediately preceding the two sample *T* test. When you choose the "Independent-Samples *T* Test" from the menu, the callout window appears that allows you to specify the variables you wish to use in the analysis, as shown in Figure 8.21.

As you can see in Figure 8.21, the dependent variable in the example problem is "Fear of Procedure." The "Options" button at the top right of the menu box allows the researcher to specify values for the CI. The default value is 95%, but you may change this depending on how you wish to balance the wider interval of the $CI_{0.99}$ procedure with the smaller interval but more precise value of the $CI_{0.95}$ procedure.

The independent variable (predictor) is placed in the "Grouping Variable:" window. This allows the researcher to identify the Practitioner and Reading groups in the database that will serve as group 1 and group 2. When you add the name of the variable to the window by using the arrow, SPSS prompts you to "Define Groups" as shown in Figure 8.22. In this example study, Practitioner is group 1 and Reading is group 2.

This procedure also allows the researcher to use continuous variables as grouping variables. Thus, if you wanted to create groups from a predictor variable like the number of jobs our applicants had held in the past, you could divide the group by specifying some value that would "cut" the subjects into two groups. The "Cut point:" button allows the researcher to specify such a value.

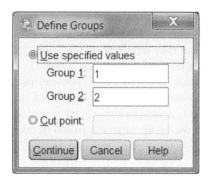

Figure 8.22 Specifying group values for the independent T test.

Group Statistics

	Group	N	Mean	Std. Deviation	Std. Error Mean
Fear of Procedure	Practitioner Session	7	11.14	4.634	1.752
	Reading Session	7	17.43	5.473	2.069

Independent Samples Test

		Levene's Test for Equality of Variances		t-test for Equality of Means					95% Confidence Interval of the Difference	
		F	Sig.	t	df	Sig. (2-tailed)	Mean Difference	Std. Error Difference	Lower	Upper
Fear of Procedure	Equal variances assumed	.228	.642	-2.319	12	.039	-6.286	2.711	-12.191	-.380
	Equal variances not assumed			-2.319	11.683	.039	-6.286	2.711	-12.209	-.362

Figure 8.23 The SPSS® output for the independent T test.

When you create the analysis by choosing "OK" as shown in Figure 8.21, SPSS creates the output showing the results of the analysis. Figure 8.23 shows the two panels of data produced in the output file. The <u>top panel is the descriptive statistics shown for each group.</u> You can compare these values to the previous manual calculations and with the Excel output.

The <u>second panel provides the specific results for the independent sample *T* test.</u> Here are some important "parts" of the analysis shown in Figure 8.23:

- I shaded the left half of the bottom panel to show that this is a <u>separate part of the analysis.</u> It is the equality of variance test or Levene's test that assesses whether we meet the assumption of equal group variances. As I discussed, if the significance is smaller than 0.05, this indicates that the equality of variance falls in the exclusion area, and you would have to conclude that the variances were not equal. However, as you can see in the panel, the significance level of 0.642 indicates that the variances are statistically equal.

- The first column of the same panel shows two "groups" of analyses: "Equal variances assumed" and "Equal variances not assumed." (I placed a line on this panel to show that they represent two different groups of findings.) These are the two possibilities for Levene's test. Since, in the current analysis, the group variances were considered equal, you can use the first row of results ("Equal variances assumed"). If Levene's test had shown a significance level smaller than 0.05, you could use the second row of results ("Equal variances not assumed") since the group variances would be considered not equal.

- Considering the first row of data, the first statistic is the calculated *t* ratio (−2.319). This value is the same as that derived from the manual calculations.

- The "Sig. (two tailed)" column indicates a significance level of .039. Remember SPSS provides the exact calculated probability of a certain finding. Therefore, this finding shows that it is well into the 0.05 exclusion area of a two-tailed test and the *T* ratio would result in a rejection of the null hypothesis. This is a finding so extreme that it could not be considered a chance finding.

- The interpretation references the group means shown in the top panel. The groups are statistically different from one another with the Practitioner group demonstrating lower FOP scores ($M = 11.14$) compared to the Reading group ($M = 17.43$).

- The standard error of difference (s_D) is provided in the next column and is the same value we calculated manually (2.711).

- The $CI_{0.95}$ values are provided in the final two columns. With the independent sample *T* test, the CI values shown are the actual interval values (lower and upper) with reference to the distribution of differences. Remember the population of mean differences is 0. The estimate of the interval shown (−12.191 to −0.380) in the last columns of the panel does not include 0. You would not expect it to contain 0 since you rejected the null hypothesis, indicating that the groups were so different that they did not belong to the same population (i.e., one in which the population of mean differences was 0). These values match the previous manual calculations.

EXCEL PROCEDURES FOR THE INDEPENDENT *T* TEST

The *T* test procedure is available in Excel from the "Data – Data Analysis" menus. Figure 8.24 shows the menu of procedures with the "t-Test: Two-Sample Assuming Equal Variances" option highlighted. Notice that another test option, directly below the highlighted selection, allows the researcher to choose the same *T* test, but one in which the variances are not assumed to be equal. Excel uses a special formula to account for the unequal variances. It is best to check that the equal variance assumption is met prior to using the *T* test (as I discussed in the previous section of this chapter); however, you can make use of this special procedure. In the current example, the homogeneity of variance assumption was met so you can choose the option shown.

In Excel, you need to create the file structure in such a way that the program will recognize the groups appropriately. If you look at Table 8.2, you will see that the data are presented in two columns. The first column entries are the raw Group 1 values (Practitioner), and the second column consists of the raw Group 2 values (Reading). When you specify the location of the data for the *T* test, be sure that you specify the columns correctly.

When you choose this option, the callout window in Figure 8.25 appears. In this window, the researcher must specify the location of both group values (in the "Input" windows), whether labels are included in the locations ("Labels" box), and which exclusion value you wish to use (in the "Alpha" window showing "0.05" in the current example). You can choose to have Excel print the output in different places ("Output options"). The default location is a separate sheet within the data file.

Figure 8.26 shows the Excel output for the *T* test of the two groups. You can compare the values with those computed manually earlier. All the values in the output match those you calculated. The "new" aspects of the output table related to the last four values. These show the probability of an extreme *t* ratio. Essentially, with these values, you do not need to make reference to a *T* table of values.

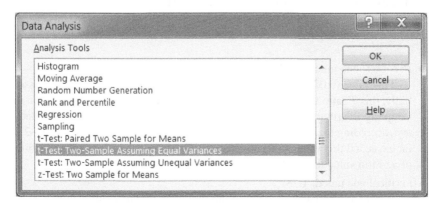

Figure 8.24 The Excel specifications for the independent *T* test.

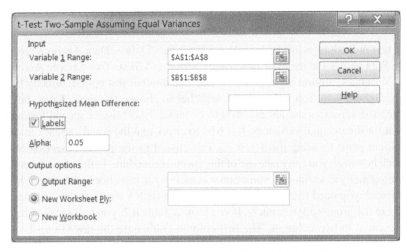

Figure 8.25   The Excel callout window for locating data.

t-Test: Two-Sample Assuming Equal Variances

	Practitioner	Reading
Mean	11.143	17.429
Variance	21.476	29.952
Observations	7	7
Pooled Variance	25.714	
Hypothesized Mean Difference	0	
df	12	
t Stat	−2.319	
P(T<=t) one-tail	0.019	
t Critical one-tail	1.782	
P(T<=t) two-tail	0.039	
t Critical two-tail	2.179	

Figure 8.26   The Excel output for the independent *T* test with equal variances.

Here are some interpretations of the results:

- *P(T <= t)* one tailed: 0.02

    This value (0.02) represents the probability of the finding ($t = -2.32$). Essentially, this *T* ratio value is the transformed mean difference score placed in the sampling distribution of differences. The exclusion value of the one-tailed *T* test, according to a table of values, is 1.783. Since the calculated value of −2.32 far exceeded this value, you can reject the null hypothesis since the probability of a *t* ratio value that high by chance alone is $p = 0.02$.

- *t* critical one tailed: 1.78

    This is a "companion" value to the immediately preceding value. It represents the exclusion value for a 0.05 one-tailed *T* test.

- $P(T <= t)$ two tailed: 0.04

  This probability is the probability of the finding using a two-tailed test. In a two-tailed (0.05) test, the calculated t ratio (-2.32) exceeded the critical tabled value of T, thus rejecting the null hypothesis. The actual probability of a t ratio value that high by chance alone is $p = 0.04$ on the two-tailed comparison chart.
- t critical two tailed: 2.18 (or 2.179 rounded)

  This value is the exclusion value for the 0.05 two-tailed test.

Taken together, the results indicate that you can reject the null hypothesis that Practitioner and Reading groups produce equal FOP scores. You can conclude that the Practitioner group produces significantly lower FOP scores than the Reading group.

As I noted earlier, CI and effect size calculations are not available in Excel. These can be easily calculated manually however. Use the formulas and procedures we discussed in the previous sections.

EFFECT SIZE FOR THE INDEPENDENT T TEST EXAMPLE

As I mentioned earlier, neither Excel nor SPSS provide Cohen's d as a measure of effect size. However, since both provide the T ratio, you can calculate the effect size manually using the "alternate" formula:

$$d = t\sqrt{\frac{n_1 + n_2}{(n_1)(n_2)}} = -2.319\sqrt{\frac{7+7}{49}} = -1.24$$

You can also calculate η^2 using the same data:

$$\eta^2 = \frac{T^2}{T^2 + df} = \frac{(-2.319)^2}{(-2.319)^2 + 12} = 0.31$$

PARTING COMMENTS

Remember that statistical tests need to be "fitted" carefully to the nature of the data and the research situation. If it is not carefully fitted, the power of the test will be diminished. Some very important things to remember in terms of the independent T test, in this regard, are that there are specific formulas to be used when the groups have *different sample sizes* and when the *sample groups are dependent, rather than independently formed*. In the former case, you learned to use a special formula for s_D that accommodated unequal sample sizes. In the latter case, you need to understand how to use the "repeated measures" T test that uses dependent samples. I will discuss this procedure in a later chapter.

You should congratulate yourself at this point. You learned about one of the most common and practically useful statistical tests available. The T test is common in all research literature, and now you will be able to understand how the results are interpreted. You also have the knowledge to assess whether test results, published or unpublished, were properly reported and used.

NONPARAMETRIC STATISTICS: THE MANN–WHITNEY *U* TEST

To this point, I have discussed *parametric statistics*, which are procedures that make reference to parameters (mean and standard deviation) of populations in helping to make statistical decisions. If you recall, I discussed the use of sampling distributions to compare sample values (i.e., means and standard deviations) to estimated population parameters. These are procedures that use interval data.

There is another "class" of statistics that do not make these assumptions. These *nonparametric* statistical procedures directly calculate test values rather than estimating parameters or referring to sampling distributions. For these reasons, they are also known as *distribution-free tests*. They typically make decisions with ordinal or nominal data.

Nonparametric procedures are also helpful for statistical decisions that involve (interval-level) sample data that do not meet certain assumptions. As we have seen, for example, the assumption of normally distributed variables is often crucial to an analysis, so much so that extremely skewed data might prevent a researcher from proceeding with a parametric procedure. With extreme violations of normally distributed data, the researcher might resort to *transforming* the skewed data (i.e., changing the skewed data so that it becomes normally distributed.) A second option for violations for normal distributions is to use nonparametric statistical tests.

There are several nonparametric statistical tests comparable to the independent sample *T* test. Possibly the most well known is the Mann–Whitney *U* test. Excel does not provide nonparametric analyses, but SPSS allows the researcher to use a variety of these tests.

As a brief (hypothetical) example, consider the data in Table 8.3. These data show the teachers' rankings of students' fear of math by the students' gender. Do male and female students evidence different levels of fear of math?

Ranked data do not have the equal interval assumption of interval data. Since the outcome data in this example are ranked (ordinal data), you cannot use the independent *T* test since that test requires at least interval data. The Mann–Whitney *U* test will help to determine whether the two sets of ranks are likely to be from the same population.

I will not detail the manual calculations for this test but rather show how to use SPSS to obtain the results. If you would like to explore this and other nonparametric tests further, you might consult Siegel and Castellan's (1988) seminal work.

As you can see from Table 8.4, the rankings are presented along with the student's gender (1 = male and 2 = female). The higher teacher ranks indicate greater math fear.

Using SPSS is straightforward. Figure 8.27 shows the specification for the test. Notice that there are two routes to conduct the test. When you choose "Nonparametric Tests," you have the option of selecting "Independent Samples" which allows you to use a template for this and related tests. However, using the second route, "Legacy Dialogs – Two Independent Samples" affords you the traditional procedure for the test specification.

Using this second route produces the menu window shown in Figure 8.28. As you can see, I specified the fear rankings as the test variable and gender as the grouping variable. At this point, I can choose the Mann–Whitney *U* as well as a number of

TABLE 8.4   Mann–Whitney
U Test Data

Fear Ranking	Gender
8	1
9	1
25	2
11	2
28	2
2	1
5	1
4	1
21	2
14	2
10	1
16	2

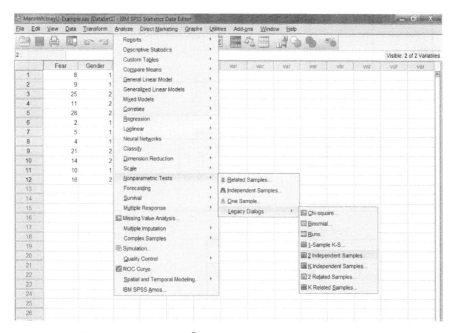

Figure 8.27   The SPSS® options for the Mann–Whitney U Test.

related tests. In the "Options" button (upper right part of the window), I chose to create descriptive statistics.

Running this test ("OK") results in the output shown in Figure 8.29. These are the primary outputs you can use to determine whether the sample groups are from different populations.

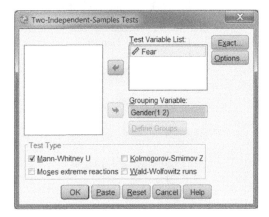

Figure 8.28   The SPSS® specification for the Mann–Whitney *U* Test.

Descriptive Statistics

	N	Mean	Std. Deviation	Minimum	Maximum
Fear	12	12.75	8.324	2	28
Gender	12	1.50	.522	1	2

Ranks

	Gender	N	Mean Rank	Sum of Ranks
Fear	1	6	3.50	21.00
	2	6	9.50	57.00
	Total	12		

Test Statistics[a]

	Fear
Mann-Whitney U	.000
Wilcoxon W	21.000
Z	–2.882
Asymp. Sig. (2-tailed)	.004
Exact Sig. [2*(1-tailed Sig.)]	.002[b]

a. Grouping Variable: Gender

b. Not corrected for ties.

Figure 8.29   The SPSS® output for the Mann–Whitney *U* Test.

The output in Figure 8.29 is in three panels. The top panel shows the descriptive statistics designed for interval data. Since the study data are in ranks, this panel will not be used. The middle panel shows the <u>average of the fear ranks</u> for both gender groups. The bottom panel shows the results of the Mann–Whitney U test. As you can see, the test resulted in a significant difference between males and females in terms of fear of math ($p = 0.004$). Female ranks were much higher on average (9.5) than those of males (3.50). Note that the Mann–Whitney U test statistic (0.000) is very low! In this test with such small samples, the lower the result, the greater the significance.

TERMS AND CONCEPTS

Between-group designs:	Those studies in which the researcher seeks to ascertain whether *entire groups* demonstrate unequal outcome measures.
Dependent samples:	Groups that have some structural linkage that affects the choice of group membership. Examples are using the same subjects (pre–post) for an experiment or comparing the results of a test using "matched groups." Tests for dependent samples are also known as "repeated measures," "within-subject," and "paired sample" tests.
η^2 **(Eta Squared)**:	η^2 creates an effect size value that expresses the amount of variation in the outcome attributed to the predictor variable.
Independent samples:	For statistical testing purposes, samples are independent if choosing the elements of one group has no connection to choosing elements of the other(s).
Matched samples:	Samples that have been intentionally created to be equivalent on one or several characteristics. Such a process affects the independence assumption of the groups. Matched groups are therefore considered "dependent" samples.
Mixed designs:	Those studies in which there are both between and within components.
Within-group designs:	Studies in which the researcher seeks to ascertain whether *subjects* in a group or matched groups change over time.

DATA LAB AND EXAMPLES (WITH SOLUTIONS)

Problem 1

Is there a difference in enrollment in AP classes depending on whether they are taught in the morning versus the afternoon? A professor wanted to compare the <u>enrollments</u>

in specialized AP seminars (12) taught by 10 colleagues: 6 who offered their seminars in the <u>morning</u> and 6 who offered their seminars in the <u>afternoon</u>. Is there a difference?

Morning enrollments: 12, 9, 9, 10, 8, 8

Afternoon enrollments: 10, 4, 7, 8, 7, 6

Directions: Calculate the following manually:

- Calculate the independent T ratio and calculate the hypothesis test.
- Calculate the effect size.
- Calculate the 0.95 CI.

Problem 2

Medical staff in a large hospital created a new procedure for a common presenting problem among patients and then trained practitioners how to use the procedure through a series of 1-week rotations. After 1 year a researcher decided to compare

TABLE 8.5   Practitioner Training and Patient Satisfaction

Satisfaction Index	Training
25	1
24	1
35	1
36	1
30	1
31	1
33	1
36	1
37	1
39	1
40	1
35	1
36	2
37	2
37	2
40	2
43	2
44	2
48	2
49	2
43	2
44	2
45	2
51	2

patient satisfaction between practitioners who had greater training with the procedure (high $= 3$–5 rotations) versus practitioners with less training (low $= 1$ or 2 rotations). Table 8.5 presents data from the study regarding patient satisfaction (higher values equal greater satisfaction on a researcher-generated survey) related to practitioner training.

Compare results in both SPSS and Excel to analyze the data and address the following:

A. Are the assumptions met for the statistical procedure you used?

B. Is there a significant difference in patient satisfaction between practitioners with low and high training?

C. What is the effect size of the finding?

D. What is the 0.95 confidence interval?

E. Comment on the research design.

F. Write a small interpretive summary of your findings.

DATA LAB: SOLUTIONS

Problem 1: Solutions 1

Calculate the independent T ratio and conduct the hypothesis test:

- $S_D = 1.022$
- Mean difference $= 2.333$.
- T ratio $= 2.283$.
- Table exclusion value $(T_{0.05,10df}) = 2.228$.
- Reject null hypothesis $(p < 0.05)$.
- Afternoon sections have greater enrollment.

Calculate the effect size:

$d = 1.32$: (Large) Sessions "move" enrollments 1.32 SDs.
$\eta^2 = 0.34$: 34% of the variation in enrollments is accounted for by morning or afternoon sessions.

Calculate the 0.95 CI:

- Lower: 0.06.
- Upper: 4.610.

- The interval does not include 0, indicating significantly different group mean of enrollment.

Problem 2: Solutions

A. Are the assumptions met for the statistical procedure you used?
- A. Yes. Interval data on Outcome variable and independent groups studied
- B. Yes. Normal distribution as measured by:
  - i. SK and KU that are in bounds for both groups
  - ii. Kolmogorov–Smirnov and Shapiro–Wilk not significant for either group
- C. Yes. Equal variance:
  - i. Levene's test ($p < 0.824$) not significant

B. Is there a significant difference in patient satisfaction between practitioners' training? Yes, independent T test ratio $= -4.762$, $p < 0.000$ (actual $= 0.000094$)[4]

C. What is the effect size of the finding?
- (i) $d = 1.94$; the difference in training results in an impact of almost 2 SDs on the sampling distribution. (You can disregard the sign as you interpret the results.)
- (ii) $\eta^2 = 0.508$; 50.8% of the variance in patient satisfaction is accounted for by the difference in training groups.

D. What is the 0.95 confidence interval?
- (i) Lower $= -13.876$.
- (ii) Upper $= -5.457$.
- (iii) This interval does not include 0, as expected since T was sig.

E. Comment on the research design.
- (i) Post facto – comparative: no randomization, study performed well after training occurred in independent groups
- (ii) Generalizability limited to the hospital sample from which the data were collected

F. Write a small interpretive summary of your findings.

A hospital study of patient satisfaction connected to training with a new procedure was significant ($T = -4.762$, $p < 0.001$). Practitioners with greater training (3–5, 1-week rotations) showed greater average patient satisfaction ($M = 43.04$, $s = 4.870$) than practitioners ($M = 33.42$, $s = 5.071$) with less training (1 or 2 1-week rotations). The study showed a large impact ($d = 1.94$) between the two groups, suggesting that training accounted for more than half ($\eta^2 = 0.508$) of the variance in patient satisfaction. The 0.95 CI was large at -13.876 to -5.57. Figure 8.30 shows the comparison on patient satisfaction by training groups.

---

[4]The SPSS® report for significance is "0.000" when the significance is this or anything beyond. If you double-click on this significance figure, the output shows the actual significance to many decimal values.

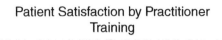

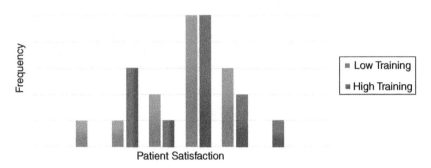

Figure 8.30   Comparison of training groups on patient satisfaction.

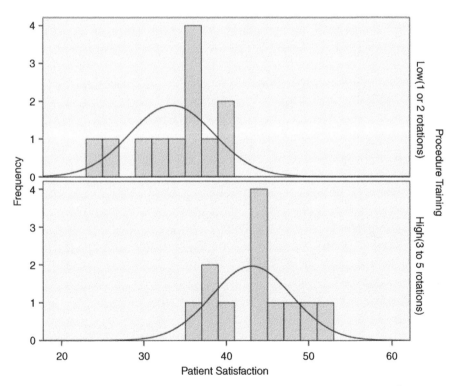

Figure 8.31   Comparison of training groups on patient satisfaction (SPSS®).

GRAPHICS IN THE DATA SUMMARY

Figure 8.31 shows the same histogram data from SPSS (use Graphs – Legacy Dialogs – Histogram menu) as Figure 8.30 in Excel. I have found it is easier to work with Excel graphics, although it takes some exploration to become familiar with the procedures. For the Excel figures, you will need to create tables of the frequencies of patient satisfaction for each of the study groups and then insert a bar graph to show the superimposed group distributions. As you can see in Figure 8.31, SPSS shows the distributions separately.

9

ANALYSIS OF VARIANCE

We now come to a very popular test with health and social science researchers. Analysis of VAriance (ANOVA) is popular because the researcher is able to compare several different groups, rather than the independent T test which only compares two groups. ANOVA is really quite an ingenious test in the way in which it allows statistical decisions by analyzing *components of the variance of the groups* to be compared.

There are several variations of this test. We will focus primarily on the "one-way" ANOVA in this chapter, but I will cover an extension of the test briefly at the end of the chapter. One-way ANOVA refers to the number of independent variables. *In research, independent variables are known as "factors."* Therefore, if you have a research problem that has several levels of one independent variable, you can use one-way ANOVA to detect any differences among the sample groups.

Chapter 10 discusses "Factorial ANOVA," which allows the researcher to analyze more than one independent variable. "Factorial" refers to the fact that there are more than one factor in the procedure. Thus, if you have two independent variables, the procedure would be known as factorial ANOVA, or a 2XANOVA.

A HYPOTHETICAL EXAMPLE OF ANOVA

In Chapter 8, I discussed an experiment I conducted on the effects of noise on human learning. Since there were only two groups to compare in that example (high vs low noise), I showed how the independent T test could be used to test the null hypothesis.

Using Statistics in the Social and Health Sciences with SPSS® and Excel®, First Edition.
Martin Lee Abbott.
© 2017 John Wiley & Sons, Inc. Published 2017 by John Wiley & Sons, Inc.

When I conducted the actual experiment however, I compared four groups on their rates of learning. Figure 9.1 shows the design of the experiment.

As you can see, there were four groups, three of which used different levels of noise and one control group with no noise present. (Recall that I used white noise in different magnitudes to distinguish the experimental groups.) The noise level in group III, 30 decibels, is comparable to quiet conversation; 60 decibels is equivalent to normal conversation; 90 decibels is equivalent to a large commercial jet landing just over a mile away. (Sustained exposure to 90 decibel noise could result in hearing loss.)

There is (still) only one independent variable (noise) in the experiment, but now there are groups in <u>four levels of the independent variable</u>. A *T* test would be inappropriate because I would need to conduct six *T* tests to compare all the group results. Why six *T* tests? Look at the comparisons in Figure 9.2.

Even if I had conducted all these *T* tests, I would have no idea of the "whole" test result. I needed the ANOVA since it conducts *all the comparisons within the same procedure at the same time*. I needed one "omnibus" answer to the question of whether noise affects human learning. If this result rejected the null hypothesis, I could then proceed to dig further into the results to examine *which* of the groups

Research Treatment Variable (Noise)			Dependent Variable (Word Recognition)
Random Selection and Assignment	No Pre-Test	Experimental Group I (90 decibels)	Outcome Test Scores (# of recognized words)
Random Selection and Assignment	No Pre-Test	Experimental Group II (60 decibels)	Outcome Test Scores (# of recognized words)
Random Selection and Assignment	No Pre-Test	Experimental Group III (30 decibels)	Outcome Test Scores (# of recognized words)
Random Selection and Assignment	No Pre-Test	Control Group (No noise level)	Outcome Test Scores (# of recognized words)

Figure 9.1   The four groups in the noise-learning experiment.

Group Comparisons
Exp. Group I Versus Exp. Group II
Exp. Group I Versus Exp. Group III
Exp. Group I Versus Control Group
Exp. Group II Versus Exp. Group III
Exp. Group II Versus Control Group
Exp. Group III Versus Control Group

Figure 9.2   The paired comparisons in the experiment with four groups.

were different from the others and therefore may have been responsible for the overall omnibus finding.

THE NATURE OF ANOVA

When a researcher conducts multiple (separate) tests on the same data in the research study, the alpha error "accumulates." This is known as *familywise error* since each comparison is part of the same "family" of tests. Thus, although it is not this simple, if you have six tests and the alpha error is 0.05 for each, you might have a 0.30 alpha error (6×0.05) in the entire family of comparisons. The more tests you conduct, the greater the likelihood that you will make alpha errors. Thus, the overall omnibus test is compromised.

The ANOVA "conducts" all these comparisons together by analyzing components of variance and therefore limits familywise error. You have seen how the T test used variance measures (i.e., sum of squares (SS)) to help detect differences between two sample groups in Chapter 8. ANOVA identifies <u>three sources of variance</u>:

- The variation that exists *within* each sample group
- The variation *between* each sample group and the overall (grand) mean
- The *total* variance from all sources

<u>Because the ANOVA process analyzes all these sources of variance simultaneously, you do not have to rely on multiple tests using the same data.</u>

The null hypothesis in the hypothetical experiment would thus be

$$H_0 : \mu_1 = \mu_2 = \mu_3 = \mu_4$$

This null hypothesis states that all four group means come from the same population; there is no difference between the group means. As you can see, there are a variety of ways in which the null hypothesis could be rejected. The following represent two of several possibilities: All the groups could be from different populations (the top example) or group 1 could be from a different population than group 2 and groups 3 and 4 could differ (the bottom example). There are several other possibilities:

$$H_A : \mu_1 \neq \mu_2 \neq \mu_3 \neq \mu_4$$
$$H_A : \mu_1 \neq \mu_2 = \mu_3 \neq \mu_4$$

If the means of the groups are markedly dissimilar to one another (in a statistically significant sense), you could reject the overall null hypothesis and conclude that at least one of the group means differs from the others. If you are able to reject the null hypothesis, the omnibus ANOVA result does not indicate which mean (or means) is different from the others. In that event, you would perform a secondary test, called a "post hoc comparison," in order to identify which of the means were significantly different from one another. I will discuss this process after I discuss the overall or omnibus ANOVA test.

THE COMPONENTS OF VARIANCE

If you recall the earlier chapters, you will remember that variance is a measure of the dispersion of scores in a distribution. Variance is a "global" measure of variation, so I will refer to it instead of the standard deviation (another measure of dispersion) as a way of determining how sample groups differ from one another. Look at Figure 9.3 to see how my experimental groups might be represented, using the noise experiment I introduced earlier.

Figure 9.3 shows the sample groups arrayed from left to right on an X-axis measuring the "number of learning errors," which is the dependent variable for this experiment. Therefore, the "no noise group" shows lower values of learning errors than any of the other groups that represent different levels of learning errors. Remember that my experimental question was whether noise affected human learning. I operationally defined learning as the number of simple words recalled during a memorization task. The experiment sought to see if different amounts of noise would decrease the number of words recalled.

Figure 9.3 shows the three sources of variance in an ANOVA analysis. The four *sample groups have their own distributions, so all their scores "spread out" around their means. This is known as "within variance"* (V_{Within}) *since the variance is measured within each sample distribution.* Figure 9.3 also shows a "shadow" distribution that represents a <u>total distribution if all the individual scores from all the sample groups were thrown into one large distribution</u>. If you were to measure *the variance of that large, composite distribution, this would constitute the "total variance"* (V_{Total}). As you can see, the composite distribution has a mean value, indicated by

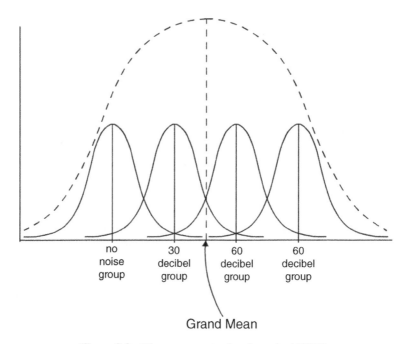

Figure 9.3   The components of variance in ANOVA.

the dashed line. This total mean is known as the "grand mean." *Between variance* (V_{Between}) *is the variation between each sample group mean and the grand mean.*

- V_{Total} is the total variance of all individual scores in all sample groups.
- V_{Between} is the variation between the sample means and the grand mean.
- V_{Within} is the variation of individual scores within their own sample groups.

THE PROCESS OF ANOVA

In effect, the ANOVA process determines *whether the sample means vary far enough from the grand mean that they could be said to be from different populations.* What makes this question difficult to determine is that within each group, the scores vary around their own group mean. If the sample group means are close enough to one another, single scores could lie within the area where the groups overlap making group identification difficult for these individual scores.

Figure 9.4 shows two possible results that illustrate the potential results of ANOVA. The top panel shows the results of an experiment in which the groups are so "squished together" that the group variances are intermingled. That is, the group means are so close together that it would be difficult to conclude that they are significantly different from the grand mean.

In the bottom panel, the group means are far enough apart that individual group variances do not have extensive overlap. That is, the variances *within* each sample group do not confuse the distance *between* the groups. If you have an actual result like the one shown in the bottom panel, you would likely determine that the group means are statistically different from one another. This might not be the case in the top panel.

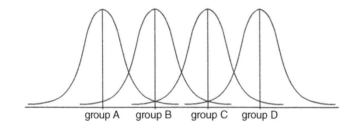

group A group B group C group D

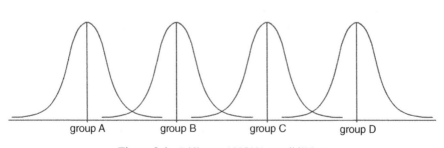

group A group B group C group D

Figure 9.4 Different ANOVA possibilities.

ANOVA seeks to determine whether the V_{Between} *would be large relative to the* V_{Within} as it appears to be the case with the bottom panel example. In the top example, the V_{Within} "muddles the picture" of how the groups relate to one another. It is for this reason that within variance is often referred to in research (and in SPSS®) as "error variance." If you want to understand how far apart the group means are from the grand mean, the error variance (V_{Within}) "gets in the way." When there is less error variance, the distance between the group means and the grand mean (i.e., the V_{Between}) becomes easier to distinguish.

CALCULATING ANOVA

The ANOVA calculation compares V_{Between} to V_{Within}. When V_{Between} is large relative to V_{Within}, there is a greater likelihood that the researcher can reject the null hypothesis. We can suggest a "conceptual equation" that expresses this relationship:

$$F = \frac{V_{\text{Between}}}{V_{\text{Within}}}$$

ANOVA uses the F distribution as a comparison distribution for the relationship of the between-to-within variance. I introduced the F test in Chapter 8 when I discussed how to test whether two sample variances were statistically equal. This same distribution (see Figure 8.16) can be used to determine where a calculated ANOVA value falls on the sampling distribution of all possible samples. After all, you are still comparing variances. But in the ANOVA test, you compare between-to-within variance, whereas in the equal variance test, you compare two sample variances.

The conceptual equation before thus expresses the relationship of between-to-within variance as a point on the F distribution of all possible samples to determine whether the sample group means are far enough from the grand mean that the calculated F ratio would fall in the exclusion area of the comparison distribution. If a researcher obtained an actual result like the bottom example in Figure 9.4, there would be a greater likelihood that the F ratio (calculated F) would fall in the exclusion area than if the top example was obtained.

Calculating the Variance: Using the Sum of Squares (SS)

The ANOVA procedure helps the researcher identify and compare all the components of variance present in the research study. Therefore, each of the variance components must be calculated in order to make a statistical decision. The Sum of Squares (SS) is used to measure the components. As I explained in past chapters, SS is a large number when the scores of a distribution are spread out and a small number when the scores are close together.

In Chapter 8, I specified the formula to calculate SS:

$$\text{SS} = \sum X^2 - \frac{\left(\sum X\right)^2}{N}$$

You can use variations of this formula to calculate each of the three sources of variance.

Calculating Components of Variance Using SS

Moving from conceptual to computational definitions, you can identify these sources as follows:

SS_T = sum of squares of the total distribution of all individual scores (V_{Total})

SS_B = sum of squares between the group means and the grand mean ($V_{Between}$)

SS_W = sum of squares within each sample group (V_{Within})

Calculating the three SS values is somewhat easier when you consider that the total variation (V_{Total}) is comprised of the between ($V_{Between}$) and within (V_{Within}) variances. Therefore,

$$SS_T = SS_B + SS_W$$

and

$$SS_W = SS_T - SS_B$$

I will introduce a simple (hypothetical) set of findings for my noise-learning experiment to demonstrate how to calculate these components. Then I will present an example with real data. Table 9.1 shows the hypothetical data for the experiment. The dependent variable is the number of learning errors.

Table 9.2 shows the data with appropriate squares to be used to calculate the sums of squares. The general SS formula follows the data; then the calculations are shown for each variance component:

$$SS = \sum X^2 - \frac{(\sum X)^2}{N}$$

Calculating SS_T

$$SS = \sum X^2 - \frac{(\sum X)^2}{N}$$

$$SS_T = (86 + 174 + 509 + 889) - \frac{(18 + 26 + 45 + 59)^2}{16}$$

$$= 1658 - 1369$$

$$= 289$$

TABLE 9.1 Hypothetical Experiment Data

Control	30 Decibels	60 Decibels	90 Decibels
5	7	12	15
4	5	11	14
3	6	10	18
6	8	12	12

TABLE 9.2   Hypothetical Experiment Data with Squared Values

	Control		30 Decibels		60 Decibels		90 Decibels	
	X_1	$X_1{}^2$	X_2	$X_2{}^2$	X_3	$X_3{}^2$	X_4	$X_4{}^2$
	5	25	7	49	12	144	15	225
	4	16	5	25	11	121	14	196
	3	9	6	36	10	100	18	324
	6	36	8	64	12	144	12	144
Σ	18	86	26	174	45	509	59	889

Calculating SS_B   Calculating SS_B uses a variation of the SS formula, but the focus is on the *deviation of each group mean from the grand mean*. Therefore, you will calculate "group means" in variance terms and subtract the variance measures from the grand mean. Here is the formula:

$$SS_B = \frac{\left(\sum X_1\right)^2}{n_1} + \frac{\left(\sum X_2\right)^2}{n_2} + \frac{\left(\sum X_3\right)^2}{n_3} + \frac{\left(\sum X_4\right)^2}{n_4} \;(-)\; \frac{\left(\sum X\right)^2}{N}$$

This equation looks intimidating, but if you look at it, the main "pieces" make sense. As you can see, a *global measure* of each group's mean ($\frac{(\sum X)^2}{n}$) results from dividing the squared group sums by the group's sample size. Then, the grand mean measure ($\frac{(\sum X)^2}{N}$) is subtracted from the total of the separate group mean measures. I shaded this portion of the equation, so you can see the components clearly. There is an important thing to note in this equation:

$$n \neq N$$

If you look carefully at the equation, you will note that the separate group mean measures have the "group sizes" (n) as the divisor. The grand mean measure at the end of the equation has the total individual score size (N) in the divisor. This is because the grand mean is calculated for all individual scores ($N = 16$), whereas the individual group mean measures are divided only by the scores that make up that group (all four sample groups have $n = 4$):

$$SS_B = \frac{\left(\sum X_1\right)^2}{n_1} + \frac{\left(\sum X_2\right)^2}{n_2} + \frac{\left(\sum X_3\right)^2}{n_3} + \frac{\left(\sum X_4\right)^2}{n_4} \;(-)\; \frac{\left(\sum X\right)^2}{N}$$

$$= \frac{324}{4} + \frac{676}{4} + \frac{2025}{4} + \frac{3481}{4} \;(-)\; \frac{(18 + 26 + 45 + 59)^2}{16}$$

$$= 81 + 169 + 506.25 + 870.25 \;(-)\; 1369$$

$$= 257.5$$

As you can see, I left the shaded portion in the equations to show that this portion is the same in the SS_T and SS_B formulas. It "represents" the grand mean, so its value will not change. In the SS_T formula, all the individual scores (X) deviate away from the (grand) mean. Thus, the shaded portion of the formula shows that this is the value from which all the scores deviate. In the SS_B formula, the shaded portion represents the grand mean as well. Here, each of the sample group means are added together and then subtracted from the grand mean. It is as if each of the group means is treated as a single score, and you are calculating the variance of the group means around the grand mean (which, of course, we are actually doing!).

Calculating SS_W   From the previous equation, you can see that if you calculate SS_T and SS_B, you can derive SS_W without additional calculations:

$$SS_W = SS_T - SS_B$$
$$= 289 - 257.5$$
$$= 31.5$$

Creating a Data Table

Now that you have calculated the key SS values, you can use a table to display the results. As you will see in the steps ahead, this is a very helpful visual step and one that both SPSS and Excel use to display the ANOVA results. You should therefore learn to use the table to keep all the calculated values in order and see how ANOVA results are reported by most all statistical software.

Table 9.3 shows the template you might use with the results thus far. As you can see the table lists the sums of squares calculated values for each "source" of variance. Remember that the SS is a measure of variance based on the raw scores in the data file.

Using Mean Squares (MS)

As you recall, inferential statistics addresses the issue of how sample values represent (or do not represent) population values. In the Z and T tests, you learned to transform sample values to points on a sampling distribution so that you could show how the calculated sample ratio compares to all possible sample values.

Treat ANOVA results in the same way. *ANOVA is also an inferential process, so you will use sample values to estimate population values.* You calculated the sample

TABLE 9.3   The ANOVA Results Table

Source of Variance	SS	df	MS	F ratio
Between	257.5			
Within	31.5			
Total	289			

(between, within, and total) variances using SS values, so you need now to use these values to estimate population (between, within, and total) variances.

This process is akin to using sample values (SD) to create an estimate (s_x) of the population standard deviation (σ_X) in the T test. In order to estimate the population standard deviation, you had to use the sample standard deviation and "adjust" it by dividing it by its degrees of freedom (in the single sample T test, the df $= N - 1$) so that it would be a better estimate of the population parameter.

With ANOVA, you use degrees of freedom to make each of the SS values better estimates of population values. These estimates are known as "mean squares" (MS) because they are created by dividing the SS by degrees of freedom, much like you create a mean by adding together the values in a sample and dividing by the number in the sample.

Degrees of Freedom in ANOVA

You can use the degrees of freedom to help estimate population values since the size of the samples greatly affects the variance estimates. By using degrees of freedom in order to obtain better estimates, you create mean squares that average out the variance regardless of sample size. Here are the degrees of freedom for each SS value:

- df_t (degrees of freedom for total SS) $= N - 1$ ($N =$ the total number of individual scores in all groups combined)
- df_b (degrees of freedom for between SS) $= k - 1$ (where $k =$ number of sample groups)
- df_w (degrees of freedom for within SS) $= N - k$

When you make specific population estimates from sample values, you use ("lose") degrees of freedom. As you see, estimating the total variance uses 1 df since you use the entire set of individual scores. Estimating the between variance uses another 1 df since you use the set of sample means. Estimating the within variance uses several more (depending on how many sample groups there are) degrees of freedom, since the sample groups are separate "sets" of scores that deviate around their respective group means.

Calculating Mean Squares (MS)

Calculating MS values is simple when you look at the ANOVA table of values in Table 9.3. Table 9.4 shows the MS values, which are derived from dividing the SS values by their respective degrees of freedom:

$$MS_B = \frac{SS_b}{df_b} = \frac{257.5}{3} = 85.83$$

$$MS_w = \frac{SS_w}{df_w} = \frac{31.5}{12} = 2.625$$

TABLE 9.4   The ANOVA Results Table with Calculated MS Values

Source of Variance	SS	df	MS	F ratio
Between	257.5	3 (k - 1)	85.83	
Within	31.5	12 (N - k)	2.625	
Total	289	15 (N – 1)	----	

You can note other features from Table 9.4:

- The between and within SS values sum to the total SS value.
- The between and within df values sum to the total df value.
- The MS_T value is not included because it is not needed to calculate the ANOVA result.

The *F* Ratio

In an earlier section of this chapter, I noted that the ANOVA process determines *whether the sample means vary far enough from the grand mean that they could be said to be from different populations.* What you need in order to determine this is a comparison of the <u>variation of the means from the grand mean</u> (MS_B), <u>relative to the variance within each of the sample groups</u> that make the earlier estimate difficult to determine (MS_W).

Here is the formula for calculating the *F* ratio. Using the values from Table 9.4, the calculated *F* ratio for this example problem is

$$F = \frac{MS_B}{MS_W} = \frac{85.83}{2.625} = 32.70$$

As you can see, the *F* ratio compares the variation of the sample means around the grand mean (MS_B) to the variation within each sample group (MS_W). I mentioned before that the within variance measure is known as "error" just for this reason. If the sample group values did not vary at all, it would be easy to see how far away the sample means vary from the grand mean! Consider the two panels in Figure 9.5.

The top panel of Figure 9.5 shows a hypothetical example of four sample groups with almost no <u>within</u> variance. In this case, it is easy to see how distinct the group means are and how clearly they differ from the grand mean. The bottom panel shows just the opposite. There is so much <u>within</u> variance that it is almost impossible to see how distinct the group means are and how they vary around the grand mean. The within variance is essentially "noise" and is therefore called error.

It is for these reasons that I said that the *F* ratio is a measure of the between variation *relative to the within variance.* That is why the *F* ratio is simply comparing the between to the within variation. When you divide the two, you would anticipate a much higher *F* ratio in the top panel than in the bottom panel since the divisor in the F ratio would be much smaller in the top panel.

In the noise example, the between variance measure was 85.83 and the within variance measure 2.625. These represent quite differing variance measures! It is fairly

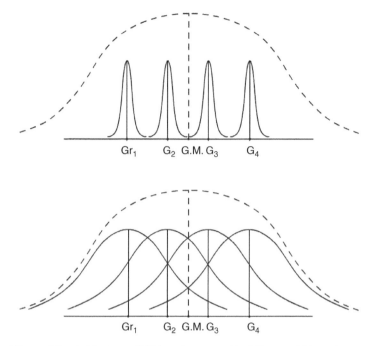

Figure 9.5   ANOVA possibilities of groups with different within variances.

TABLE 9.5   The Final ANOVA Results Table

Source of Variance	SS	df	MS	F ratio
Between	257.5	3	85.83	32.70
Within	31.5	12	2.625	
Total	289	15	----	

easy to assume that the resulting F ratio (32.70) represents a situation where the sample group means are quite spread out around the grand mean. The question is, how far from the grand mean do the sample means have to vary before they could be said to represent different populations? This is the essence of the ANOVA hypothesis test.

Table 9.5 shows the final ANOVA table with the F ratio included. The structure of the table allows you to "see" how the calculation for the F ratio was performed. I divided the between MS (85.83) by the within MS (2.625) to yield 32.70.

The F Distribution

Figure 8.16 shows that the F distribution does not appear to be similar to the Z or T distributions. Remember I mentioned in Chapter 8 that the F distribution is a sampling distribution of *variances*, not means. In the F test for equal variances, most group variances hover around 1 when the variances are equal (since if we divide similar variance measures, the ratio will be close to 1.00).

TABLE 9.6   The *F* Table of Values Exclusion Areas

			df in the Numerator (between)			
		Exclusion Level	**1**	**2**	**3**	**4**
df in the Denominator	1	0.05	161	200	216	225
		0.01	4052	4999	5403	5625
	2	0.05	18.51	19.00	19.16	19.25
		0.01	98.49	99.00	99.17	99.25
		--------------	--------------	-------	-------	-------
				-------	--------	------
	10	0.05	4.96	4.10	3.71	3.48
		0.01	10.04	7.56	6.55	5.99
	11	0.05	4.84	3.98	3.59	3.36
		0.01	9.65	7.20	6.22	5.67
	12	0.05	4.75	3.88	3.49	3.26
		0.01	9.33	6.93	5.95	5.41
	13	0.05	4.67	3.80	3.41	3.18
		0.01	9.07	6.70	5.74	5.20

Critical (Exclusion) Values for the Distribution of F

In the ANOVA test, you do not compare two group variances but between-to-within variance. When you compare these measures, the resulting F ratio is often much larger than 1. Thus, *the F distribution is directional.* Together with the fact that variance measures cannot be negative (they can be very small but not negative), the researcher needs to <u>compare a calculated F ratio with a tabled value of F</u> that represents all possible samples of variance.

The F distribution is therefore the sampling distribution of comparison. F tables of values identify the exclusion values at 0.05 and 0.01 probability, for example. The table is complex because it takes into account the degrees of freedom of both the between and the within measures since sample size is so critical to the analyses.

Table 9.6 shows a portion of the F table from the F table of values in the appendices. In the noise example, the tabled value of F at 0.05 with df's for between (3 – in the column) and within (12 – in the rows) variance measures identifies an exclusion value of 3.49 (shaded value) at the 0.05 level.[1] Thus, 3.49 is the value on the F distribution that defines the exclusion area. If the calculated F value exceeds this tabled value, you can reject the null hypothesis. In this example, the calculated $F = 32.70$ far exceeds the tabled value of F. Therefore, you can conclude that the finding ($F = 32.70$) falls in the 0.05 exclusion area of 3.49 and is therefore not likely a chance finding, $p < 0.05$ (i.e., it is a statistically significant finding).

---

[1]Note that the table also includes the 0.01 level of exclusion along with the 0.05 level for each critical value of F chosen.

If the example values represented the data in my experimental study, I could reject the null hypothesis. This would mean that, taken together, the means of the group noise levels vary so greatly around the grand mean that the groups represent different populations of students.[2]

EFFECT SIZE

Like the other statistical analyses, you can create an effect size that shows the "impact" of the independent (predictor) variable on the dependent (outcome) variable. In the case of my noise example, the effect size concern could be asked, "how much does the *grouping on the independent variable* affect the outcome measure?" By this question, I would be trying to determine how much noise impacts learning by measuring how much the specific noise groupings (0, 30, 60, and 90 decibels) push the group outcome measures (learning errors) apart.

So far, I have discussed effect size in terms of Cohen's *d* measures where I analyzed the difference between two groups (independent *T* test) or between a group and a population (single sample *T* test). The ANOVA determines the significance of group differences by examining variance, so you can <u>use a variance measure to express effect size</u>.

The Greek symbol for eta square "η^2" is the symbol that refers to effect size in ANOVA. *It refers to the proportion of variance in the outcome measure explained by the grouping on the independent variable.* I discussed this in Chapter 8 with reference to an effect size formula for independent *T* Test (see "The Eta Squared Method"). This is an easy calculation from the ANOVA table using the following formula:

$$\eta^2 = \frac{SS_{Between}}{SS_{Total}}$$
$$= \frac{257.5}{289}$$
$$= 0.89$$

Thus, 89% of the variance in learning errors is due to assigning subjects to four different noise levels. The effect size is very large (only 100% is possible, obviously), but this is probably due to the fact that I had very small sample group sizes (four per group), and this is a hypothetical example.

How large is large? That is, how large does η^2 have to be before you would say it is "meaningful"? That is a question for which there are many answers! The reason

[2]By the way, the actual outcome of my experiment was interesting! I found no significant differences between the groups. My speculation as to why was that I was using white noise rather than "real" noise (like different kinds of music, street noise, people yelling, etc.). I didn't take into account what the subjects were <u>used to</u> (i.e., they were all different coming in to the experiment; some were used to studying with music and others weren't, etc.), and they were all trying really hard to do well on the "test." The research literature on this issue is very interesting. My undergraduate experiment as yet has not won any prizes for original research!

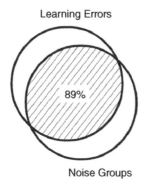

Figure 9.6   Venn diagram showing effect size.

it has many answers is that it depends on the sample sizes, number of groups, etc., I alluded to power analysis in earlier chapters. Statisticians have constructed tables that take into account factors that would have an impact on the size of the effect size value. For example, there are tables for the 0.05 level of significance and the group size as considerations in judging effect size (see Cohen, 1988).

There are therefore many standards offered by statisticians and researchers for judging effect size meaningfulness. I tend to take two approaches to this question. First, I suggest the same guidelines I offered in Chapter 8 as benchmark comparisons: 0.01 (small), 0.06 (medium), and 0.14 (large). These are ballpark figures because the next approach is the most crucial.

The second approach to the question is <u>allowing the researcher to judge the meaningfulness of the effect size by the nature of the problem studied.</u>   It   would therefore have a lot to do with the subject. If I am studying a hypothetical research question with very small sample sizes (as I did in the noise-learning example), I would not be very excited about a very large effect size (and in our study, 0.89 far exceeded the 0.15 guideline for "large effect size"). However, if I am studying a new drug that can lessen the death rate from AIDS, I would be ecstatic to find an effect size of 0.03 even though it might be judged "small" by the earlier benchmarks.

One way to visually understand effect size as "explained variance" is to use Venn diagrams. Look at Figure 9.6. The top circle represents the outcome measure of learning errors. The bottom circle represents the noise groups. Effect size is represented in the portion of the top circle with diagonal lines. The 89% refers to the η^2 value of 0.89. If the top circle represents all the variation of learning errors, I can <u>reduce</u> that variance by 89% just by knowing the different noise conditions. That would only leave 11% of the variance in learning errors unexplained.

POST HOC ANALYSES

<u>If an ANOVA analysis results in the rejection of the null hypothesis,</u> the next consideration is which specific group mean variation(s) from the grand mean might be responsible for the overall size of the F ratio? Stated differently, are all the sample

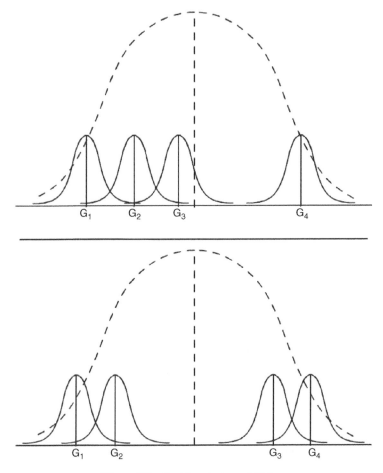

Figure 9.7   Post hoc test possibilities.

means similar in producing learning errors (obviously not since we rejected the null hypothesis), or are some group means much more responsible for affecting the F ratio? What configuration of group mean differences affected the overall F ratio?

Figure 9.7 shows two possibilities of group differences that might produce a significant F ratio. The top panel shows that the first three noise level groups are similar in producing learning errors, but the subjects in the fourth noise level are much more likely to produce learning errors than the other three. The bottom panel of Figure 9.7 shows that the first two groups are similar, but both are very different from the third and fourth groups (which are similar to one another). There can be other combinations of findings as well.

"Varieties" of Post Hoc Analyses

Post hoc analyses look at group comparisons within the overall ANOVA (significant) result to detect where sample group comparisons may be so large that they cannot be said to belong to the same population. The process is similar to individual T tests of pairs of samples within the overall ANOVA study. If you recall, I mentioned earlier in this chapter that my ANOVA study would consist of six separate T tests if I wanted to conduct paired comparisons. Since I could not do this without creating family-wise error, I performed the ANOVA test which compared all the sources of variance at once.

After the overall (omnibus) test of ANOVA is found to be significant, you must "return" to the initial question about which paired differences may be responsible for the ANOVA result. In order to avoid familywise error with the paired comparisons, statisticians have created processes for identifying paired sample differences that limit the overall error measures. Many are specially designed to fit specific research designs. Here are some examples of procedures used for "unplanned" comparisons (paired comparisons not identified before the study):

- Scheffe's test – A conservative post hoc analysis that works well with uneven group sizes and uses stricter decision criteria.
- Tukey's HSD – This Honestly Significant Difference procedure is used when the researcher wants to compare all possible pairs of samples.
- Dunnett – This test is used only with single comparisons, usually comparing a control and experimental group(s).

There are several other post hoc analyses available for use depending on the nature of the research issues. I will demonstrate the most common post hoc analysis for unplanned comparisons, Tukey's HSD. Statistical programs such as SPSS provide results for this and other post hoc analyses, so you can expand your range of under-standing and expertise of post hoc analyses as you pursue further research.

The Post Hoc Analysis Process

The general process researchers follow after concluding that the omnibus (overall) ANOVA test is significant is as follows:

1. Calculate the Tukey HSD critical value.
2. Create a comparison table that includes all the group means.
3. Compare each mean difference to the critical HSD value to determine which of the pairs are significantly different from one another.
4. Conclude the post hoc analysis with a general summary of results.

Tukey's HSD (Range) Test Calculation

This test is also called Tukey's Range Test since it requires the use of the "Studentized Range Table" (shown in the appendix) to help identify a critical value of compari-son. In essence, the HSD *is a critical value of exclusion* since it is based on a set of probabilities that define extreme values on a distribution that takes into account the degrees of freedom in the overall study and the number of groups in the analysis.

Thus, *this approach uses a formula to determine the value beyond which the paired group differences in the study would be considered extreme.*

The Tukey HSD formula is as follows:

$$\text{HSD} = q_{(\text{Range})} \sqrt{\frac{\text{MS}_w}{n}}$$

The "pieces" of the formula are the following:

- HSD is the calculated point on the comparison distribution that identifies extreme values; any test value that is calculated to be larger than this value is considered extreme and would result in the rejection of the hypothesis that a specific pair of group means was equal.

- $q_{(\text{Range})}$ is the value obtained in the Studentized Range Table that helps to establish the exclusion value. I will use the example of the 0.05 level of exclusion, but you can establish the value for 0.01 or other levels of exclusion. If I do not specify otherwise in the examples that follow, you can assume I am using the 0.05 level.

- MS_w is the <u>Mean Square within</u> value found in the ANOVA table. In the example earlier it is equal to 2.625. Recall that I mentioned that the ANOVA within measures were known as "error." Thus, in the formula, the error measure is "adjusting" the critical value of exclusion. If the error is large, it will have a marked impact on the exclusion area.

- n is the group size used in the comparison(s). In my example, all the groups were $n = 4$. Thus, you can use this formula to establish a single HSD critical value for each of the six paired comparisons.

- If the sample group sizes are unequal, you would need to create more than one HSD value for the paired comparisons. The SPSS program adjusts for unequal group sizes.

Using the range table is straightforward if you remember that it is adjusted based on the ANOVA error measure (within group MS). Table 9.7 shows a small part of a Range Table (see the appendix for the complete table) to give you an example of how to use it.

As you recall, I had four noise groups in the experiment, and the MS_W degrees of freedom was 12 (see Table 9.5). Based on these values, I shaded the relevant columns

TABLE 9.7   Example of Values from a Studentized Range Table

MS_W df	Number of Sample Groups						
	2	3	4	5	6	7	8
11	3.115	3.822	4.258	4.575	4.824	5.03	5.203
12	3.083	3.775	4.200	4.509	4.752	4.951	5.12
13	3.057	3.736	4.152	4.454	4.691	4.885	5.05

and rows in the Range Table in Table 9.6. The number of sample groups is the "4" column, and the MS_W df is the "12" row. Where these intersect is the $q_{(Range)}$ value used in the HSD calculation:

$$HSD = q_{(Range)} \sqrt{\frac{MS_w}{n}}$$

$$= HSD = 4.20 \sqrt{\frac{2.625}{4}}$$

$$= 3.40$$

Mean Comparison Table

Once the HSD critical value is calculated, you can proceed to examine how the group means differ. If you refer to Figure 9.2, you will see the six group comparisons that are necessary when there are four sample groups. In order to see what the group differences are between the paired groups, it is a simple matter of subtracting the group means. Table 9.8 lists the means of each of the four sample groups.

You could calculate the six paired sample differences by subtracting each pair of means as follows:

$$M_1 - M_2 = -2.00$$
$$M_1 - M_3 = -6.75$$
$$M_1 - M_4 = -10.25$$
$$M_2 - M_3 = -4.75$$
$$M_2 - M_4 = -8.25$$
$$M_3 - M_4 = -3.50$$

Doing the comparisons this way would yield the appropriate paired mean differences. Notice in the list, however, that if you subtract the higher group means (e.g., M_4) from the lower (e.g., M_1), the values are negative. In these paired comparison tests, you are interested only in the magnitude of the difference, not the sign. You can interpret the overall results by referring to the size of the means, but the paired tests do not use the sign. Therefore, you can subtract the smaller group means from the larger to get positive values.

TABLE 9.8 The Group Means

Groups	Means
M_1	4.50
M_2	6.50
M_3	11.25
M_4	14.75

TABLE 9.9   Matrix of Group Means

	M_1 (4.5)	M_2 (6.5)	M_3 (11.25)	M_4 (14.75)
M_1 (4.5)	---	2.00	6.75	10.25
M_2 (6.5)		---	4.75	8.25
M_3 (11.25)	-6.75		---	3.50
M_4 (14.75)				---

Another method for doing this is to create a "matrix" of group means. A matrix is simply a table constructed of rows and columns. You will see arrays of data in matrix form later in the book, so it is a good idea to use them to display data. SPSS uses matrix arrays for some outputs including the post hoc analysis.

Table 9.9 shows the group means in a matrix display. Previously, I calculated the difference of M_1 and M_3 to be −6.75. I placed this value in the matrix under column M_1 and row M_3. Thus, when I subtract 11.25 from 4.5, I get −6.75.

However, I can obtain positive values by subtracting the lower mean values from the higher. I have shown these values in the table. For example, subtracting 4.5 (M_1) from 11.25 (M_3) results in a value of 6.75, which is located in the M_3 column and the M_1 row. Notice that the matrix is symmetrical. The same values will appear in the lower "triangle" that appear in the upper "triangle" (I shaded the upper triangle) in Table 9.9. I left the −6.75 in both the lower and upper triangles to show the symmetry of the table.

Compare Mean Difference Values from HSD

The next step in the post hoc analysis is to compare the group mean differences (from Table 9.9) to the HSD value of 3.40. If any of the group mean differences <u>exceed</u> the HSD value, you would consider those two means *significantly* different. As you can see from the table, all the mean pairs exceed HSD except the $M_1 - M_2$ difference (2.00).

Post Hoc Summary

The ANOVA post hoc analysis showed that all paired comparisons showed significant differences except the group 1 (control group)–group 2 (30 decibels) comparison. Figure 9.8 shows how the groups might be arrayed to yield this finding.

ASSUMPTIONS OF ANOVA

As with the other statistical tests I discussed, the researcher needs to assess whether the conditions of the data are appropriate for the ANOVA test. Here are the primary assumptions, although ANOVA is also somewhat robust with respect to slight variations of assumptions:

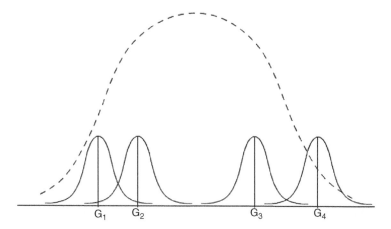

Figure 9.8 The post hoc summary for the example.

1. Population is normally distributed.
2. Population variances are equal. This assumption refers to the variance of each of the sample groups. You should make sure that the groups (in our case the noise conditions) have equal variance on the outcome measure (in our case, learning errors). (This is the homogeneity of variance assumption.)
3. Samples are independently chosen.
4. Interval data on the dependent variable.

ADDITIONAL CONSIDERATIONS WITH ANOVA

I will have more to say about these procedures, but here are some things to keep in mind if you use one-way ANOVA:

1. You can still use ANOVA ("the F test") even if the study only uses two group means. In this case, remember that there is a relationship between F and T such that $F = T^2$.
2. The effect size is critical, as you learned with the other tests I covered. You learned to calculate η^2 which indicates the strength of the effects of F. <u>Effect size is always calculated, even if the omnibus F test does not result in the reject of the null hypothesis.</u> Simply because a study finding is (or is not) statistically significant does not indicate how much of a *practical impact* it has. *Statistical significance and effect size are separate considerations.*
3. ANOVA like the T test can be used in experimental contexts (where you consciously change the value of an independent variable to see what effects this has on a dependent variable) and for post facto situations (where you simply try to determine if there are existing differences among several sample groups

without changing the value of the independent variable). In my example of noise and learning, I used ANOVA experimentally, since I directly "manipulated" or changed the value of the independent variable (noise level), to see if this affected the dependent variable (errors in learning performance).

4. Be sure to meet the assumptions of the test before you use it:
   - Populations are normally distributed.
   - Population variances are equal.
   - Independent selection.
   - Interval data on the dependent variable.

THE HYPOTHESIS TEST: INTERPRETING ANOVA RESULTS

This section presents another example of ANOVA showing the complete process of analysis and hypothesis testing. Although it is a hypothetical example, it reflects recent questions about the impact of sleep deprivation on health. Table 9.10 presents the data for health measures (diagnosis report with higher numbers indicating better health) according to three hourly amounts of sleep. There are obviously categories of sleep other than 6, 7, or 8 hours, but this study treats sleep as a categorical independent variable since the 6, 7, and 8 represent self-reported sleep amounts. In an actual study, you might measure sleep as a continuous variable. I am using the categories here as an example of ANOVA. In the extended example that follows, I will use Excel and SPSS to analyze the question, "does different amounts of sleep affect health?"

ARE THE ASSUMPTIONS MET?

Before proceeding to the manual calculations for this example problem, you need to examine the assumptions for ANOVA. Are the data appropriate for the one-way ANOVA?

TABLE 9.10 The Data for One-Way ANOVA Example

	SLEEP		
	6 Hrs.	7 Hrs.	8 Hrs.
HEALTH	4	13	12
	10	11	13
	8	12	11
	6	6	10
	2	8	17
	4	4	9

Is Population Normally Distributed?

As you recall from Chapter 3, I mentioned that skewness and kurtosis are good indicators to help assess normal distributions. For ANOVA, you need to make sure that the outcome data are normally distributed for each of the level of the independent variable. In this case, there are three independent variable levels: 6, 7, and 8 hours of sleep. Are the health data normally distributed? Use the results in Figure 9.9 to check this assumption.

The Excel output in Figure 9.9 indicates that all three groups are fairly normally distributed as determined by the similarity of mean and median values. The skewness and kurtosis figures appear within boundaries of normal. Use SPSS to investigate the skewness and kurtosis further since the standard errors are reported for skewness and kurtosis. Figure 9.10 shows the descriptive values that include skewness and kurtosis standard errors (using "Analyze – Compare Means – Means"), and Figure 9.11 shows the histograms for the groups.

As you can see, skewness and kurtosis for all groups of sleep are within bounds when the Sk and Ku values are divided by their standard errors. The histograms in

	6 Hrs	7 Hrs.	8 Hrs.
Mean	5.67	9.00	12.00
Standard Error	1.20	1.46	1.15
Median	5.00	9.50	11.50
Mode	4	#N/A	#N/A
Standard Deviation	2.94	3.58	2.83
Sample Variance	8.67	12.80	8.00
Kurtosis	−0.86	−1.72	1.67
Skewness	0.42	−0.35	1.19
Range	8	9	8
Minimum	2	4	9
Maximum	10	13	17
Sum	34	54	72
Count	6	6	6

Figure 9.9 The descriptive output (Excel) to test the normal distribution assumption.

Report

Health

SleepHours	Mean	N	Std. Deviation	Kurtosis	Std. Error of Kurtosis	Skewness	Std. Error of Skewness	Variance
6 Hours	5.67	6	2.944	−.859	1.741	.418	.845	8.667
7 Hours	9.00	6	3.578	−1.721	1.741	−.354	.845	12.800
8 Hours	12.00	6	2.828	1.669	1.741	1.193	.845	8.000
Total	8.89	18	3.969	−.492	1.038	.029	.536	15.752

Figure 9.10 SPSS® descriptive output for normal distribution assumption.

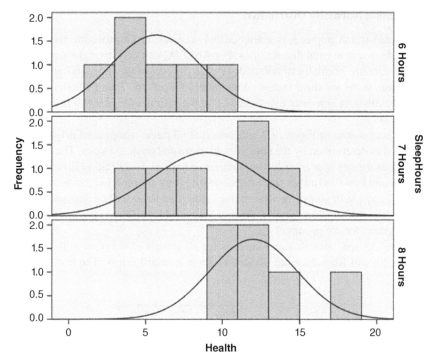

Figure 9.11   SPSS® graphs for FR groups.

Figure 9.11 show differences between the groups but due to low sample size are not definitive "evidence" of normal distributions.

If the researcher determined skewness and kurtosis values were excessive, they could make a number of choices:

- Choose not to use ANOVA.
- Transform the outcome measure so it conforms to normal bounds.
- Examine and possibly eliminate the outliers which may change the distribution configuration, according to some research criterion.
- Proceed with the analysis and note the concerns in the conclusions.

By the way, I used the "Analyze – Compare Means – Means" menus in SPSS to generate the values in Figure 9.10. I could have used the "Analyze – Descriptive Statistics – Frequencies" menus as I have in past chapters, but I wanted to show this useful function. Figure 9.12 shows the menus and choices for this procedure. List the dependent variable on the "Means" menu (under "Dependent List"), and specify the groups of the independent variable ("SleepHours" in this example) in the "Independent List" window. As you can see, I specified means, kurtosis, skewness, standard errors, etc., for the SleepHours groups.

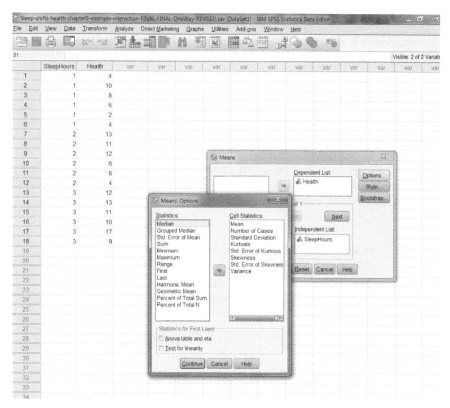

Figure 9.12 The SPSS® means procedure.

Are the Variances Equal?

This second assumption is important for ANOVA since it relies on comparisons of variance measures. Excel does not have a good way to assess equal variances for multiple groups. As we saw in Chapter 11 with the T test, Excel's "F-Test Two-Sample for Variances" analysis tool is very helpful for two sample groups, but not more than two. In Chapter 8, I discussed the SPSS Levene's test output that is included with the T test. You can use the same process to test for equal variances in the ANOVA sample groups. In the sections that follow, I will examine the Levene's test results for ANOVA.

Are the Samples Independently Chosen?

This assumption is met if the subjects identified to provide (sleep hours and health) data were randomly chosen and not placed in groups due to any structurally linking criteria. The result would be that the groups are occupied by different subjects without any relationship between them.

Does the Dependent Variable Consist of Interval Data?

This assumption is met. Health scores are presumably interval data resulting from a standardized diagnosis instrument (since this is a hypothetical study).

Manual Calculations

Before I demonstrate SPSS and Excel procedures, I will show the manual calculations for comparison. Table 9.11 shows the data with key sums for the ANOVA calculations.

You can use the formulas I presented earlier to "populate" the ANOVA summary table. The calculations for SS_T, SS_B, and SS_W follow. Table 9.12 shows the values in the completed ANOVA summary table.

TABLE 9.11   The ANOVA Example Database with Calculation Values

	SLEEP HOURS					
	6 Hours		**7 Hours**		**8 Hours**	
	X_1	X_1^2	X_2	X_2^2	X_3	X_3^2
	4	16	13	169	12	144
	10	100	11	121	13	169
	8	64	12	144	11	121
	6	36	6	36	10	100
	2	4	8	64	17	289
	4	16	4	16	9	81
ΣX	34		54		72	
ΣX^2		236		550		904
$(\Sigma X)^2$	1,156		2,916		5,184	
N	6		6		6	
MEANS	5.67		9.00		12.00	

TABLE 9.12   The Completed ANOVA Summary Table for the Extended Example

Source of Variance	SS	df	MS	F ratio
Between	120.447	2	60.223	6.131
Within	147.33	15	9.822	
Total	267.78	17	----	

Calculating SS_T ($SS_T = 267.78$):

$$SS_T = \sum X^2 - \frac{(\sum X)^2}{N}$$

$$= (236 + 550 + 904) - \frac{(34 + 54 + 72)^2}{18}$$

$$= 1690 - 1422.22$$

Calculating SS_B ($SS_B = 120.447$):

$$SS_B = \frac{(\sum X_1)^2}{n_1} + \frac{(\sum X_2)^2}{n_2} + \frac{(\sum X_3)^2}{n_3} (-) \frac{(\sum X)^2}{N}$$

$$= \frac{1156}{6} + \frac{2916}{6} + \frac{5184}{6} (-) \frac{(34 + 54 + 72)^2}{18}$$

$$= 192.667 + 486 + 864 (-) 1422.22$$

Calculating SS_W ($SS_W = 147.333$):

$$SS_W = SS_T - SS_B$$

$$= 267.78 - 120.447$$

The hypothesis test:

Null hypothesis: H_0: $\mu_1 = \mu_2 = \mu_3 = \mu_4$.

Alternate hypothesis: H_A: $\mu_1 \neq \mu_2 \neq \mu_3 \neq \mu_4$.

Critical value of exclusion: $F_{(0.05, 2, 15)} = 3.68$.

Calculated F: 6.131.

Decision: Reject the null hypothesis.

This test is significant at or beyond $p < 0.05$. The calculated F ratio was so large it surpassed the 0.05 exclusion value of 3.68 and therefore lies in the extreme portion of the comparison distribution.

Interpretation: The omnibus test indicates that different sleep hour groups show different mean health values. Health increases as the hours of sleep increase.

Effect size: $\eta^2 = 0.45$.

The effect size is an easy calculation using the ANOVA summary table of values. As the calculation indicates, 45% of the variance in health values is accounted for by the different hours of sleep groupings. This value far exceeds the 0.15 guideline for a high effect size indicating a strong influence of sleep on health.

$$\eta^2 = \frac{SS_{Between}}{SS_{Total}}$$
$$= \frac{120.444}{267.778}$$

Post Hoc Analysis

Using the Tukey Range test, you can create the HSD critical comparison value to compare the mean differences of health by groupings of sleep. The Tukey Range table of values identifies $q_{(Range)} = 3.67$. I identified this value in the table by viewing the groups $= 3$ column and the MS_W df row $= 15$. (Recall that this formula requires the sample sizes to be equal.)

$$HSD = q_{(Range)} \sqrt{\frac{MS_w}{n}}$$
$$= 3.67 \sqrt{\frac{9.822}{6}}$$
$$= 4.70$$

Table 9.13 continues the post hoc analysis by presenting group mean differences to compare with the HSD value. As you can see, sleep group 6 is significantly different from sleep group 8 since the mean difference (6.33) exceeds the HSD value of 4.70. I highlighted this difference in the table by placing an asterisk next to the significant value. Sleep groups for 6 and 7 hours and groups for 7 and 8 hours did not significantly differ from one another.

Figure 9.11 shows how these group means appear as you examine the histograms for each group. Figure 9.13 shows the groups graphed together. You can see that the health values are comparatively highest for the 8 hour sleep group.

USING SPSS® AND EXCEL WITH ONE-WAY ANOVA

The manual calculations for the ANOVA problem can be checked by using the SPSS and Excel programs for the one-way ANOVA.

TABLE 9.13   The Group Mean Difference Matrix

	6 Hrs. (5.67)	7 Hrs. (9.00)	8 Hrs. (12.00)
6 Hrs. (5.67)	---	3.33	**6.33***
7 Hrs. (9.00)		---	3.00
8 Hrs. (12.00)			---

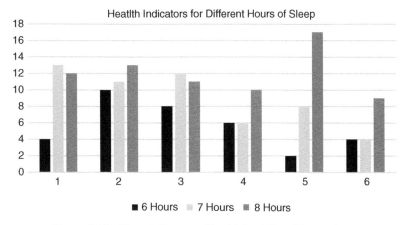

Figure 9.13   Three indicators of health by 6, 7, or 8 hours sleep.

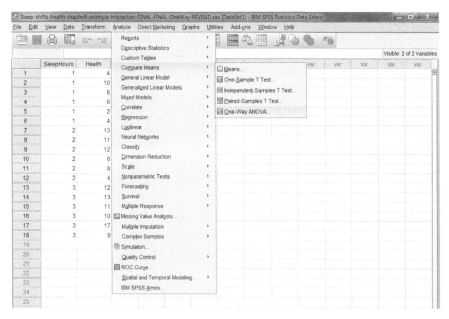

Figure 9.14   The SPSS® menu options for accessing the one-way ANOVA.

SPSS® Procedures with One-Way ANOVA

The one-way ANOVA procedure in SPSS is easy to create and thorough in what it reports. Figure 9.14 shows the menu choices for the one-way ANOVA procedure. As you can see, it is in the same menu group that includes the single sample *T* test and the independent samples *T* test, which I discussed in previous chapters. This menu also includes the Means procedure I used before to create the descriptive data for the three SleepHour groups.

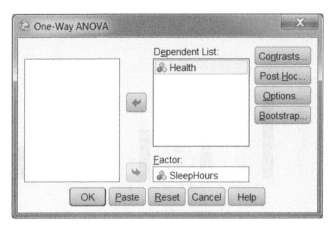

Figure 9.15   The one-way ANOVA specification windows.

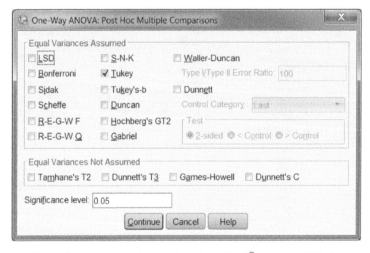

Figure 9.16   The post hoc choices from SPSS® one-way ANOVA.

When you select the one-way ANOVA procedure, the window shown in Figure 9.15 appears that allows the researcher to specify the analysis. As you can see, I specified the Health variable as the outcome measure and SleepHours as the grouping variable ("Factor"). The buttons on the top right of the screen can be used for further specification.

Figure 9.16 shows the choices available from selecting the "Post Hoc" button from the one-way ANOVA menu. As you can see, the menu lists several post hoc procedures available for inclusion in the analysis. I selected the Tukey procedure to demonstrate the results alongside the manual calculations of the Tukey Range Test. Notice that the post hoc procedures are "grouped" according to whether equal variances (of the SleepHour sample groups) are assumed or not. There are post hoc procedures available if you find the group variances to be unequal.

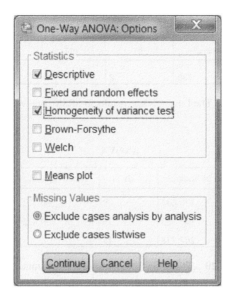

Figure 9.17 Options for SPSS one-way ANOVA.

Descriptives

Health

	N	Mean	Std. Deviation	Std. Error	95% Confidence Interval for Mean		Minimum	Maximum
					Lower Bound	Upper Bound		
6 Hours	6	5.67	2.944	1.202	2.58	8.76	2	10
7 Hours	6	9.00	3.578	1.461	5.25	12.75	4	13
8 Hours	6	12.00	2.828	1.155	9.03	14.97	9	17
Total	18	8.89	3.969	.935	6.92	10.86	2	17

Figure 9.18 The descriptives report in SPSS® one-way ANOVA.

If you select the "Options" button from the one-way ANOVA menu (Figure 9.15), you can select several important procedures to use in the analysis. Figure 9.17 shows these choices. As you can see, I chose "Descriptive" procedures to derive the group means and related data and the "Homogeneity of variance test" option which will produce Levene's test for equality of variance. This test allows the researcher to assess the equal variance assumption for one-way ANOVA that I discussed in the earlier section on the assumptions for ANOVA.

Figures 9.18–9.21 show the output resulting from these specifications. The descriptive values are reported in Figure 9.18, and Figure 9.19 follows with Levene's test results.

As you see, the Levene's test was *not significant* since the "Sig." reported is $p = 0.543$. Therefore, the test statistic did not land in its exclusion region, or it would have reported a much smaller chance probability (i.e., $p < 0.05$). Since Levene's test was not significant, the sleep groups can be considered to have equal variance in

Test of Homogeneity of Variances

Health

Levene Statistic	df1	df2	Sig.
.636	2	15	.543

Figure 9.19   The Levene's test results in SPSS® one-way ANOVA.

ANOVA

Health

	Sum of Squares	df	Mean Square	F	Sig.
Between Groups	120.444	2	60.222	6.131	.011
Within Groups	147.333	15	9.822		
Total	267.778	17			

Figure 9.20   The SPSS® one-way ANOVA summary table.

Multiple Comparisons

Dependent Variable: Health

Tukey HSD

(I) SleepHours	(J) SleepHours	Mean Difference (I-J)	Std. Error	Sig.	95% Confidence Interval	
					Lower Bound	Upper Bound
6 Hours	7 Hours	−3.333	1.809	.190	−8.03	1.37
	8 Hours	−6.333*	1.809	.009	−11.03	−1.63
7 Hours	6 Hours	3.333	1.809	.190	−1.37	8.03
	8 Hours	−3.000	1.809	.253	−7.70	1.70
8 Hours	6 Hours	6.333*	1.809	.009	1.63	11.03
	7 Hours	3.000	1.809	.253	−1.70	7.70

*. The mean difference is significant at the 0.05 level.

Figure 9.21   The Tukey post hoc results in the SPSS® one-way ANOVA procedure.

their health scores. That is, since the test was not significant, the null hypothesis of equal variances among sample groups *was not rejected*. This is the finding that confirms the equal variance assumption is met for one-way ANOVA and that allows the researcher to continue with the ANOVA analysis.

If Levene's test would have shown a significant result, the "Sig." value would be smaller than 0.05, indicating that its calculated test value would have fallen in the exclusion area. Under this circumstance, the researcher would need to decide how to proceed since one of the ANOVA assumptions would not have been met.

The next panel of the results is the ANOVA summary table shown in Figure 9.20. This table is identical to the summary table based on the manual calculations earlier with one additional column. The "Sig." column (0.011) indicates that the calculated F value exceeds the F table cutoff value (3.68) and is therefore considered significant.

SPSS calculates the exact probability of a finding (0.011), but you can report the significance on the hypothesis test as "$p < 0.05$" since this is an indication that the overall exclusion level of 0.05 is exceeded.

SPSS does not routinely produce η^2 but you can confirm the effect size is the same as our manual calculation ($\eta^2 = 0.45$) by dividing the appropriate values from the ANOVA summary table. The same interpretation follows: 45% of the variation in health is accounted for by grouping sleep into these three categories.

The final panel of the SPSS output is the post hoc analysis specified in Figure 9.16. The results are shown in Figure 9.21. I highlighted the row showing the significant difference between the 6 and 8 hours of sleep groups. The first row of data compares the 6 and 7 hour groups with the result of no difference (Sig. = 0.190). The second row compares the 6 and 8 hours of sleep groups indicating a significant difference (Sig. = 0.009). The additional columns show the results of the paired comparisons.[3]

The Tukey report in Figure 9.21 is arranged a bit differently than the group mean matrix I presented previously. However, you can see that both negative and positive values are reported depending on which value is reported first. As with my matrix, the interpretation of the values depends on the context of the research question. In this study, the group means indicate mean health values of respondents in the 6, 7, and 8 hour sleep groups. Positive values indicate higher health values, so you might use the positive values from the table in a summary report if the group means (see Figure 9.18) support this finding.

General Linear Model (GLM) Approach to Analyzing ANOVA

SPSS provides another method for calculating ANOVA (including one-way ANOVA). The General Linear Model (GLM) is a way of calculating the linear relationships among independent variables and a dependent variable (univariate) or multiple dependent variables (multivariate) through a set of related procedures. I will discuss the SPSS GLM to analyze ANOVA procedures in the next chapter (addressing Factorial ANOVA). You can use the GLM process for one-way ANOVA analyses, but the one-way procedure I outlined earlier is a simple way to understand the ANOVA results.

Excel Procedures with One-Way ANOVA

In order to use one-way ANOVA in Excel, the data need to be arrayed like the data table in Table 9.10. Show three columns, one for each of the sleep hour groups, and populate the rows with health values for each of the respondents.

Simply select the entire set of data, including the labels in the first row, and use the "Data – Data Analysis" menus to bring you to the screen shown in Figure 9.22. As you can see, there are three choices for ANOVA. The one-way ANOVA uses a single factor (one independent variable), so the top choice is the option you need for the analysis.

---

[3] Note that the output does not specify the HSD value of comparison (4.70) but indicates significant group differences by including an "*."

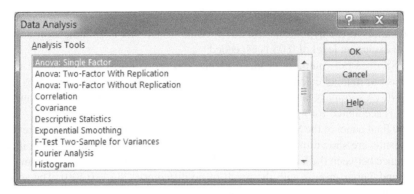

Figure 9.22 The single factor ANOVA menu option in Excel.

Anova: Single Factor

Groups	Count	Sum	Average	Variance
6 Hours	6	34	5.67	8.67
7 Hours	6	54	9.00	12.80
8 Hours	6	72	12.00	8.00

ANOVA

Source of Variation	SS	df	MS	F	P-value	F crit
Between Groups	120.444	2	60.222	6.131	0.011	3.682
Within Groups	147.333	15	9.822			
Total	267.778	17				

Figure 9.23 The Excel single factor ANOVA output.

When you run this procedure (after specifying the location of the data in a separate screen), Excel returns the output shown in Figure 9.23. The top panel is the descriptive statistics showing the means and variances of health values for each sleep hour group. The "Average" column is helpful when you create the mean difference matrix for the post hoc analysis.

The bottom panel of Figure 9.23 shows the ANOVA summary table. This is the same table you created by manual and the same as the SPSS summary table. It shows the sources and measures of variance and the calculated F ratio (6.131). Excel also reports the exact probability of the F ratio like SPSS in the "P-value" column.

The "F crit" (or, critical value for F) value in the summary table indicates the point value on the F distribution that defines the exclusion area. The calculated F ratio of 6.131 well exceeds this value (3.682), resulting in the p-value less than 0.05.

Notice that the Excel output does not include information about effect size. However, you can calculate eta squared η^2 easily from the summary table as you did in the manual calculations. Recall that $\eta^2 = 0.45$ calculated as follows:

$$\eta^2 = \frac{SS_{Between}}{SS_{Total}}$$
$$= \frac{120.444}{267.778}$$

Because the omnibus test was significant (i.e., the null hypothesis is rejected), you can perform the post hoc analysis. However, no provision is made in Excel to create the post hoc analysis. You can perform it as you did in the manual calculations or using SPSS.

THE NEED FOR DIAGNOSTICS

Every researcher knows that real data can be problematic. Not all sample group data conform to perfect distributions. Sometimes, even small discrepancies in the data or data entry errors can have a huge effect on the results of an analysis. Ordinarily, I include a section on "Diagnostics" when I write about statistical procedures (e.g., see Abbott, 2010) because this is such an important, but often overlooked, consideration. I will discuss these issues as we encounter them in this text.

Before you begin an analysis, pay attention to the assumptions for the procedure you are using, and examine the data to ensure there are no issues that may lead to invalid results. Simply looking at the data can sometimes identify potential problems (excessive values, missing data, etc.). You may be surprised what your eyes pick up that the analyses do not!

Often, a few or even a single extreme case can dramatically affect results. If you identify extreme cases you are faced with the question of what to do. Should you eliminate the case(s)? Transform the cases to a mean value? Or leave the case if you are assured that it is a valid score? *There can be a fine line between using diagnostic procedures to eliminate cases that should be eliminated and simply eliminating cases because it makes the results better*! Keep or eliminate cases based on the nature of the study and the research study guidelines.

The researcher is ultimately in charge of the nature of the research and producing meaningful results. Statistical procedures can help to make sense out of data and help to make statistical decisions, but the researcher is ultimately the most important part of the process for conducting a study and making conclusions.

NON-PARAMETRIC ANOVA TESTS: THE KRUSKAL–WALLIS TEST

As I discussed in Chapter 8, there are non-parametric tests that correspond to the parametric tests that I cover in this book. One of the "parallel" non-parametric tests for the independent sample T Test is the Mann–Whitney U that I discussed in Chapter 8. There are non-parametric tests that are similar to the ANOVA test as well.

**TABLE 9.14   Hypothetical Data
for Kruskal–Wallis Test**

Meters	Ease-of-Use Ratings
1	10
1	9
1	9
1	9
2	1
2	3
2	2
2	2
3	5
3	4
3	3
3	4

The Kruskal–Wallis test is one of the parallel non-parametric tests for one-way ANOVA. Like the Mann–Whitney U, this test uses ranks and determines whether groups of dependent variable ranks are different from one another.

The data in Table 9.14 are hypothetical data that compare ease-of-use ratings of three types of glucose meters by a sample of 12 patients recently diagnosed with type II diabetes. Ratings are based on a scale of 1–10 with a value of 10 being the easiest to use.

Like the ANOVA test, the research question is whether the ratings of the three meter groups are equivalent or statistically different. The Kruskal–Wallis test uses ranks to make the determination since the ease-of-use ratings are subjective.

Using SPSS to specify the Kruskal–Wallis test is a similar process to the one I used for the Mann–Whitney U in Chapter 8. Figure 8.27 (see Chapter 8) shows the process for choosing the Mann–Whitney U test. You use the same menu selection for the Kruskal–Wallis test except that you choose "K Independent Samples" rather than "Two Independent Samples" since Kruskal–Wallis tests the differences among more than two groups.

When you choose this option, you will see the window in Figure 9.24. As you can see, I specified "Usage" variable as the test variable (dependent variable) and entered the three "Meter" groups in the "Grouping Variable" window. Notice that you can choose other tests of this type in the "Test Type" box, but I will only show the results for the Kruskal–Wallis test.

Figure 9.25 shows the result output for the Kruskal–Wallis test in two panels. The top panel shows the mean ranks by meter group and the bottom panel shows the test statistics that determine whether there are significant differences in ease-of-use ratings between the meter groups. As you can see from the results, I can reject the null hypothesis at the $p < 0.007$ level. There are significant ease-of-use rating differences between the meter groups.

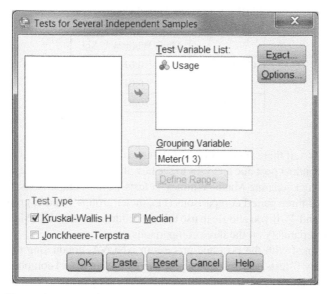

Figure 9.24   The specification window for the Kruskal–Wallis test.

Ranks

	Meter	N	Mean Rank
Usage	1.00	4	10.50
	2.00	4	2.63
	3.00	4	6.38
	Total	12	

Test Statistics[a,b]

	Usage
Chi-Square	9.788
df	2
Asymp. Sig.	.007

a. Kruskal Wallis Test

b. Grouping Variable: Meter

Figure 9.25   The output for the Kruskal–Wallis test.

**TABLE 9.15   The Paired Comparison
Results**

	Mann Whitney U Sig.
Groups 1 - 2	0.017
Groups 1 - 3	0.017
Groups 2 - 3	0.027

Like ANOVA, if there are significant differences between the different groups, you may wish to conduct post hoc analyses to see how the groups differ. One way of doing this is to conduct separate Mann–Whitney U tests for all comparisons. In this case, there would be three paired comparisons (i.e., meter groups 1 and 2, groups 1 and 3, and groups 2 and 3). If you choose to use this procedure, use the SPSS Mann–Whitney U procedure separately on the three comparisons.

As I explained with the post hoc process in ANOVA, conducting three separate Mann–Whitney U tests may result in a problem since this would compound the overall alpha error. However, you can still use this process by using a "correction" to the alpha exclusion area. The Bonferroni method specifies that you can divide the overall alpha level (0.05) by the number of paired comparisons in order to create an appropriate target significance area for each. Since there are three comparisons, using the 0.05 level of significance, this technique would specify a new region of rejection at $p < 0.0167$ ($0.05/3 = 0.017$) for the comparisons.

This procedure creates a conservative estimate of the significance of paired comparisons. In the current example, the overall Kruskal–Wallis results indicated a significant finding at $p < 0.007$. If you were to conduct all three comparisons using the exclusion values before (0.017), you would find the results shown in Table 9.15. As you can see, the first two comparisons were significant at $p < 0.017$. If you were more selective in the comparisons, you could specify only one or possibly two comparisons, but beyond this, you would not have confidence in the differences.

There are other methods for creating corrected rejection regions for paired comparisons. The Bonferroni method is very conservative; other methods might show that the final comparison (groups 2–3) was also significant.

One further warning is in order for both the Mann–Whitney U and Kruskal–Wallis tests. If you have several tied ranks, the results may be somewhat compromised, but the SPSS program will help to account for this.

TERMS AND CONCEPTS

ANOVA:	The ANalysis Of VAriance test that assesses the extent to which the variance between group means and the grand mean of a distribution is large relative to the variance of individual scores of different sample groups. This test is typically used with three or more sample groups.

Bonferroni method:	A pairwise comparison procedure that divides the overall alpha level (0.05) of a test by the number of paired comparisons in order to create more conservative target significance areas for each.
***F* Test**:	The statistical test comparing the between and within variances in an ANOVA test. The calculated ratio of between-to-within variance is compared to the exclusion values of the *F* distribution.
Familywise error:	The inflation of alpha error due to conducting multiple post hoc comparison tests.
Kruskal–Wallis test:	The non-parametric test comparable to ANOVA based on rank/ordinal data.
Levene's test:	The statistical test assessing the assumption of homogeneity of variance.
Post hoc analyses:	Individual comparison tests conducted among sample group values subsequent to a significant ANOVA finding.
Variance between:	The variation of group means around the grand mean in an ANOVA analysis.
Variance total:	The total variation (between and within) in an ANOVA analysis resulting from all individual scores varying around the grand mean.
Variance within:	The variation of scores around their own group means in an ANOVA analysis. Also known as "error."

DATA LAB AND EXAMPLES (WITH SOLUTIONS)

Problem 1

Calculate the one-way ANOVA by manual on the following values, conduct the hypothesis test, calculate effect size, and perform the post hoc analysis if warranted:

    Group A: 5, 9, 6, 8, 7
    Group B: 1, 4, 3, 2, 2
    Group C: 9, 8, 9, 4, 4

Problem 2

The data in Table 9.16 shows the (hypothetical) self-reported blood sugar levels of workers who are paid in three different ways: by salary, by hourly, and by commission. Is there a difference in blood sugar readings among the different payment methods? Conduct all appropriate tests with the data in Table 9.16 (if warranted).

TABLE 9.16   Blood Sugar: Pay Method Data

Blood Sugar Level (Self-Reported)		
Salary	Hourly	Commission
78	99	88
99	108	92
87	111	91
75	114	87
66	106	91
82	120	92
101	135	87
79	100	88
73	97	96
81	95	80

DATA LAB: SOLUTIONS

Problem 1

Calculate the one-way ANOVA by manual:

SS_B	67.60	MS_B	33.8	F ratio	9.657143
SS_W	42.00	MS_W	3.5		
SS_T	109.60				

Conduct the hypothesis test:

F ratio	9.66
$F_{(0.05, 2, 12)}$	3.88
Decision	Reject the null hypothesis, $p < 0.05$
Interpretation	At least one of the group means is different from the others

Calculate effect size: $\eta^2 = 67.6/109.6 = 0.617$. This is a large effect size. 61.7% of the variance in the values is accounted for by the three groupings (A, B, C).

Perform the post hoc analysis if warranted:

$$HSD = q_{(Range)} \sqrt{\frac{MS_w}{n}} = 3.77\,(0.775) = 2.92$$

Findings: Group B is different from both groups A and C; groups A and C are not different from each other (see Table 9.17).

TABLE 9.17   Post Hoc Analysis for Problem 1

	Group A (7.00)	Group B (2.40)	Group C (6.80)
Group A (7.00)	---	**4.60***	0.20
Group B (2.40)		---	**4.40***
Group C (6.80)			---

Problem 2

Are the assumptions met for ANOVA? Normal distribution of groups. The panels of Figure 9.26 show that skewness and kurtosis are within normal bounds (panel 1) and that the K–S and S–W are both non-significant (panel 2).

Are the assumptions met for ANOVA? Equal variance across groups. Panel 3 of Figure 9.26 shows that results for Levene's test are non-significant (panel 3) indicating equal variance in groups.

Report

Blood

Payment	Mean	Kurtosis	Std. Error of Kurtosis	Skewness	Std. Error of Skewness
Salary	82.10	−.049	1.334	.660	.687
Hourly	108.50	1.208	1.334	1.117	.687
Commission	89.20	1.783	1.334	−.763	.687
Total	93.27	1.024	.833	.742	.427

Tests of Normality

		Kolmogorov-Smirnov[a]			Shapiro-Wilk		
	Payment	Statistic	df	Sig.	Statistic	df	Sig.
Blood	Salary	.204	10	.200*	.929	10	.438
	Hourly	.156	10	.200*	.913	10	.300
	Commission	.204	10	.200*	.926	10	.412

*. This is a lower bound of the true significance.

a. Lilliefors Significance Correction

Test of Homogeneity of Variance

		Levene Statistic	df1	df2	Sig.
Blood	Based on Mean	2.781	2	27	.080
	Based on Median	2.344	2	27	.115
	Based on Median and with adjusted df	2.344	2	20.072	.122
	Based on trimmed mean	2.615	2	27	.092

Figure 9.26   The data to check for normal distribution.

Blood

ANOVA

	Sum of Squares	df	Mean Square	F	Sig.
Between Groups	3732.867	2	1866.433	19.330	.000
Within Groups	2607.000	27	96.556		
Total	6339.867	29			

Figure 9.27 The ANOVA results for Problem 2.

Multiple Comparisons

Dependent Variable: Blood

Tukey HSD

(I) Payment	(J) Payment	Mean Difference (I-J)	Std. Error	Sig.	95% Confidence Interval	
					Lower Bound	Upper Bound
Salary	Hourly	−26.400*	4.394	.000	−37.30	−15.50
	Commission	−7.100	4.394	.256	−18.00	3.80
Hourly	Salary	26.400*	4.394	.000	15.50	37.30
	Commission	19.300*	4.394	.000	8.40	30.20
Commission	Salary	7.100	4.394	.256	−3.80	18.00
	Hourly	−19.300*	4.394	.000	−30.20	-8.40

*. The mean difference is significant at the 0.05 level.

Figure 9.28 The post hoc analysis for the ANOVA result.

Are the assumptions met for ANOVA? Assumptions #3 (independent selection) and #4 (interval data) are met.

ANOVA results? Figure 9.27 shows the results for the ANOVA test. Based on the analysis ($F = 19.33$), reject the null hypothesis, $p < 0.05$.

Effect size? $\eta^2 = 3732.867/6339.867 = 0.589$

- Large effect size.
- 58.9% of the variance in blood glucose reading is accounted for by the method of payment for work.

Post hoc analyses? Figure 9.28 shows the Tukey post hoc analysis. The results indicate that hourly payment indicates the highest mean blood reading and that it is significantly different from payment by either salary or commission.

10

FACTORIAL ANOVA

In Chapter 9, I discussed the one-way analysis of variance (ANOVA) research study that included one independent variable and one dependent variable. The designation "one-way" ANOVA makes reference to the independent variable. I will extend these procedures by adding a second (or more) independent variables to the design. This is known as *factorial* ANOVA because the focus is how multiple factors (i.e., independent variables) affect an outcome variable. When a second independent variable is added, the procedure is known as a "two-way ANOVA." A shorthand identification of factorial ANOVA is "2XANOVA" indicating that there are two independent variables (a 3XANOVA has three independent variables).

Before I discuss factorial ANOVA, I want to mention briefly some extensions of the ANOVA procedure. I will not explore these in this book, but you will see how adaptable ANOVA is to different research situations.

EXTENSIONS OF ANOVA

There are several ANOVA procedures for special research designs and situations. The basic ANOVA design is very flexible in that it can admit several different sources of variance to compare at the same time.

Within-Subjects ANOVA

An ANOVA procedure designed for use with *repeated measures* is known as within-subjects ANOVA. These are designs that use two or more measures from

Using Statistics in the Social and Health Sciences with SPSS® and Excel®, First Edition.
Martin Lee Abbott.
© 2017 John Wiley & Sons, Inc. Published 2017 by John Wiley & Sons, Inc.

the same subjects or from matched group subjects. (I will briefly examine one of these, within-subjects ANOVA, in a later chapter.) An example might be an ANOVA design with only one group of subjects that is measured more than once, perhaps as a "before–after" design or "pretest–posttest" design.

In these designs, the two measures of the dependent variable are highly related to one another because they measure the same person(s) twice. Thus, you need a statistical procedure that will take this relationship into account as the overall ANOVA is calculated.

Two-Way Within-Subjects ANOVA

If the ANOVA design has more than one independent variable on which the same group or subjects are measured twice, the researcher can use this two-way within-subjects ANOVA. These research situations call for procedures that help suss out the differences among repeated measures. For example, suppose I used pre–postcomparisons on the noise-learning subjects (within subjects), but I also tested them under "non-white noise" and "white noise" conditions. In this case, there is more than one independent variable on whose levels the same subjects are measured twice.

ANCOVA

A very useful ANOVA design that researchers use to control extraneous influences is *analysis of covariance* or ANCOVA. If the researcher cannot truly randomize in the study, ANCOVA might be helpful as a way of limiting the influence of a variable or variables "outside" the design (known as "covariates") that might affect the results.

As an example, if I had not been able to randomly select and assign subjects to the noise-learning experiment, I might be concerned that variables other than noise might affect the outcome measure (learning). In this case, I might use some existing measure of "learning ability" (GPA, achievement test score) as a "control" on learning so that the posttest measure would measure only the effects of the noise, not the individual subjects' *ability to learn*. A pretest score is a popular covariate.

ANCOVA procedures are controversial when the researcher relies on them rather than randomization for producing valid and meaningful results. Randomization provides the greatest confidence that all the extraneous variables are controlled in a research situation. However, the researcher may not have the luxury of full randomization. In these cases, particularly in quasi-experimental designs, ANCOVA is a helpful tool.

ANCOVA procedures are also (perhaps especially) useful in post facto designs when there is no manipulation of the independent variable. The researcher attempts to control as many additional influences as possible on the outcome measure and ANCOVA can be very helpful. ANCOVA is also used in procedures that are not ANOVA based, like multiple regression procedures.

Multivariate ANOVA Procedures

The procedures I cover in this book are *univariate* procedures. This means that there is only one dependent or outcome variable in the research design. Advanced statistical measures use *multivariate* procedures that have <u>more than one outcome variable.</u> MANOVA and MANCOVA are two examples of multivariate procedures.

MANOVA

When a researcher adds one or more *dependent* variables to an ANOVA design, the procedure is called MANOVA or multivariate analysis of variance. To extend my noise experiment example, I could have added another dependent variable such as performance on a visual recognition task. Thus, I would have had one independent variable (noise) and two dependent variables (learning performance and visual recognition). I would use MANOVA with this design since all the sources of error are contained when you examine all the statistical tests at the same time. (I discussed this in earlier chapters as familywise error.)

MANCOVA

Of course, the statistical procedures can become increasingly sophisticated along with the sophistication and complexity of the design. Multivariate analysis of covariance (MANCOVA) is the extension of ANCOVA to designs with *multiple dependent variables*.

FACTORIAL ANOVA

The factorial ANOVA performs the single ANOVA procedure twice (or as many times as there are independent variables in the design) within the same analysis. In this way, the familywise error is contained. In the output, you will learn to recognize the separate effects of these two independent variables (called *main effects*).

INTERACTION EFFECTS

The factorial ANOVA also performs an additional analysis of the *interaction effects*. As I have stated elsewhere, *an interaction is present when the relationship between one predictor and the outcome variable changes at different levels of another predictor variable* (Abbott, 2010). The key feature of an interaction effect is that both independent variables <u>have effects on each other as well as the dependent variable;</u> different levels of one independent variable affect the levels of the other independent variable.

An Example of 2XANOVA

To take an example, suppose that in the noise-learning example, I was interested in the difference between men and women as well as the difference between noise conditions in producing learning errors. This 2XANOVA would include the following primary analyses:

- Main effect 1: Do noise conditions differ in number of learning errors?
- Main effect 2: Do men and women differ in number of learning errors?

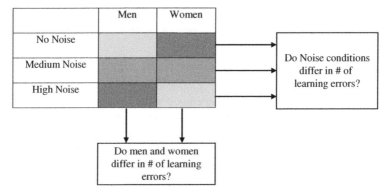

Figure 10.1   Main effects analyses in 2XANOVA.

- Interaction effect: Do men and women produce different learning errors under different noise conditions?

Figure 10.1 shows the design of an experiment in which I added a second independent variable (men vs women) to the earlier noise-learning design. (In Figure 10.1 you can see that I created three groups of noise rather than the previous four groups to create a clearer example.) As you can see, there are two <u>main effects</u> indicated by the analyses between rows (noise) and between columns (men vs women). The dependent variable learning errors is represented by the shaded areas where they would be entered according to the independent variable categories.

The other analysis in 2XANOVA is the <u>interaction effect</u>, represented by the different shades in Figure 10.1. The darker the shade, the higher the learning errors. In Figure 10.1, men and women differ in their patterns of errors under different noise conditions. This is an interaction effect. Figure 10.2 shows how the interaction effect appears with a line chart.

As you can see, Figure 10.2 shows that men produce more errors as the noise levels increase. Women show a different pattern. Their highest errors are produced under no noise conditions with lower numbers of errors in medium- and high-noise conditions. This is a hypothetical example, so I cannot draw conclusions about the nature of noise and sex on learning errors. However, the example provides insight into the fact that 2XANOVA conducts several analyses simultaneously. The interaction effect is shown separately in the 2XANOVA output.

Charting Interactions

When the interaction graph shows that the lines from different groups do not cross or intersect, the researcher would not expect a significant interaction. In these cases, the groups may be different on the dependent variable, but the values of one independent variable are consistently parallel across values of the other independent variable.

There are different kinds of interactions that you will recognize by graphing them.

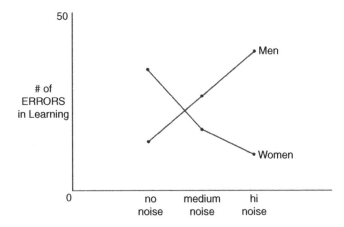

Figure 10.2 The interaction effect of sex and noise conditions.

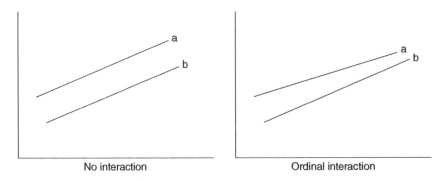

Figure 10.3 Ordinal interaction patterns compared to no interaction.

Disordinal interactions are those in which the lines cross in the plotted graph. Figure 10.2 is an example of the disordinal interaction.

Ordinal interactions are those in which the lines may not cross within the plotted graph, but they are not parallel. In these cases, the lines could intersect or cross if they were carried out beyond the plotted area of the graph. (In these cases, the researcher would need to decide if the extension of the analyses would not be of interest to the research question.) Figure 10.3 shows examples of an ordinal interaction and a study with no interaction.

SIMPLE EFFECTS

Generally, a significant interaction effect in the 2XANOVA takes precedence over the main effects findings. If there is a significant interaction, the main effects dynamics "hide" the unequal cell findings across the factors. Looking at Figure 10.1, for example, you could not detect the different ways men and women are affected by noise conditions if you were simply comparing the total of men versus women. The different shades would be mixed together and indistinguishable. Likewise, if you were just considering noise differences, the men's and women's shades would be mixed together.

The interaction effects allow you to "disaggregate" or take the findings apart in such a way that you can see the differences in one variable at each level of the other. *Simple effects* are the ways you can detect all these nuances. Simple effects show the differences in categories of one independent variable within single categories of the other independent variable.

In Figure 10.2, both the men's and women's lines represent the separate simple effects of sex in the noise groups. The figure shows that, if you focus only on men, you can see that the errors increase across noise conditions. For women, the effects of noise are inconsistent on their error production.

There are separate calculations for simple effects that researchers learn to calculate in advanced statistics books or through SPSS® and other statistical programs. I will demonstrate these procedures briefly.

2XANOVA: AN EXAMPLE

The data I use for this procedure is an extension of the sleep–health data example I developed in Chapter 9. Table 9.10 showed the data for a one-way ANOVA in which health measures differed by the number of hours each respondent slept. If you recall, the results of that study found that differences in sleep mattered to health and that sleeping 8 hours was connected to the greatest health values.[1]

Table 10.1 shows the database similar to that shown in Table 9.10 with some different values. The primary difference is that this study introduces a second factor "SEX" to show how ANOVA can be useful in analyzing data with more than one independent variable.

TABLE 10.1   The Data for the Sleep–Sex Impact on Health

	Sleep		
	6 HRS.	7 HRS.	8 HRS.
SEX: Male	4	17	12
	10	18	13
	9	15	11
SEX: Female	6	6	10
	2	8	17
	4	4	9

[1] Please recall that this is a hypothetical example. Current research suggests that sleep and health are connected, but this small example is used for illustration only of the ANOVA procedure.

CALCULATING FACTORIAL ANOVA

The factorial ANOVA has several comparisons that recognize the complexity of the data. There are three primary comparisons:

- "Main effects" (two comparisons)
  - Row effects (male or female in Table 10.1)
  - Column effects (hours of sleep in Table 10.1)
- "Interaction effects" (one comparison)

Calculating factorial ANOVA begins by calculating the total, between, and within sums of squares as you did with the one-way ANOVA. These are the "building blocks" of the 2XANOVA calculations. With the one-way ANOVA, recall that the <u>total SS</u> is the measure of variation of all the individual scores around the grand mean. The <u>between SS</u> is the measure of variation between the group means and the grand mean.

TABLE 10.2 Data Summaries for 2XANOVA Calculations

	6 HOURS		7 HOURS		8 HOURS			
	X	X^2	X	X^2	X	X^2		
MALE	4	16	17	289	12	144		
	10	100	18	324	13	169		
	9	81	15	225	11	121		
ΣX	23		50		36		$\Sigma X_{(row)}$	109
ΣX^2		197		838		434	$\Sigma X^2_{(row)}$	1469
n	3		3		3		$n_{(row)}$	9
FEMALE	6	36	6	36	10	100		
	2	4	8	64	17	289		
	4	16	4	16	9	81		
ΣX	12		18		36		$\Sigma X_{(row)}$	66
ΣX^2		56		116		470	$\Sigma X^2_{(row)}$	642
n	3		3		3		$n_{(row)}$	9
$\Sigma X_{(col)}$	35		68		72			
$\Sigma X^2_{(col)}$		253		954		904		
$n_{(col)}$	6		6		6			

The within SS (the error measure) is the measure of variation of the group scores around their own group means.

The "new" measures represent the following sources of variation:

- Row SS measure the variation of the row means (shift level means in the example) in reference to the grand mean.
- Column SS measure the variation of the column means (hours of sleep means in the example) in reference to the grand mean.
- Interaction SS measures the variations of row means at levels of the column means in reference to the grand mean.

Table 10.2 shows the data in Table 10.1 with the key calculations needed for the 2XANOVA. As you can see, there are totals for the individual cells as well as separate summaries for columns and rows.

Calculating SS_T (all six "cells" are included in the equation):

$$SS = \sum X^2 - \frac{(\sum X)^2}{N}$$

$$SS_T = (197 + 838 + 434 + 56 + 116 + 470)(-)\frac{(23 + 50 + 36 + 12 + 18 + 36)^2}{18}$$

$$= 2111 - 1701.39$$

$$SS_T = \mathbf{409.61}$$

Calculating SS_B (including the six cell means):

$$SS_B = \frac{(\sum X_1)^2}{n_1} + \frac{(\sum X_2)^2}{n_2} + \frac{(\sum X_3)^2}{n_3} + \frac{(\sum X_4)^2}{n_4} + \frac{(\sum X_5)^2}{n_5}$$

$$+ \frac{(\sum X_6)^2}{n_6} (-) \frac{(\sum X)^2}{N}$$

$$SS_B = \frac{(23)^2}{3} + \frac{(50)^2}{3} + \frac{(36)^2}{3} + \frac{(12)^2}{3} + \frac{(18)^2}{3} + \frac{(\sum 36)^2}{3}$$

$$(-) \frac{(23 + 50 + 36 + 12 + 18 + 36)^2}{18}$$

$$= 2029.67(-) 1701.39$$

$$SS_B = \mathbf{328.28}$$

Calculating SS_W (including the six cell values):

$$SS_W = SS_T - SS_B$$

$$= 409.61 - 328.28$$

$$SS_W = \mathbf{81.33}$$

Calculating the $SS_{(Rows)}$ (the main effect of sex):

$$SS_{(Rows)} = \frac{\left(\sum row1\right)^2}{n_1} + \frac{\left(\sum row2\right)^2}{n_2} (-) \frac{\left(\sum X\right)^2}{N}$$

$$= \frac{(109)^2}{9} + \frac{(66)^2}{9} (-) 1701.39$$

$$= 1804.111 (-) 1701.39$$

$$SS_{(Rows)} = \mathbf{102.72}$$

Calculating the $SS_{(columns)}$ (the main effect of sleep hours):

$$SS_{(columns)} = \frac{\left(\sum col1\right)^2}{n_1} + \frac{\left(\sum col2\right)^2}{n_2} + \frac{\left(\sum col3\right)^2}{n_3} (-) \frac{\left(\sum X\right)^2}{N}$$

$$= \frac{(35)^2}{6} + \frac{(68)^2}{6} + \frac{(72)^2}{6} (-) 1701.39$$

$$= 1838.83 (-) 1701.39$$

$$SS_{(columns)} = \mathbf{137.44}$$

Calculating the interaction:

Like the SS_W you can calculate the interaction SS (symbolized as SS_{rXc}) by subtracting the SS for rows and columns from the overall SS between as follows:

$$SS_{rXc} = SS_B - (SS_{(Rows)} + SS_{(columns)})$$

$$= 328.28 - (102.72 + 137.44)$$

$$SS_{rXc} = \mathbf{88.12}$$

The 2XANOVA Summary Table

Just as you did with the one-way ANOVA, you can now create the ANOVA summary table for the 2XANOVA. It has two rows to show each of the main effects and a separate row to show the interaction effect, but it is otherwise the same as the one-way table. Table 10.3 shows the summary table with the calculated SS values included.

Recall that the ANOVA is an inferential process, so you need to estimate the population variances (MS values) from the sample variances (SS values). You need the degrees of freedom to create the estimates appropriately. These are a bit different from the one-way ANOVAs since you are estimating different values, but the basics are the same. Here are the ways to calculate the various degrees of freedom:

$df_{Total} = N - 1$ (the overall number of observations minus 1)
$df_{Row} = r - 1$ (the number of rows minus 1)
$df_{Col} = c - 1$ (the number of columns minus 1)

$df_{rxc} = (r-1)(c-1)$ (i.e., (number of rows -1) $\times$ (number of columns -1); or,
$df_{Row} \times df_{Col}$)
$df_W = N -$ the number of cells

TABLE 10.3   The 2XANOVA Summary Table

Source of Variance	SS	df	MS	F
Between	328.28			
Row Main Effect (Sex)	102.72			
Column Main Effect (Sleep)	137.44			
Interaction Effect (Sex X Sleep)	88.12			
Within (Error)	81.33			
Total	409.61			

Creating the MS Values

In the one-way ANOVA, you used the following formula to calculate the F ratio:

$$F = \frac{MS_B}{MS_W}$$

This formula simply compared the between to the within sums of squares in order to see if the group means were far apart relative to the (error) variance within each of the sample groups. With 2XANOVA, you do the same thing, except that you calculate the F values for each of the three effects (main effects and interaction effect) by dividing each by the overall MS_W:

$$F_{row} = \frac{MS_{row}}{MS_W}; \quad F_{col} = \frac{MS_{col}}{MS_W}; \quad F_{rxc} = \frac{MS_{rxc}}{MS_W}$$

Table 10.4 shows the completed 2XANOVA summary table with the values calculated earlier. Using the F ratios for the various components of the study, you can proceed with hypotheses tests to determine whether the F ratios are in the exclusion area of the comparison distribution and therefore not likely to occur by chance.

THE HYPOTHESES TEST: INTERPRETING FACTORIAL ANOVA RESULTS

Table 10.4 shows the F table values in the last column. These values indicate the 0.05 exclusion region. Thus, any F ratio larger than the tabled values would be considered significant at the $p < 0.05$ level. According to the table, the omnibus test, the main effects and the interaction effect are all significant. Thus, their F ratio values are too high to be expected to occur by chance (at the 0.05 level).

TABLE 10.4   The Completed 2XANOVA Summary Table

Source of Variance	SS	df	MS	F
Between	328.28	5	65.66	9.68*
Row Main Effect (Sex)	102.72	1	102.72	15.15*
Column Main Effect (Sleep Hours)	137.44	2	68.72	10.14*
Interaction Effect (Sex X Sleep)	88.12	2	44.05	6.50*
Within (Error)	81.33	12	6.78	
Total	409.61	17		

*Indicates the value is significant beyond $p < .01$.

The Omnibus F Ratio

When I tested the one-way ANOVA, I created the omnibus F ratio, a transformed ratio of the sample values applied to the comparison distribution in order to assess whether the sample values were likely a chance finding. In 2XANOVA, the focus is on the <u>F ratios of the specific row, column, and interaction effects</u> to determine the same thing. That is why they can be computed by adding the SS values for the main effects and the interaction effects. This will provide an overall $SS_{Between}$ value that can yield the omnibus F ratio. Thus,

$$SS_{Between} = SS_{row} + SS_{col} + SS_{r \times c}$$

$$= 102.72 + 137.44 + 88.12$$

$$SS_{Between} = 328.28$$

The $MS_{Between}$ can then be calculated by dividing the $SS_{Between}$ by its df measure (in this example, it is 5 since it combines the df measures for the three effects):

$$MS_{Between} = \frac{SS_{Between}}{df_{Between}}$$

$$= \frac{328.28}{5}$$

$$MS_{Between} = 65.656$$

The omnibus F ratio can be calculated by using the $MS_{Between}$ value divided by the MS_{Within} value as in the one-way ANOVA:

$$F = \frac{MS_B}{MS_W}$$

$$= \frac{65.656}{6.78}$$

$$F = 9.68$$

EFFECT SIZE FOR 2XANOVA: PARTIAL η^2

Just as with one-way ANOVA, you need to understand the effect size of the study. With one independent variable, it was a simple matter to calculate η^2, which expresses the proportion of the total variance in the outcome variable explained by the independent variable groups:

$$\eta^2 = \frac{SS_{Between}}{SS_{Total}}$$

You can calculate the "omnibus" effect size as follows:

$$\eta^2 = \frac{SS_{Between}}{SS_{Total}}$$
$$= \frac{328.28}{409.61}$$
$$\eta^2 = 0.80$$

This value expresses the combined impact of the groups of sex and sleep hours on the health measure. Thus the combined groupings explain 80% (expressing 0.80 as a percentage) of the outcome measure of health.

Since the study added another independent variable, however, you can "break the overall explained variance down" into its specific proportions. The procedure creates three proportions of the total variance that can be so measured. The effect size for 2XANOVA is therefore known as "Partial Eta Squared" or "Partial η^2." It is partial because it is not an overall measure. Rather, it "partials out" the overall variance so that *only the contribution of the specific main effect (or interaction effect) is measured on the total variance explained.*

Since the SS_W is the error measure in ANOVA, you have to take it into account in the overall assessment of calculating the F ratios and the effect sizes as well. The following is a "conceptual equation" explaining how effect size works for partial effects:

$$\text{Partial } \eta^2 = \frac{SS_{Effect}}{SS_{Effect} + SS_W}$$

As you can see, the SS measure for the specific effect (main effect and/or interaction effect) is divided by the same SS measure plus the SS_W. The reasoning is that the bottom part of the equation constitutes the *total SS for the particular effect under consideration.* Thus, the formula yields a *percentage of variance explained in the dependent variable that is provided by the proportion of the specific effect relative to its error measure.*

Here is how Partial η^2 is calculated for each main effect:
Effect size for row main effect (sex):

$$\text{Partial } \eta^2_{row} = \frac{SS_{row}}{SS_{row} + SS_W}$$
$$= \frac{102.722}{102.722 + 81.333}$$
$$\text{Partial } \eta^2_{row} = 0.558$$

Effect size for column main effect (sleep):

$$\text{Partial } \eta^2_{\text{col}} = \frac{SS_{\text{col}}}{SS_{\text{col}} + SS_W}$$

$$= \frac{137.44}{137.44 + 81.33}$$

$$\text{Partial } \eta^2_{\text{col}} = 0.628$$

Effect size for interaction effect (sex × sleep):

$$\text{Partial } \eta^2_{r \times c} = \frac{SS_{r \times c}}{SS_{r \times c} + SS_W}$$

$$= \frac{88.11}{88.11 + 81.33}$$

$$\text{Partial } \eta^2_{r \times c} = 0.52$$

The question of the effect size "meaningfulness" is a matter for the researcher to decide. The following guidelines can be used for assessing η^2: 0.01 (small), 0.06 (medium), and 0.15 (large). Since these are measures for the "omnibus" effect size, they may be too large for the partial measures. However, they do provide some benchmark for judging the magnitude of partial η^2 results.

DISCUSSING THE RESULTS

As you saw in Table 10.4, the omnibus test, the main effects for both sex and sleep, and the interaction effect are all significant. Thus, sex and sleep taken together significantly affect the health measure (since the omnibus test was significant). The results are inconsistent among the various groups of the factors however. The researchers task is now to "dig deeper" into the findings to understand the specific contributions of each of the levels of the factors upon the outcome measure.

I mentioned earlier that *when there is a significant interaction effect in the 2XANOVA, this finding takes precedence over the main effects findings.* Since there are inconsistent values of one variable on values of the other variable (as indicated by the significant interaction), you need to examine the interaction findings before other values. The two ways to do this are by graphing the interaction and examining simple effects. I will show one of the plots from the SPSS analysis that shows the interaction, and then I will discuss the simple effects findings in a separate section in the following when I discuss the SPSS output.

Figure 10.4 shows the three sleep lines for both males and females. As you can see, there is a disordinal interaction between these two factors on the outcome measure of health values. The three sleep categories are different for males than they are for females. We will disentangle the statistical findings for these differences in the following, but you can see that the males' health values are almost evenly divided among the sleep levels while females appear to indicate differences from between 6 hours and both of the other sleep hour levels.

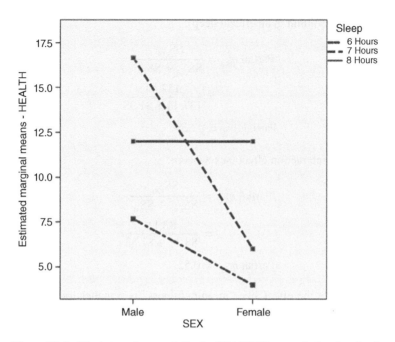

Figure 10.4 The interaction graph for the 2XANOVA example (sex by sleep).

The simple effects analyses are produced by SPSS, but you can view the plots for each. The simple slope questions for males and females health scores among the different sleep categories are:

- Are the health differences among 6, 7, and 8 hours of sleep among males large enough to be considered statistically significant? If so, which?
- Are the health differences among 6, 7, and 8 hours of sleep among females large enough to be considered statistically significant? If so, which?

The trends among both males and females appear to show differences depending on the category of sleep. But are they "different enough" to be considered significant? You could calculate the simple effects manually, but most researchers rely on statistical programs to help assess all the findings for 2XANOVA.

Excel does not have a straightforward method for assessing 2XANOVA. One procedure exists for "ANOVA: Two-Factor Without Replication," but there is no provision for examining interaction effects.

SPSS has a straightforward way to create the complete 2XANOVA procedure including interaction effects. Examining simple effects is not immediately apparent through the main menus however. The researcher must rely on "syntax" statements that create the appropriate output for simple effects. Syntax is akin to programming within SPSS. It is not as intimidating as it sounds because the program includes "macro-like" statements that the researcher can use to create custom output. I will discuss the syntax statements for simple effects in the following section.

USING SPSS® TO ANALYZE 2XANOVA

Figure 10.5 shows the data file structure for the SPSS 2XANOVA analysis. As you can see, the dependent variable (HEALTH) is listed with its raw score values in the third column, and the first two columns show the two study factors (i.e., independent variables). The SES categories are 1 = male and 2 = female. Sleep categories are 1 = 6 hours, 2 = 7 hours, and 3 = 8 hours.

The data file is laid out in such a way that SPSS will analyze the data as I have shown it in the manual calculations. Taking the first three cases as an example, the health outcomes of 4, 10, and 9 are associated with the group of scores in the male category with 6 hours of sleep (see Table 10.2).

Once the file is created, you can access the 2XANOVA through the Analyze menu. Figure 10.6 shows the choices leading to the appropriate ANOVA. As you can see, the "General Linear Model" menu is chosen first. This general category includes procedures that allow the researcher to examine the linear effects of one or more independent variables on dependent variable(s). By choosing "Univariate" you specify procedures that include only one dependent variable.

You will note that this procedure is different from the procedure I discussed in Chapter 9 for one-way ANOVA. That procedure ("Explore – Compare Means – One-Way ANOVA" – see Figure 9.14) is a basic analysis designed only for one independent variable. The procedure I specified in Figure 10.6 is for multiple independent variables but only a single dependent variable. It can be used for a much more comprehensive analysis as you will see in the following.

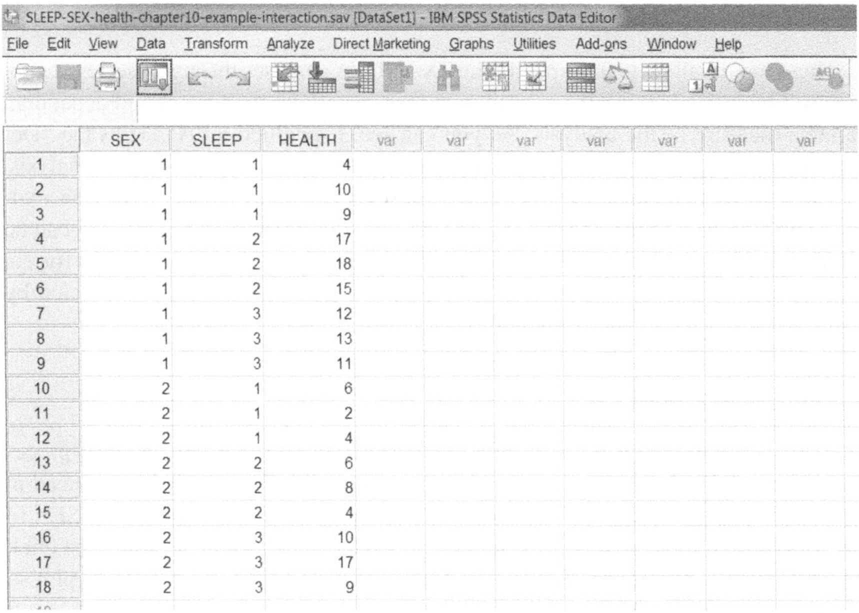

	SEX	SLEEP	HEALTH	var	var	var	var	var	var	var
1	1	1	4							
2	1	1	10							
3	1	1	9							
4	1	2	17							
5	1	2	18							
6	1	2	15							
7	1	3	12							
8	1	3	13							
9	1	3	11							
10	2	1	6							
11	2	1	2							
12	2	1	4							
13	2	2	6							
14	2	2	8							
15	2	2	4							
16	2	3	10							
17	2	3	17							
18	2	3	9							

Figure 10.5 The SPSS® data file for the 2XANOVA example.

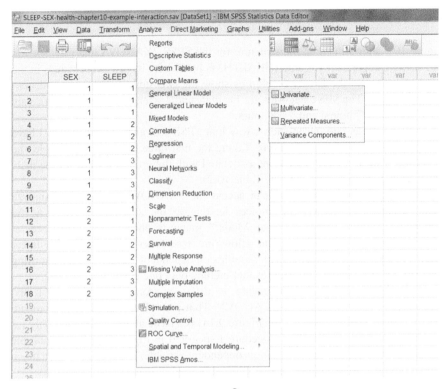

Figure 10.6   The SPSS® 2XANOVA menus.

These menus allow you to specify the 2XANOVA analyses through a series of sub-menus. Figure 10.7 shows the overall menu for specifying the factors and dependent variable measure of the analysis. As you can see, I specified HEALTH as the "Dependent Variable" and both SEX and SLEEP as the "Fixed Factor(s)" in this analysis.

The Univariate menu allows the researcher several choices for specifying the analysis. The buttons on the upper right side of the callout window in Figure 10.7 can be used to customize the output. In what follows, I will show a series of callouts for the 2XANOVA procedure for our example. More complex analyses can be created by researchers who gain experience with 2XANOVA.

The "Plots" Specification

This choice allows you to create plots of the factors and is a very helpful procedure. Figure 10.8 shows how to use the menus to specify the plot that I produced in Figure 10.4. As you can see, I created the "SEX*SLEEP" plot by specifying SEX in the "Horizontal Axis" and SLEEP in the "Separate Lines" window. You must click the "Add" button (located just above the Plots window) once you specify the plot so that it shows up in the Plots window.

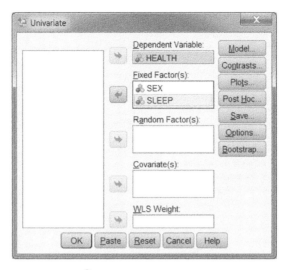

Figure 10.7   The SPSS® menus for specifying the 2XANOVA procedure.

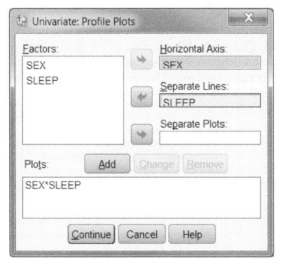

Figure 10.8   The Plots window that specifies the results graph.

The "Post Hoc" Specification

You can choose the next button "Post Hoc" from the Univariate window if you wish to examine the group differences. Figure 10.9 shows that I specified the Tukey test for sleep since it had more than two categories. This will be a helpful information; however many researchers prefer the simple effects analyses since there is a significant interaction.

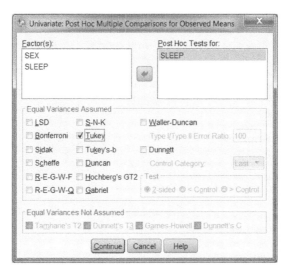

Figure 10.9   The "Post Hoc" window specifying the Tukey analysis for sleep.

The "Options" Specification

The "Univariate: Options" button is important for specifying further the kinds of output you wish to see. Figure 10.10 shows some of the choices you can make. For this example, I specified descriptive statistics and effect size estimates, along with the homogeneity test for equal variances. The "Estimated Marginal Means" shown in the upper part of the panel are *estimated population means for the cells*. This menu would help with the simple effects analyses.

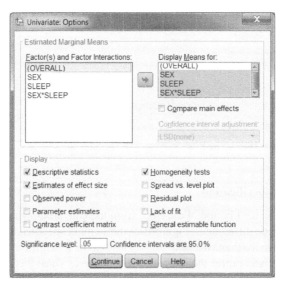

Figure 10.10   The choices in the "Univariate: Options" window.

Simple Effects

SPSS does not list simple effects analyses in the specification menu. Researchers must use SPSS "syntax" (a series of preprogrammed commands) in conjunction with the 2XANOVA procedure. The following syntax specification must be added to the procedure syntax in order to produce simple effects output (readers unfamiliar with SPSS syntax may want to note these for further study):

/EMMEANS = TABLES (SEX*SLEEP) comp (SEX)
/EMMEANS = TABLES (SLEEP*SEX) comp (SLEEP)

These statements enable the researcher to see two simple effects plots. The first shows sex and sleep on the same graph with separate lines for sex. The second shows separate lines for sleep. The latter is shown in Figure 10.4.

After the foregoing choices are made, the researcher can create the 2XANOVA by choosing "OK" on the main Univariate menu. In what follows, I will present some of the main parts of the SPSS output relevant to our example. Figure 10.11 shows the main summary table. You can compare the values in this table to the values I calculated manually earlier.

Omnibus Results

As you can see in Figure 10.11, two columns are added to the summary table that we did not include in the manual calculations. The "sig." column specifies whether, and how far, the transformed F ratio value falls into the comparison distribution. Thus, sig. values beyond 0.05 (i.e., less than 0.05) indicate that the F results fall further into

Tests of Between-Subjects Effects						
Dependent Variable: HEALTH						
Source	Type III Sum of Squares	df	Mean Square	F	Sig.	Partial Eta Squared
Corrected Model	328.278*	5	65.656	9.687	.001	.801
Intercept	1701.389	1	1701.389	251.025	.000	.954
SEX	102.722	1	102.722	15.156	.002	.558
SLEEP	137.444	2	68.722	10.139	.003	.628
SEX * SLEEP	88.111	2	44.056	6.500	.012	.520
Error	81.333	12	6.778			
Total	2111.000	18				
Corrected Total	409.611	17				

*R Squared = .801 (Adjusted R^2 = .719).

Figure 10.11   The SPSS® 2XANOVA summary table.

the exclusion region and are considered significant. All the F ratio study values are significant (main effects: SEX and SLEEP, and the interaction (SEX*SLEEP) effect).

The "Partial η^2" values match those I calculated manually. One note here is that the Partial Eta Squared for the Corrected Model (0.478) shown in Figure 10.11 is actually the omnibus η^2. The "Corrected Model" results represent the omnibus between variance measures. The "Corrected Total" variance measure represents the Total variance measure.

Figure 10.11 results indicate that the significant interaction will take precedence in the discussion and findings of these data. Had the interaction not been significant, you could have proceeded to examine the results for each main effect separately. In what follows, I will discuss the simple effects findings since the interaction was significant.

Simple Effects Analyses

When you include the appropriate syntax instructions for simple effects, SPSS produces simple effects tables showing separate F tests for each level of one variable across the levels of the second factor. Figure 10.12 shows the simple effects table for sex within each of the sleep levels Each row of this table represents a separate F test of sex within that particular level.

As you can see from Figure 10.12, the category of findings for 7 hours assesses whether male and female health values differ for those reporting 7 hours of sleep. The F ratio (25.180) is significant ($p = 0.000$), which indicates that males and females are significantly different in health values among those reporting 7 hours of sleep.[2] Male

Univariate Tests							
Dependent Variable: HEALTH							
SLEEP		Sum of Squares	df	Mean Square	F	Sig.	Partial Eta Squared
6 HOURS	Contrast	20.167	1	20.167	2.975	.110	.199
	Error	81.333	12	6.778			
7 HOURS	Contrast	170.667	1	170.667	25.180	.000	.677
	Error	81.333	12	6.778			
8 HOURS	Contrast	.000	1	.000	.000	1.000	.000
	Error	81.333	12	6.778			

Each F tests the simple effects of SEX within each level combination of the other effects shown. These tests are based on the linearly independent pairwise comparisons among the estimated marginal means.

Figure 10.12 The SPSS® simple effects table for levels of schools on subject areas.

---

[2]Remember that a significance level of "0.000" as reported by SPSS is shorthand for a very small "actual" probability. You may want to simply report "$p < 0.001$" to indicate a very small chance probability.

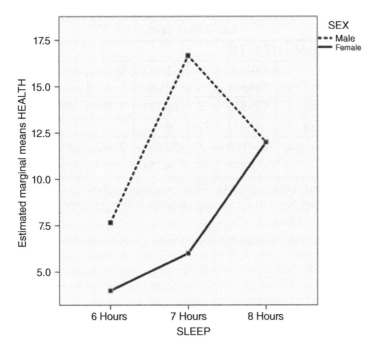

Figure 10.13 The simple effects graph for the 2XANOVA example (sleep by sex).

and female health values are not significantly different from each other among those reporting either 6 or 8 hours of sleep.

The plot in Figure 10.13 shows these simple effects results. Like the plot in Figure 10.4, this figure shows how the dependent variable (Health) scores on each level of one factor change across levels of the other factor. In Figure 10.13, the plot provides a visual description of the simple effects reported in Figure 10.12. The health values for males and females is furthest apart (significantly so) within the 7 hours category whereas they are equivalent in the 8 hours category, and relatively close within the 6 hours category.

Figure 10.14 shows the other simple effects analysis. In this table, both the uni-variate tests for sleep levels within sex categories are significant (male: $F = 8.967$, $p = 0.004$; female: $F = 7.672$, $p = 0.007$). This analysis indicates that the different sleep levels appear to show significantly different health scores within male and female categories.[3] Separate tables in the SPSS output allow you to pinpoint the pairwise differences.

Figure 10.4 is a plot of this simple effect analysis. As you can see, males show health values for 6-, 7-, and 8-hour categories that appear almost equidistant from one another. Females indicate large health differences between those reporting 8 hours versus those reporting either 6 or 7 hours.

[3]The differences between 6 and 8 hours for males is $p < 0.06$, not significant, but nearly so.

Univariate Tests							
Dependent Variable: HEALTH							
SEX		Sum of Squares	df	Mean Square	F	Sig.	Partial Eta Squared
MALE	Contrast	121.556	2	60.778	8.967	.004	.599
	Error	81.333	12	6.778			
FEMALE	Contrast	104.000	2	52.000	7.672	.007	.561
	Error	81.333	12	6.778			

Each F tests the simple effects of SLEEP within each level combination of the other effects shown. These tests are based on the linearly independent pairwise comparisons among the estimated marginal means.

Figure 10.14   The SPSS® simple effects table for sleep within male and female categories.

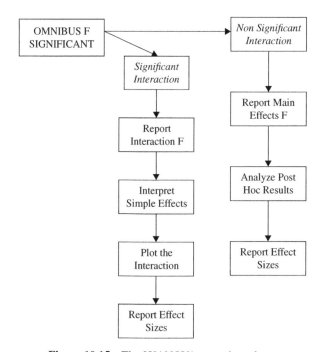

Figure 10.15   The 2XANOVA procedure chart.

SUMMARY CHART FOR 2XANOVA PROCEDURES

The procedures for 2XANOVA may seem complex compared to those for one-way ANOVA, but they are straightforward. SPSS provides a thorough series of output to help with the simple effects analyses, which seem to be the most time-consuming aspects. Figure 10.15 is a procedural flow chart for 2XANOVA that you might consider as you prepare to use the procedure with your data.

TERMS AND CONCEPTS

Analysis of covariance (ANCOVA):	An ANOVA-type design that limits the influence of a variable or variables outside the design (known as "covariates") that might affect the results.
Disordinal interactions:	Interactions indicated by graph lines that cross in the plot area.
Factorial ANOVA:	A designation indicating an ANOVA with more than one independent variable (i.e., factor).
Interaction effects:	When *the relationship between one predictor and the outcome variable changes at different levels of another predictor variable* (see Abbott, 2010).
MANCOVA (multivariate ANCOVA):	The statistical procedure that uses ANCOVA with multiple dependent variables.
MANOVA (multivariate ANOVA):	The statistical procedure that uses ANOVA with multiple dependent variables.
Multivariate:	The designation in statistical analyses indicating more than one dependent variable.
Ordinal interactions:	Interactions that may not cross in the plot area but which may cross if the lines were continued outside the plot area.
Partial η^2:	The effect size measure expressing the proportion of the total variance explained by an independent variable when other influences are controlled.
Simple effects:	Differences (outcome) in the categories of one variable within single categories of another variable.
SPSS® syntax:	Preprogrammed commands used in SPSS procedures.
Univariate:	The designation in statistical analyses indicating one dependent variable.
Within-subjects ANOVA:	Indicating an ANOVA used for repeated measures, either the same group of subjects or subjects in matched groups.

DATA LAB AND EXAMPLES (WITH SOLUTIONS)

Problem 1

Is patient satisfaction different for two medical conditions when attended by different providers? Table 10.5 shows the satisfaction ratings of patients (scale: 0–10, with higher numbers indicating greater satisfaction) for two different medical conditions (coronary artery disease and diabetes) among different medical providers (APN, MD, and PA).

Directions:

- Calculate the factorial ANOVA manually and interpret findings.
- Report and interpret effect size.

TABLE 10.5   Patient Satisfaction Ratings of Providers and Medical Conditions

	Provider		
	APN	MD	PA
Coronary Artery Disease	2	9	5
	5	8	7
Diabetes	9	2	5
	9	3	6

Problem 2

Use SPSS to analyze the data presented in Problem 1. Use the General Linear Model – Univariate program to present and discuss the following:

- Simple effects tests for both factors
- Pairwise comparisons for both simple effects analyses
- Profile plots for both simple effects

DATA LAB: SOLUTIONS

Problem 1

Solutions

Manual Calculations: Tables 10.6 and 10.7 show the manual calculations and ANOVA summary table, respectively, for Problem 1. As you see, the omnibus F (10.15) is significant indicating some significant differences among the data. Also, there is a significant interaction ($F = 24.812$), which takes precedence in the interpretation.

TABLE 10.6 Manual Calculations for Problem 1

		APN		MD		PA			
		X	X^2	X	X^2	X	X^2		
Coronary Artery Disease		2	4	9	81	5	25		
		5	25	8	64	7	49		
	ΣX	7		17		12		$\Sigma X_{(row)}$	36
	ΣX^2		29		145		74	$\Sigma X^2_{(row)}$	248
	n	2		2		2		$n_{(row)}$	6
Diabetes		9	81	2	4	5	25		
		9	81	3	9	6	36		
	ΣX	18		5		11		$\Sigma X_{(row)}$	34
	ΣX^2		162		13		61	$\Sigma X^2_{(row)}$	236
	n	2		2		2		$n_{(row)}$	6
$\Sigma X_{(col)}$		25		22		23			
$\Sigma X^2_{(col)}$			191		158		135		
$n_{(col)}$		4		4		4			

Calculating SS_T (all six "cells" are included in the equation):

$$SS_T = \sum X^2 - \frac{\left(\sum X\right)^2}{N}$$

$$= (484)(-)\frac{(70)^2}{12}$$

$$= 484 - 408.33$$

$$SS_T = 75.67$$

Calculating SS_B (including the six cell means):

$$SS_B = \frac{\left(\sum X_1\right)^2}{n_1} + \frac{\left(\sum X_2\right)^2}{n_2} + \frac{\left(\sum X_3\right)^2}{n_3} + \frac{\left(\sum X_4\right)^2}{n_4} + \frac{\left(\sum X_5\right)^2}{n_5}$$

$$+ \frac{\left(\sum X_6\right)^2}{n_6}(-)\frac{\left(\sum X\right)^2}{N}$$

$$= \frac{(7)^2}{2} + \frac{(17)^2}{2} + \frac{(12)^2}{2} + \frac{(18)^2}{2} + \frac{(5)^2}{2} + \frac{(11)^2}{2}(-)\frac{(70)^2}{12}$$

$$= 476 \, (-) \, 408.33$$

$$SS_B = 67.67$$

Calculating SS_W (including the six cell values):

$$SS_W = SS_T - SS_B$$

$$= 75.67 - 67.67$$

$$SS_W = 8.00$$

Calculating the $SS_{(Rows)}$ (the main effect of condition):

$$SS_{(Rows)} = \frac{\left(\sum row1\right)^2}{n_1} + \frac{\left(\sum row2\right)^2}{n_2} (-) \frac{\left(\sum X\right)^2}{N}$$

$$= \frac{(36)^2}{6} + \frac{(34)^2}{6}(-)408.33$$

$$= 408.67 \, (-)408.33$$

$$SS_{(Rows)} = 0.334$$

Calculating the $SS_{(columns)}$ (the main effect of provider):

$$SS_{(columns)} = \frac{\left(\sum col1\right)^2}{n_1} + \frac{\left(\sum col2\right)^2}{n_2} + \frac{\left(\sum col3\right)^2}{n_3} (-) \frac{\left(\sum X\right)^2}{N}$$

$$= \frac{(25)^2}{4} + \frac{(22)^2}{4} + \frac{(23)^2}{4} \, (-) \, 408.33$$

$$= 409.50 \, (-) \, 408.33$$

$$SS_{(columns)} = 1.17$$

$$SS_{r \times c} = SS_B - (SS_{(Rows)} + SS_{(columns)})$$

$$= 67.67 - (0.334 + 1.17)$$

$$SS_{r \times c} = 66.17$$

TABLE 10.7   ANOVA Table for Problem 1

Source of Variance	SS	df	MS	F
Between	67.67	5	13.53	10.15*
Row Main Effect (Condition)	.33	1	.33	.25
Column Main Effect (Provider)	1.17	2	.58	.436
Interaction Effect (Cond. X Prov.)	66.17	2	33.08	24.87*
Within (Error)	8.00	6	1.33	
Total	75.67	11		

*Significant at or beyond p < .001.

Problem 1

Effect Size

$$\eta^2 = \frac{SS_{Between}}{SS_{Total}}$$

$$= \frac{67.67}{75.67} = 0.894$$

The <u>omnibus effect size</u> of 0.894 indicates that 89.4% of the variance in patient satisfaction is due to the combination of condition and provider. The <u>partial effect sizes</u> are

Effect size for row main effect (condition):

$$\text{Partial } \eta^2_{\text{row}} = \frac{SS_{\text{row}}}{SS_{\text{row}} + SS_W}$$

$$= \frac{0.333}{0.333 + 8.00}$$

$$\text{Partial } \eta^2_{\text{row}} = 0.04$$

Effect size for column main effect (provider):

$$\text{Partial } \eta^2_{\text{col}} = \frac{SS_{\text{col}}}{SS_{\text{col}} + SS_W}$$

$$= \frac{1.167}{1.167 + 8.00}$$

$$\text{Partial } \eta^2_{\text{col}} = 0.127$$

Effect size for interaction effect (condition × provider):

$$\text{Partial } \eta^2_{r\times c} = \frac{SS_{r\times c}}{SS_{r\times c} + SS_W}$$

$$= \frac{66.167}{66.167 + 8}$$

$$\text{Partial } \eta^2_{r\times c} = 0.892$$

Problem 2: Solutions

Simple Effects Tests for Both Factors

These tests are based on adding the following syntax statements to the specification for the General Linear Model – Univariate procedure:

Univariate Tests							
Dependent Variable: Satisfaction							
Provider		Sum of Squares	df	Mean Square	F	Sig.	Partial Eta Squared
APN	Contrast	30.250	1	30.250	22.688	.003	.791
	Error	8.000	6	1.333			
MD	Contrast	36.000	1	36.000	27.000	.002	.818
	Error	8.000	6	1.333			
PA	Contrast	.250	1	.250	.188	.680	.030
	Error	8.000	6	1.333			

Each F tests the simple effects of Condition within each level combination of the other effects shown. These tests are based on the linearly independent pairwise comparisons among the estimated marginal means.

Pairwise Comparisons							
Dependent Variable: Satisfaction							
Provider	(I) Condition	(J) Condition	Mean Difference (I-J)	Std. Error	Sig.[b]	95% Confidence Interval for Difference[b]	
						Lower Bound	Upper Bound
APN	Coronary Artery Disease	Diabetes	-5.500*	1.155	.003	-8.325	-2.675
	Diabetes	Coronary Artery Disease	5.500*	1.155	.003	2.675	8.325
MD	Coronary Artery Disease	Diabetes	6.000*	1.155	.002	3.175	8.825
	Diabetes	Coronary Artery Disease	-6.000*	1.155	.002	-8.825	-3.175
PA	Coronary Artery Disease	Diabetes	.500	1.155	.680	-2.325	3.325
	Diabetes	Coronary Artery Disease	-.500	1.155	.680	-3.325	2.325

Based on estimated marginal means.

*The mean difference is significant at the .05 level.

[b] Adjustment for multiple comparisons: Least Significant Difference (equivalent to no adjustments).

Figure 10.16   The simple effects analyses for condition.

/EMMEANS = TABLES (Condition*Provider) comp (Condition)
/EMMEANS = TABLES (Provider*Condition) comp (Provider)

Simple Effects Tests and Pairwise Comparisons for Both Simple Effects Analyses (with Profile Plots)

Figure 10.16 shows the simple effects of condition within each level combination of the other factor. As you can see, both APN and MD show significant differences between the condition levels of CAD and diabetes.

The pairwise comparison output in Figure 10.16 shows the following:

- Diabetes satisfaction is higher for APN.
- CAD satisfaction is higher for APN.

These findings are evident in the plot shown in Figure 10.17.

Figure 10.18 shows the simple effects analyses for provider within the categories of condition. As you can see, both APN and MD show significant differences in the CAD condition, whereas all the providers are different from one another in the diabetes condition.

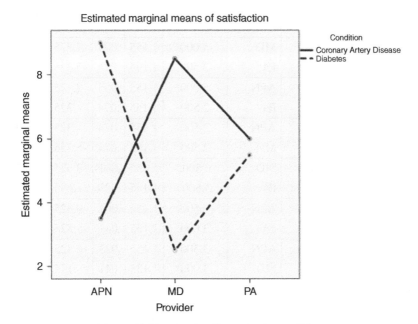

Figure 10.17   Simple effects plot for condition.

Univariate Tests							
Dependent Variable: Satisfaction							
Condition		Sum of Squares	df	Mean Square	F	Sig.	Partial Eta Squared
Coronary Artery Disease	Contrast	25.000	2	12.500	9.375	.014	.758
	Error	8.000	6	1.333			
Diabetes	Contrast	42.333	2	21.167	15.875	.004	.841
	Error	8.000	6	1.333			

Each F tests the simple effects of Provider within each level combination of the other effects shown. These tests are based on the linearly independent pairwise comparisons among the estimated marginal means.

Pairwise Comparisons							
Dependent Variable: Satisfaction							
Condition	(I) Provider	(J) Provider	Mean Difference (I-J)	Std. Error	Sig.[b]	95% Confidence Interval for Difference[b]	
						Lower Bound	Upper Bound
Coronary Artery Disease	APN	MD	-5.000*	1.155	.005	-7.825	-2.175
		PA	-2.500	1.155	.074	-5.325	.325
	MD	APN	5.000*	1.155	.005	2.175	7.825
		PA	2.500	1.155	.074	-.325	5.325
	PA	APN	2.500	1.155	.074	-.325	5.325
		MD	-2.500	1.155	.074	-5.325	.325
Diabetes	APN	MD	6.500*	1.155	.001	3.675	9.325
		PA	3.500*	1.155	.023	.675	6.325
	MD	APN	-6.500*	1.155	.001	-9.325	-3.675
		PA	-3.000*	1.155	.041	-5.825	-.175
	PA	APN	-3.500*	1.155	.023	-6.325	-.675
		MD	3.000*	1.155	.041	.175	5.825

Based on estimated marginal means.
*The mean difference is significant at the .05 level.
[b]Adjustment for multiple comparisons: Least Significant Difference (equivalent to no adjustments).

Figure 10.18   Simple effects analyses for provider.

The pairwise comparison output in Figure 10.18 shows the following:

- MDs show higher CAD satisfaction than APNs.
- APNs show highest satisfaction ratings for diabetes, followed by PAs and then MDs.

These findings are evident in the plot shown in Figure 10.19.

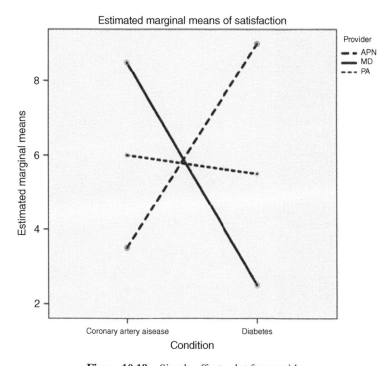

Figure 10.19 Simple effects plot for provider.

11

CORRELATION

Correlation has an intuitive appeal. Most everyone understands that correlation is concerned with whether changes in one thing are linked to changes in something else. Thus, for example, you may observe that wealthier people seem to have better overall health than those with lower wealth levels. Or, stated differently, as wealth increases, health increases as well.

Correlation is a way of understanding the association between two variables. What does association mean? It refers to "relatedness" or the extent to which two events "vary with one another." To use this language with the wealth–health example just cited, you might say that the increase in wealth (however it is measured) is accompanied by increases in health (according to its measures). In a general sense, you can say that the values of the one variable (health) change positively as the values of the other variable (wealth) increase. Thus, the values of both variables increase together, or "covary."

Not every correlation is what it seems, however. There may be additional variables not taken into account in the analysis that give the original two variables the "appearance of covarying." This possibility of spuriousness (see Chapter 2) hints at the complexity of a seemingly obvious relationship. Is it really wealth that results in health, or is it something (or things) else? In this and the following chapters on regression, I intend to explore this question further.

Using Statistics in the Social and Health Sciences with SPSS® and Excel®, First Edition.
Martin Lee Abbott.
© 2017 John Wiley & Sons, Inc. Published 2017 by John Wiley & Sons, Inc.

THE NATURE OF CORRELATION

I will examine correlation in some depth in this chapter. It is a useful procedure for many reasons, and several methods of calculating correlations exist that are adapted to the different natures of possible research questions.

Explore and Predict

Evaluators use correlation to *explore* the relationships among a series of variables they suspect may be important to a research question. Other evaluators may use correlation to help *predict* an outcome knowing that the predictor and the outcome variables are related. Explanation and prediction are two important uses of correlation.

Different Measurement Values

Correlation is somewhat unusual in that the researcher can assess the relationship between two variables that have widely differing values. For example, a researcher may operationally define "wealth" as simply income and health as the number of visits a person makes to the doctor in a year. These measures create two different sorts of scores. The wealth values, as income, may range from (theoretically) 0$ to millions, while health values typically range from none to an upper number of less than 100.[1]

Different Data Levels

In the foregoing example, the researcher can measure the association between two differently measured variables because they assess how one score changes as the other score changes. Thus, both variables do not have to be measured with the same *values*. Correlation measures are so powerful that a researcher can also calculate the correlation of two variables measured with different *levels of data* (i.e., interval, ordinal, or nominal). A researcher might correlate wealth as income (ratio level) to self-reported health on a questionnaire (ordinal level) as "A Lot, Some, A Little, or None."

Correlation Measures

In this chapter, I discuss correlation measures that can be used with two interval- or ratio-level variables. Table 11.1 shows some *additional* correlation measures that can be calculated with variables of different levels of data. There are many others, but this should help you appreciate the flexibility of the procedure.

As you can see, there are several measures of correlation that can be "customized" for the specific nature of the researcher's study question. The first three columns of Table 11.1 show measures of correlation that use different levels of data. The italicized correlation measures are those that use "artificial" measures. For example, the

---

[1] Typically, according to the BRFSS database.

TABLE 11.1   Measures of Correlation

Correlation Measures			
Nominal Level Data	**Ordinal Level Data**	**Nominal by Ordinal**	Proportional Reduction in Error (PRE)
Contingency Coefficient	Spearman's Rho	*Biserial*	η^2 Partial η^2 r^2
Phi Coefficient	Kendall's Tau	Point Biserial	Gamma
Cramer's V			(Cohen's) Kappa
Tetrachoric			

tetrachoric correlation measures two continuous (interval-level) variables that have been *dichotomized*. A researcher may use this procedure by categorizing income as high, medium, or low and also measuring health as "weak" or "strong." Both of these are continuous variables, but some researchers dichotomize them for various reasons (despite the fact that it isn't a good idea!). Tetrachoric correlation might measure the relationship between these two variables or other dichotomized variables.

Table 11.1 also shows a column (the fourth column) of measures known as proportional reduction in error (PRE) measures. I have already discussed some of those measures at the interval level (η^2 and partial η^2), but there are several others at different levels of data (indicated in Table 11.1 in different shades), for example, gamma for ordinal and Cohen's kappa for nominal data. These are measures in which correlation is used to "reduce error." You saw in Chapter 9 (one-way ANOVA) that η^2 is a measure of how much variance in the outcome variable is explained by the categories of the predictor variable. That is, how much variation (error) is <u>reduced</u> by knowing the relationship between the two variables? Eta square and other such measures are expressed in the amount of *variance explained*.

We cannot hope to cover all of these in this book. I wanted you to see the tremendous variety of correlation measures; and there are yet more measures I didn't include in Table 11.1. I will discuss Pearson's correlation coefficient in this chapter which is the most common correlation procedure with interval data.

THE CORRELATION DESIGN

The correlation study is a post facto design since the researcher is *relating* two sets of scores that have been gathered on an individual case. You would not use correlation in an experimental design since in the latter, you attempt to detect *differences* in group scores after an intervention. Correlation measures "sameness" and an experiment measures "difference." Multiple regression procedures, which are based on correlation, can be used in experimental designs under certain circumstances (see Abbott, 2010).

PEARSON'S CORRELATION COEFFICIENT

Named after Karl Pearson, Pearson's correlation coefficient, symbolized by "r," is used to measure the relationship between two interval-level variables. I used the example earlier of wealth and health to show how this method can be quite versatile and helpful.

Interpreting Pearson's Correlation

When you calculate Pearson's r, you need to know what it means! Pearson's r is a number that varies from -1.0 to $+1.0$. The closer the r value is to 0, the less the two variables are related to one another. Here are the two primary "dimensions" of Pearson's r that are helpful for interpreting the relationship:

- Strength: *The closer the r value gets to either −1 or +1, the stronger the correlation between two variables.* An r value of 1.00 would indicate that every time one variable increased by one unit, the second variable increased by one unit. It is also the case that a value of 1.00 would indicate that each time a variable decreases by one unit, the second variable also decreases by one unit.
- Direction: *When the variables change their values in the same direction, the r is a positive correlation. Whenever the variables change in opposite directions, the r value is negative.* "Positive" and "negative" do not mean "good" and "bad"; they simply indicate the direction of change in both variables. Negative correlations are also called *inverse correlations* since one variable is going up as the other is going down in value.

Figure 11.1 shows some examples of the different possibilities of weak and strong and positive and negative r values. Keep in mind these r values are not real. I simply wanted to show that an r value can take different values and have different "signs." I will discuss later how to calculate Pearson's r and how to determine whether the r value is strong or weak.

I used shading in Figure 11.1 to indicate strength of relationship. The "Weak" column thus shows lighter shading and correlations (both positive and negative) that are close to 0. The "Strong" column has a darker shade indicating stronger correlations (both positive and negative) closer to 1.00 and -1.00. The arrows in the cell indicate direction, whether positive (both arrows pointing in the same direction) or negative (arrows pointing in opposite directions). You can see from these features that a negative correlation closer to -1.00 is considered strong even though it is an inverse relationship. Remember that negative does not mean bad, just opposite direction.

The (Hypothetical) Example

I use a hypothetical example in what follows to demonstrate how to calculate Pearson's r. Table 11.2 shows the data which generally addresses the relationship between wealth and health. These data are modeled after variables from the GSS database that describe respondents' opinions of their health and how their family income compares to other family incomes. As you can see, the variables are "Income Opinion" (IncomeOP), measuring respondents' appraisal of their income to other

		STRENGTH	
		WEAK	STRONG
DIRECTION	POSITIVE	r = 0.02	r = .85
		↑ Storks--Babies ↑	↑ Family Income--Student Achievement ↑
		There is very little (non-spurious) relationship between the number of storks and the number of babies being born	As we have seen, schools with wealthier families have higher aggregate achievement scores
	NEGATIVE	r = −.10	r = −.73
		↑ Noise--Human Learning ↓	↑ Lattes Consumed—Success at Threading a Sewing ↓ Needle
		In my undergraduate experiment, the data only weakly reported an association of increasing noise and decreasing learning	Generally, as people ingest more caffeine, they are less dexterous!

Figure 11.1   Examples of Pearson's *r* values.

TABLE 11.2   Data for Correlation Example

Income Opinion	*Health Opinion*
3	3
5	4
5	5
3	3
3	2
2	3
2	3
3	3
2	2
4	2
3	4
1	1

families' incomes, and "Health Opinion" (HealthOP), a subjective appraisal of their own health. Both variables have values ranging from 1 to 5, with higher values indicating greater subjective income (in the former variable) and greater health (in the latter variable).[2] The research question is whether there is a correlation between opinions of income and health.

[2]These variables are modeled after the GSS variables "finrela" and "health1." I changed some values for heuristic reasons, so the conclusions cannot be taken as reflecting the findings from a similar study using the overall database. However, the trends are the same for the overall database: a small but positive relationship between opinions of income and health.

Assumptions for Correlation

As with other statistical procedures, there are assumptions that must be met before you can use Pearson's r correlation with confidence. The primary assumptions are as follows:

- Randomly chosen sample.
- Variables are interval level (for Pearson's r).
- Variables are independent of one another. This assumption is somewhat difficult to understand, but it deals with "autocorrelation" which is the tendency for one set of scores to be linked to a second set in a series, like time-related measures. If you measure daily crime rates, for example, there will be a "built-in" correlation since each day is most often related to the next. With correlation, you need to make sure that there are no such "linkages" like a time series in the data.
- Variables are normally distributed.
- Variances are equal. Pearson's r is robust for these violations unless one or both variables are significantly skewed.
- Linear relationship. The two variables must display a "straight line" when plotting their values. Thus, for example, if you were correlating the age of a car with the value of a car, the correlation would probably be a straight line (in a downward direction, indicating an inverse relationship). Violations of this assumption might include "curvilinear" relationships in which plotted data appear to be in the form of a "U" pattern. For example, with the age and value of a car, the linear relationship might change over time since really old cars *increase* in value. You can see this pattern in a *scattergram*, which I will discuss later. Formally, you can detect "curvilinear" relationships through SPSS®.

It should be noted that correlation is a robust test, which means that it can provide meaningful results even if there are some slight violations of these assumptions. However, some assumptions are more important than others in this regard, as you will see.

PLOTTING THE CORRELATION: THE SCATTERGRAM

I mentioned the scattergram in discussing the assumption of linearity earlier. Variously known as "scatter diagram," "scatterplot," "scatter graph," or simply "scattergram," you can create a visual graph that shows the relationship between two variables.

Figure 11.2 shows the scattergram between the two example variables, IncomeOP and HealthOP. As you can see, the dots on the graph are displayed from the lower left side of the plot to the upper right side. This pattern indicates a positive correlation because the values of one variable increase in value as the values of the other variable increase.

Reading the plot is straightforward. The values in the table of data are presented in pairs with each pair representing a single respondent's values on both variables. Thus,

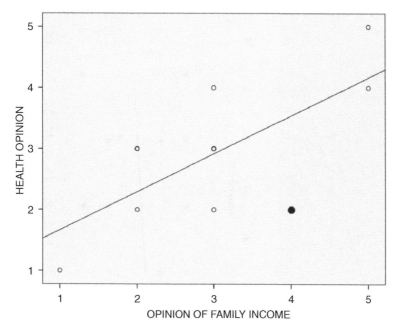

Figure 11.2 The scattergram between health and income.

the top pair of values in Table 11.2 indicates a respondent who indicated opinions that their income was average (value of 3) and that their health was good (value of 3). I filled in the dot in Figure 11.2 to show the pair of scores for the tenth respondent in Table 11.2 (the respondent indicating above average income and fair health).

As you can see, the pairs of scores are entered into the plot simultaneously so that each dot represents the pair of scores of an individual respondent. Typically, the outcome variable is placed on the Y-axis and the predictor variable is placed on the X-axis.

In correlation designs it is not always apparent which variable is the outcome and which is the predictor; you simply have to understand which is which from the research question. The "inherent" research question in this example study is whether income (opinion) influences health (opinion). Therefore, income is the predictor variable (X) in this study. It could just as easily be the other way around! A researcher could posit that health statuses influence a person's income level.

Patterns of Correlations

Correlations can be positive like the one in Figure 11.2, or they can be negative and even nonlinear. Figure 11.3 shows some of the possibilities for correlation patterns in scattergrams. The upper left panel in Figure 11.3 shows the positive correlation with the actual data in Figure 11.2. However, the results could have been different. The upper right panel shows a negative (or inverse) correlation in which health decreases with higher income. The lower left panel shows a curvilinear relationship in which health is better at middle income levels but lower when income is either lower or

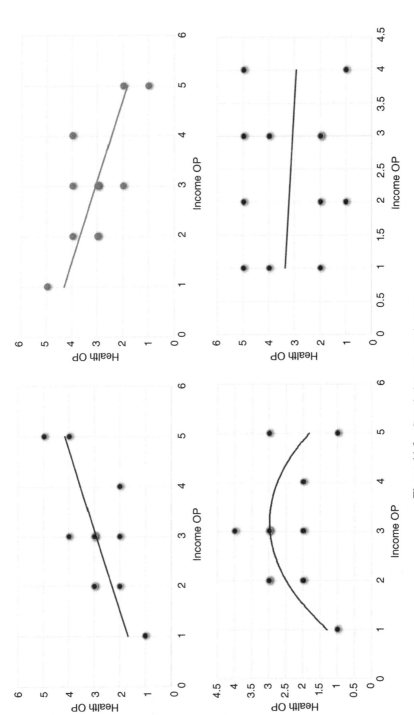

Figure 11.3 Correlation patterns in scattergrams.

higher. The bottom right panel shows no correlation at all; the scores do not fall into a recognizable pattern, as indicated by a "flat" trend line. These panels are only to show the correlation possibilities that might be produced in an actual study.

Strength of Correlations in Scattergrams

The correlation panels in Figure 11.3 showed correlations with different directions or patterns. The dots could "extend upward to the right" (positive correlation), "downward to the right" (negative correlation), or in other patterns. Figure 11.4 shows scattergrams that indicate the *strength* of the correlation.

The top two panels represent positive correlations. The dots are arrayed from bottom left to upper right. But notice that the *extent of the scatter around the line* is different. I use a line to represent the scatter and pattern of the dots (in a later chapter, I will discuss how to calculate the equation for this "line of best fit"). When the dots have a wide scatter, like the scattergram in the top right panel, the correlation is weaker. This would indicate that as values of one variable (books read) increase, the values of the other also increase, but not consistently. The upper left panel shows a positive correlation with a tighter pattern of dots that indicate more of a consistent increase in the values of both variables. I use the darker color to show stronger correlations.

The lower panels of Figure 11.4 show negative correlations. In the bottom right panel, the correlation is inverse in that as one variable increases in value, the other decreases, but the values do not change consistently. The negative correlation in the bottom right panel shows a much higher correlation since the dots are very close to the line indicating a more consistent change in values.

The panels underscore the fact that "negative" correlations are not necessarily bad since negative only refers to direction. As you can see in the bottom left panel of Figure 11.4, this negative correlation is very strong.

You can easily freehand draw a scattergram with pairs of data. However, both SPSS and Excel provide simple procedures to create the graphs.

USING SPSS® TO CREATE SCATTERGRAMS

SPSS has a straightforward way to create scattergrams using the main Graphs menu. Figure 11.5 shows how to create the scattergram through the "Graph – Legacy Dialogs – Bar" path of menu choices. Near the bottom of the list is "Scatter/Dot" which will produce a specification box that allows you to design your scattergram. In this system, you do not need to move the data columns so that one of the variables is listed first, as in Excel.

When you choose "Scatter/Dot," the menu box in Figure 11.6 appears. This box allows you to choose the scattergram that matches the complexity of the research data. For my fictitious example, the "Simple Scatter" choice is appropriate.

Choosing "Simple Scatter" produces a specification window like the one shown in Figure 11.7. As you can see, I specified that income opinion should be placed on the X-axis since I might hypothesize that income differences give way to different

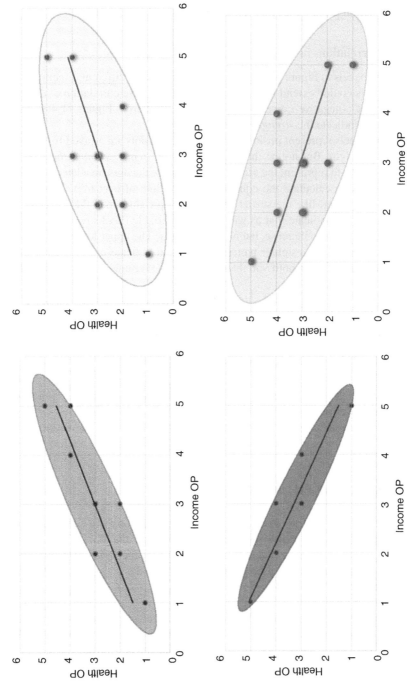

Figure 11.4 Strength of correlations in the scattergram.

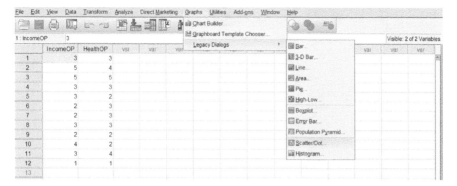

Figure 11.5   The SPSS® graph menu for creating scattergrams.

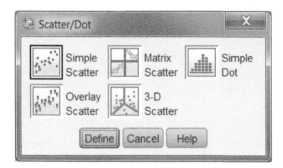

Figure 11.6   The Scatter/Dot menus.

health statuses. Health opinion is placed in the *Y*-axis. I can select the "Titles" and "Options" buttons in the upper right corner of the window to further specify the graph, but I prefer to edit the scattergram once it is produced.

When you choose "OK" from the window in Figure 11.7, SPSS produces a graph in the output file like the one shown in Figure 11.2. If you double-click on the graph, you can make a series of edits using the available menu screens. I added the line to the "basic" scattergram to produce the graph in Figure 11.2.

USING EXCEL TO CREATE SCATTERGRAMS

With the table of data entered in an Excel spreadsheet, simply highlight the entire table (including labels) and choose the "Insert" menu from the main menu list. Figure 11.8 shows this selection with the example data. As you can see, I highlighted the table of values and chose Insert. I then clicked on the Scatter icon listed among the other graph icons. At that point, I could choose several scattergram types in a drop-down menu. For the simple linear correlation, the upper left choice is appropriate. As the data increase in complexity, you can experiment with the other scattergram choices.

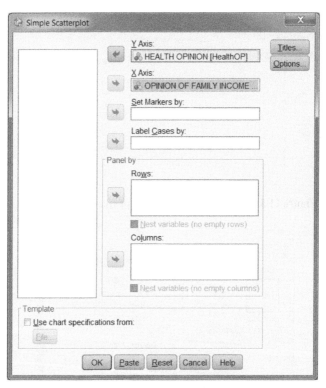

Figure 11.7   The scattergram specification window in SPSS®.

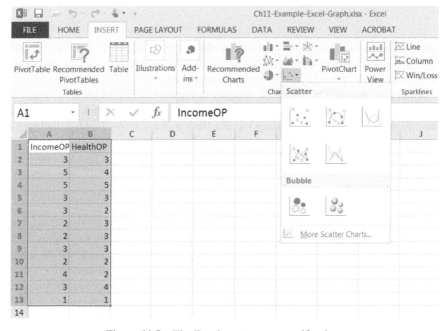

Figure 11.8   The Excel scattergram specification.

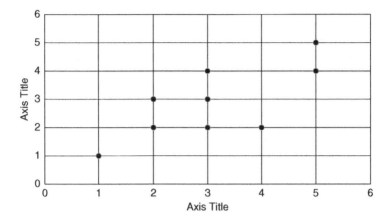

Figure 11.9   The Excel scattergram.

Figure 11.9 shows the scattergram created by the menu choices earlier. As you can see, the dots are displayed according to the pairs in the data table. One note here is that you must add the axis titles to the scattergram by editing it using the small icons that appear to the right of the graph when you select it. This is important to do since you want to make sure the variables are specified on the appropriate axes. As you can see in Figure 11.9, the axes are not titled, so you need to add the titles. In this case, the first variable (IncomeOP) in the Excel data table (see Figure 11.8) is placed on the *X*-axis as is appropriate.

The scattergram in Figure 11.9 is the "plain" graph that Excel produced using the specifications earlier. *You can edit the graph by double-clicking on parts of the graph and then right-clicking for edit choices.* A simple way to make edits is to use the main menu bar when you have the graph selected. The "Chart Tools" menu provides several different ways that you can make the graph appear. For example, one choice includes axis titles, another includes the raw data table, and so on. You can include the Trendline through the data using these methods.

CALCULATING PEARSON'S *r*

There are several ways to calculate Pearson's *r* manually. Formulas exist using the "deviation" method or the "calculation method" or even the "Z score method." I will present two formulas in this book since both point out different facets of Pearson's *r*.

The Z score method appears to be the most simple until you realize that, in order to use it, you have to transform every score to a Z score. The calculation method is my preferred method since it uses symbols and formulas I introduced in past chapters and includes a simple data table of values.

THE Z SCORE METHOD

The many formulas for calculating Pearson's r manually result from measuring various elements that express different components of the correlation relationship.

The Z score formula is as follows:

$$r_{XY} = \frac{\sum Z_X Z_Y}{N}$$

In this formula, the correlation between two variables X and Y (symbolized by r_{XY}) is calculated by *summing the products* of the X_Z scores and the Y_Z scores and then dividing by the number of pairs (*in correlation, the N indicates pairs, not the total set of scores*). In order to carry out this formula, z scores for each of the X and Y values must be created using the formula I discussed in Chapter 4:

$$Z = \frac{X - M}{SD}$$

Creating z scores manually is tedious, especially with many pairs of scores. On the other hand, creating the z scores in an Excel spreadsheet is quite simple, as I discussed in Chapter 4. Table 11.3 shows the values as I created them in an Excel spreadsheet using the embedded z formula. I first calculated the mean and SD values for both variables as shown.

Once these calculations are made, the following Z score formula will calculate Pearson's r (using the relevant calculations in the final column of Table 11.3):

$$r_{XY} = \frac{\sum Z_X Z_Y}{N}$$
$$= \frac{8.39}{12}$$
$$= 0.699$$

Note: Be careful with the calculation of the numerator of the formula. It is <u>not</u> the sum of the Z scores for the IncomeOP column (0) times the Z score sum of the HealthOP column (0). This mistake would look like the following:

$$r_{XY} = \frac{\left(\sum Z_X\right)\left(\sum X_Y\right)}{N}$$

The reason that this is inappropriate is that the sums of these particular columns would be equal to 0! Like the deviation method for calculating SD that we discussed earlier, there will be an equal number of negative and positive z scores in a normally distributed set of scores. Therefore, you must *multiply each pair of Z scores* to arrive at the values in the last column of Table 11.3. Otherwise, this is the result:

$$r_{XY} = \frac{(0)(0)}{12}$$
$$= 0$$

TABLE 11.3   The Data Table Showing Z Scores

	IncomeOP	Z(Income)	HealthOP	Z(Health)	Z_X*Z_Y
	3	0.00	3	0.08	0.00
	5	1.74	4	1.04	1.82
	5	1.74	5	2.01	3.49
	3	0.00	3	0.08	0.00
	3	0.00	2	−0.88	0.00
	2	−0.87	3	0.08	−0.07
	2	−0.87	3	0.08	−0.07
	3	0.00	3	0.08	0.00
	2	−0.87	2	−0.88	0.77
	4	0.87	2	−0.88	−0.77
	3	0.00	4	1.04	0.00
	1	−1.74	1	−1.85	3.21
Σ		0.00		0.00	
Mean	3.00		2.917	Σ ZX*ZY	8.39
SD	1.15		1.037	r	0.699

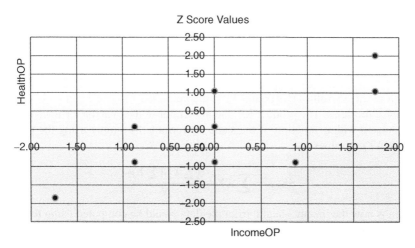

Figure 11.10   The Z score scattergram in Excel.

The reason to use the Z score formula is to use the transformed X and Y values as Z scores that present the X and Y values in the same scales. This will become more apparent when I discuss regression procedures, but for now, look at Figure 11.10 that presents the scattergram with Z score values for both the X and Y raw score values. The X-axis is the Z score values of IncomeOP and the Y-axis represents the Z values of the HealthOP.

As you can see, all the values of the two scores are now expressed *in the same scale*, as Z score values the majority of which (over 99%) range between −3.00 and +3.00.

Whereas in Figure 11.9 the values were expressed in *raw score units* (i.e., the units of the original scores), the transformed scores are expressed in *z score units*. To take an example, the lower left dot expressed in Figure 11.9 is (IncomeOP= 1, HealthOP = 1). In Figure 11.10, the Z scores are (IncomeOP = −1.74, HealthOP = −1.85).

Using Z scores creates the same scale for raw score variable units of any magnitude. This does not change the correlation or the placement of the dots in the scattergram.

THE COMPUTATION METHOD

There are several computation formulas for Pearson's r. I prefer the following because it uses the sum of squares (SS) measures that I have used throughout former chapters. The overall formula looks straightforward. Conceptually, the formula expresses correlation ("r") as the proportion of the "cross product" SS (or the SS of the $X*Y$ pairs) to the square root of the overall product of the X and Y sums of squares[3]:

$$r_{XY} = \frac{SS_{XY}}{\sqrt{(SS_X)(SS_Y)}}$$

Recall that the SS is a general (unstandardized) variance measure of the population of scores. The computation formula thus includes variance (SS) measures of the XY products as well as the individual X and Y SS values. The formula for SS we discussed in Chapter 3 is

$$\sum X^2 - \frac{(\sum X)^2}{N}$$

Each of the SS values (for X and Y) in the Pearson's r formula can be computed with these formulas. The product SS (the numerator in the Pearson's r formula) can be calculated with a variation of the same SS formula by simply using the product column (XY) of values:

$$SS_{XY} = \sum XY - \frac{(\sum X)(\sum Y)}{N}$$

Here is how the income–health example data would be computed using the computation formula:

The SS_{XY}

$$SS_{XY} = \sum XY - \frac{(\sum X)(\sum Y)}{N}$$

$$SS_{XY} = 115 - \frac{(36)(35)}{12}$$

$$SS_{Income \times Health} = \textbf{10.00}$$

---

[3]This makes conceptual sense if you recognize the denominator as a combined variance measure of X and Y together, since each SS is multiplied and transformed to a combined variance measure. Thus, the formula expresses the "variance" of the XY product measures as a proportion of the overall variance of both sets of scores. This is conceptually what ANOVA does – compares variance components.

The SS_Y

$$SS_Y = \sum Y^2 - \frac{(\sum Y)^2}{N}$$

$$SS_{Health} = 115 - \frac{1225}{12}$$

$$\mathbf{SS_{Health} = 12.92}$$

The SS_X

$$SS_X = \sum X^2 - \frac{(\sum X)^2}{N}$$

$$SS_{Income} = 124 - \frac{1296}{12}$$

$$\mathbf{SS_{Income} = 16.00}$$

Pearson's *r*

$$r_{XY} = \frac{10.00}{\sqrt{(16.00)\,(12.92)}}$$

$$= \frac{10.00}{14.38}$$

$$= 0.695$$

As you can see, the resulting Pearson's *r* of 0.695 is equivalent to the *r* value computed with the *Z* score formula (with minor rounding differences). Both formulas yield the same value.

THE HYPOTHESIS TEST FOR PEARSON'S *r*

What does the Pearson's *r* value indicate? Recall that the study asked if income was correlated to health. The scattergrams presented strong visual evidence that there was a relationship, but how can the resulting *r* of 0.695 help to judge the strength of the relationship?

The *r* of 0.695 is certainly closer to 1.00 than it is to 0, so you can use this as one gauge of its meaningfulness. However, like the other statistical tests I have discussed, you assess the statistical significance of a test ratio by comparing it to a sampling distribution.

Therefore, the first way to determine whether the *r* value is significant is to perform the hypothesis test as I have with other statistical procedures. If the calculated value exceeds the tabled value (i.e., if the calculated value is further out in the tail of the exclusion area), you can conclude that the test value is statistically significant.

Use the same steps as you did with other statistical tests:

1. The null hypothesis (H_0): $\rho = 0$
   The null hypothesis states that the correlation between the variables in the population from which the sample values came (symbolized by the parameter value of rho or ρ) is 0.

2. The alternative hypothesis (H_A): $\rho \neq 0$
   The alternative hypothesis states that the population correlation is not 0.

3. The critical value $r_{df(0.05)}$
   The comparison value for the value of r that defines the exclusion area at a given probability level (I used 0.05 in the above value) is determined by a table of values as are other statistical procedures. The tables for correlation are extensive and detailed. The critical values for correlation table, which lists exclusion values for Pearson's r, is found in the Appendix.

   Like other statistical procedures, testing the null hypothesis for correlation uses degrees of freedom since you estimate a population parameter from a sample statistic. The degrees of freedom for correlation is $N - 2$, where N is the number of pairs. You "lose" two degrees of freedom since you are estimating a population value with two sample sets of values.

   The table for correlation specifies that the two-tailed 0.05 critical (exclusion) value for r at 10 degrees of freedom (12 pairs minus $2 = 10$) is $r_{df(0.05)} = 0.576$. Values that are greater than 0.576 would therefore be considered statistically significant.

4. The calculated value of $r = 0.695$

5. Statistical decision
   You reject the null hypothesis since the calculated value (0.695) exceeded the critical value of exclusion (0.576). *A significant correlation indicates that a calculated value with this magnitude is unlikely to occur by chance if there is no correlation in the population.*

6. Interpretation
   You can consider the calculated r of 0.695 to be statistically significant. This indicates that it is likely not a chance finding. In the words of the example question, respondents' opinions of their incomes and their health statuses are positively correlated.

The Comparison Table of Values

Because the correlation tables are so extensive and because I will discuss SPSS and Excel results, I do not include comprehensive correlation tables in this book. However, there is an alternate way to identify the critical values by using the T table of values which is included. Cohen (1988) provides the following formula that you can use in the T tables as a comparison value. In effect, you "transform" the r value into a t ratio that you can then compare against the critical values of T in the T table (using $N - 2$ degrees of freedom in the table):

$$t = \frac{r\sqrt{N - 2}}{\sqrt{1 - r^2}}$$

Therefore, in the present example

$$t = \frac{0.695\sqrt{12 - 2}}{\sqrt{1 - 0.483}}$$
$$= 3.057$$

The r value of 0.695 is "transformed" to a t ratio of 3.057. When you consult the T table of values using $N - 2$ degrees of freedom, you note that the critical value of $t_{0.05,10} = 2.228$. Therefore, the calculated r is significant since it resulted in a t score that exceeded the critical T value.

EFFECT SIZE: THE COEFFICIENT OF DETERMINATION

A second way to judge the meaningfulness and strength of a correlation beyond the hypothesis is the effect size. I have shown with every statistical procedure ways to measure the "impact" of a relationship. With correlation, you can judge the strength of the relationship by the *coefficient of determination* or r^2. *This value is simply the square of r and refers to the amount of variance in one variable explained by the other.* What this means is this: you can consider the fact that a distribution of scores (e.g., health opinion values) vary a certain amount or are spread out around a mean score.

The question is <u>why</u> do health opinion values vary? In a world where every person was the same, there would be no variance – everyone would offer the same health opinion. But we don't live in that kind of world, so something or things are responsible for people getting different health opinion values. Figure 11.11 shows how the example study variables relate to one another in terms of "explaining variance."

If you establish that a correlation is significant (i.e., between income and health opinions), the variables' measures overlap (like the Venn diagram in Figure 11.11), and you can understand this overlap to be the amount of variance in the outcome measure (health opinions) that is accounted for by the predictor variable (income opinion). Thus, knowing a respondent's income opinion is a partial explanation of their health opinions. The income opinion does not explain all the variation in health opinion, since there is still a lot of "unexplained variance" (the amount of the health opinion circle in Figure 11.11 not overlapping with income opinion circle), but it "chips away" at the overall spread of the scores. The r^2 value is this explained variance.

Figure 11.12 shows another way to visualize effect size in correlation. The overall distribution represents the entire variability of health opinion values. With a correlation of 0.695, the r^2 of 0.483 reduces the amount of "unexplained variance" in reading

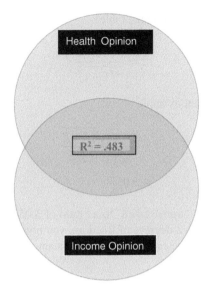

Figure 11.11   The effect size of correlation–explaining variance.

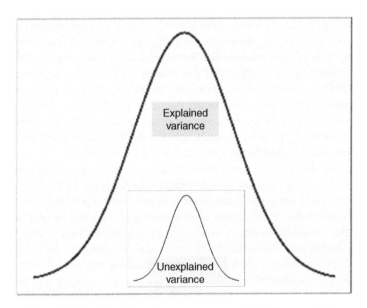

Figure 11.12   The effect size components produced by correlation.

to $(1.00 - 0.483 = 0.517)$. Thus, other variables not in the analysis might help further to "explain away" the remaining unexplained variation.

I will discuss further insights into r^2 in the chapters on regression. *For now you can understand it as the percentage of the variance in one variable (outcome) contributed by another (predictor).* Knowing how much variance is explained is helpful to the researcher, but what guidelines exist that might help judge the extent of the explained variance? Cohen (1988) provides the following conventions for the r^2:

Small effect size: $r^2 = 0.01$ ($r = 0.10$)
Medium effect size: $r^2 = 0.09$ ($r = 0.30$)
Large effect size: $r^2 = 0.25$ ($r = 0.50$)

These r^2 size conventions may appear to be small, and for some studies they may not be appropriate. The researcher must ultimately decide the meaningfulness of the correlation effect size since it is tied to the nature of the research question. Thus, I might not be excited about an r^2 of 0.09 in a small exploratory study of the relationship between income and health among electronics workers, but I might be very excited about the same effect size in a study of this relationship in a large national study relating total wealth measures to specific health behaviors.

The r^2 is one of the PRE methods I mentioned at the opening of this chapter. If you look at Figure 11.1, r^2 is listed in the last column with the other PRE methods that I discussed in the ANOVA chapters. All these are related measures in that they focus on explaining variance. I will develop this notion further in discussing regression methods.

DIAGNOSTICS: CORRELATION PROBLEMS

Several factors affect the size of a correlation and therefore its power (i.e., the ability to reject the null hypothesis when it should be rejected). The following are several such factors.

Correlations and Sample Size

As I stressed in previous chapters, hypothesis tests establish whether a finding is likely a chance finding. (We just discussed the effect size, which is distinguished from the statistical rejection of the null hypothesis.) Be aware that *the sample size dramatically affects the size of Pearson's r.*

For example, with 15 cases, the researcher can reject the null hypothesis (two-tailed test at 0.05) with $r = 0.514$. With a sample of 30, the researcher can reject the null hypothesis when $r = 0.361$. With a sample of 102, the researcher can reject the null hypothesis at 0.195. It only takes an $r = 0.098$ to reject the null hypothesis with $N = 402$! *Therefore, with the same study variables, but simply larger samples, the researcher will reject the null hypothesis more easily.*

Correlation Is Not Causation

I noted this injunction previously. The problem with discovering correlations is the temptation to assume that the variables are *causally* related. Thus, you might be tempted to assume that in the example study I have been using, income opinions cause health opinions to increase. A correlation cannot make this claim. There are many things that are related to opinions about one's health other than opinions about one's income – and some of them may be better explanations of increases in scores. What are some? If you were to list other *potential* causes, you could probably produce a long list (e.g., health behavior practices, diet, exercise, genetic predispositions, etc.).

Restricted Range

The strength and size of a correlation is dramatically affected by "restricted range," or the selection of scores that do not display full variability. Figure 11.13 shows this problem with a scattergram. If a study sample is relatively homogenous on the variables (e.g., all the subjects appear to be similar in IncomeOP and HealthOP), the resulting correlation can appear to be very low. In the top panel of Figure 11.13, respondents of all different income and health opinions were plotted, indicating a strong correlation. If the study were to be restricted to respondents who were very similar to one another, like those respondents enrolled in health clubs, the resulting correlation would be less pronounced and perhaps not significant. The power of a correlation is related to the variability of the study variables.

Extreme Scores

"Outlier" scores can have a dramatic effect on the calculated r. Often, deleting only a single extreme score has a surprisingly marked effect on the results. With correlation, extreme scores, especially in studies with small sample sizes, can be problematic.

I offer the same suggestion with correlation studies as with studies using other statistical procedures. The researcher must use their understanding of the data and

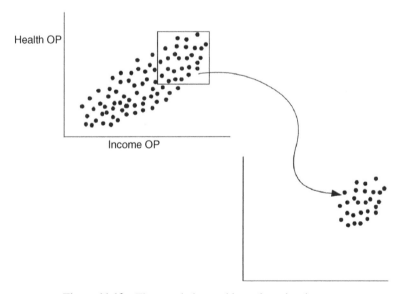

Figure 11.13   The correlation problem of restricted range.

the research situation in order to manage extreme scores. They can transform such scores, delete them, or retain them as legitimate depending on their understanding.

The first step in limiting the effects of extreme scores is to detect them! In other works (e.g., Abbott, 2010), I devote significant attention to diagnostic procedures for correlation and regression studies. The serious researcher should seek these works out before engaging in a correlation study.

Heteroscedasticity

This essentially refers to violating the equal variance assumption among study variables. Homoscedasticity is the condition in which an outcome variable has equal variation across the levels of the predictor variable. If this condition is not present as, for example, if the scores of one study variable were markedly skewed, the correlation would show a distortion (heteroscedasticity). Figure 11.14 shows the two conditions of homoscedasticity (top panel) and heteroscedasticity (bottom panel). The top panel of Figure 11.14 shows that the values of one variable are distributed evenly across the values of the other variable (homoscedasticity). The bottom panel shows unevenness of the values of one variable across the other variable (heteroscedasticity) indicated by the different sized circles encompassing the scatter of dots on the graph. In some cases, heteroscedasticity may result in a departure from linearity.

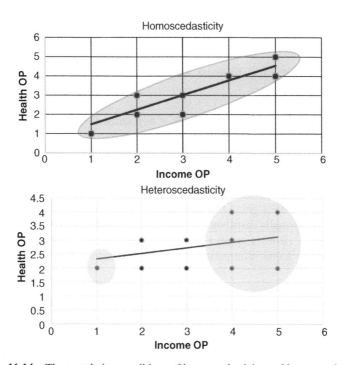

Figure 11.14 The correlation conditions of homoscedasticity and heteroscedasticity.

Curvilinear Relations

I showed an example of a curvilinear relationship in Figure 11.3 (bottom left panel). In these types of relationships, the pattern of the data may extend in one direction and then break in a different direction creating a nonlinear path. In Abbott (2010), I discussed diagnosis of curvilinear relationships in great detail. These are often not easy to detect, but SPSS has a straightforward procedure that helps to make the assessments about whether the linearity assumption is violated in a study. I will develop this procedure in the chapters dealing with bivariate regression.

CORRELATION USING SPSS® AND EXCEL

In this section, I will analyze the example database with both SPSS and Excel. In doing so, I will use the steps I discussed earlier as the process for performing the correlation analysis and making conclusions:

1. Check assumptions.
2. Calculate Pearson's r.
3. Evaluate Pearson's r using:
   a. Hypothesis test
   b. Effect size

Assumptions for Correlation

I can use SPSS and Excel to assist with the assumptions. Some do not require additional analyses:

Randomly chosen sample: My example is hypothetical, so I will assume random selection of respondents.

Variables are interval level: I use self-report responses similar to those in GSS. While the data are not strictly interval level, researchers often treat them as such, especially if they are repeatedly used with consistent results.

Variables are independent of one another: The variables are not linked.

Variables are normally distributed: Figure 11.15 (SPSS) shows the descriptive information (from Explore) in two panels. Figure 11.16 (Excel) shows much of the same information, but does not include the additional tests of normality.

The variables appear to be normal from these results. The SPSS report includes the standard error for skewness and kurtosis, so you can confirm that the values for both variables lay within the boundaries we discussed for both measures. The Kolmogorov–Smirnov test for IncomeOP is significant ($p < 0.037$), but other measures disagree. The more important matter is that the outcome variable (HealthOP) is normally distributed.

Descriptives

			Statistic	Std. Error
HEALTH OPINION	Mean		2.92	.313
	95% Confidence Interval for Mean	Lower Bound	2.23	
		Upper Bound	3.61	
	5% Trimmed Mean		2.91	
	Median		3.00	
	Variance		1.174	
	Std. Deviation		1.084	
	Minimum		1	
	Maximum		5	
	Range		4	
	Interquartile Range		2	
	Skewness		.192	.637
	Kurtosis		.219	1.232
OPINION OF FAMILY INCOME	Mean		3.00	.348
	95% Confidence Interval for Mean	Lower Bound	2.23	
		Upper Bound	3.77	
	5% Trimmed Mean		3.00	
	Median		3.00	
	Variance		1.455	
	Std. Deviation		1.206	
	Minimum		1	
	Maximum		5	
	Range		4	
	Interquartile Range		2	
	Skewness		.373	.637
	Kurtosis		−.160	1.232

Tests of Normality

	Kolmogorov-Smirnov[a]			Shapiro-Wilk		
	Statistic	df	Sig.	Statistic	df	Sig.
HEALTH OPINION	.219	12	.115	.939	12	.487
OPINION OF FAMILY INCOME	.250	12	.037	.910	12	.212

a. Lilliefors Significance Correction

Figure 11.15 The SPSS® descriptive output for the study variables.

Figures 11.17 and 11.18 show the histograms for the outcome variable HealthOP. In both cases, the histograms indicate distributions that appear normal, despite small sample sizes.

Variances are equal: You can assume equal variance since neither variable is *markedly* skewed.

Linear relationship: Figure 11.2 shows the SPSS scattergram between the example study variables. Figure 11.19 shows the Excel scattergram between Math and FR. As you can see, the pattern of the dots is fairly evenly distributed around the line, and the overall shape of the dots is in a straight line.

	IncomeOP	HealthOP
Mean	3.00	2.92
Standard Error	0.35	0.31
Median	3.00	3.00
Mode	3.00	3.00
Standard Deviation	1.21	1.08
Sample Variance	1.45	1.17
Kurtosis	−0.16	0.22
Skewness	0.37	0.19
Range	4.00	4.00
Minimum	1.00	1.00
Maximum	5.00	5.00
Sum	36.00	35.00
Count	12.00	12.00

Figure 11.16 The Excel descriptive statistics.

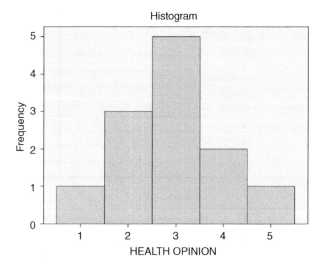

Figure 11.17 The SPSS® histogram for HealthOP.

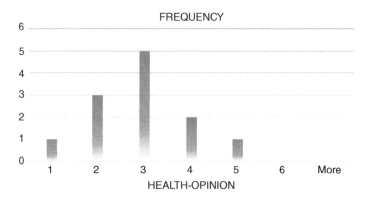

Figure 11.18 The Excel histogram for HealthOP.

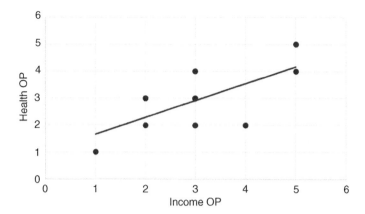

Figure 11.19   The Excel scattergram between IncomeOP and HealthOP.

Computation of Pearson's *r* for the Example Data

See the manual calculations for the example data in the section "THE COMPUTA-TION METHOD."

Correlation Using SPSS®

Figure 11.20 shows the SPSS correlation menu. Note that it is called "Bivariate" because you use the program to specify a two-variable correlation ("bi" – two). When you make this choice, you are presented with the specification menu shown in Figure 11.21.

As you can see in Figure 11.21, I included both variables in the "Variables:" window. The default values for this specification window are shown. The analysis will produce Pearson's *r* (this is the only value produced in the default analysis), and SPSS will create a ("Two-tailed") hypothesis test and "Flag significant correlations" according to the default checks.

If you select the "Options" button in the upper right part of the window, you can request means, standard deviations, and cross-product values. The latter are helpful if you wish to compare the values with those you calculated manually. For this example, I did not select the options.

Choosing "OK" will produce the correlation matrix shown in Figure 11.22. The outputs of the SPSS matrix are helpful because they provide the values you need for the hypothesis test. As you can see, the correlation significance level ("$p = 0.012$") is listed, which indicates that the correlation is in the exclusion area and therefore considered a significant correlation. The calculated r fell so far into the exclusion region that it has an extremely small probability of representing a chance finding.

As with other output I presented, SPSS lists the *exact probability* of the finding. When you create hypotheses tests using correlation tables to specify exclusion values, you would report significance as "$p < 0.05$," indicating that the calculated value fell into the exclusion area beyond the boundary of the 0.05 level of probability.

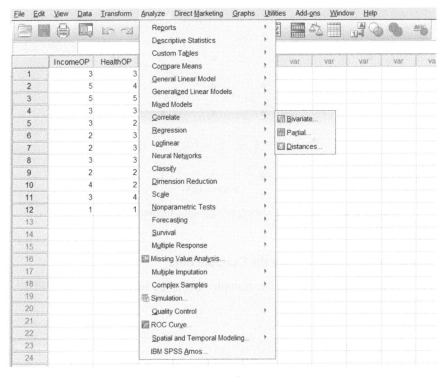

Figure 11.20   The SPSS® Correlation menu.

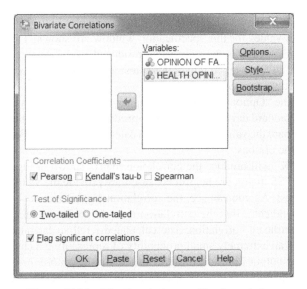

Figure 11.21   The Correlation specification window.

Correlations

		OPINION OF FAMILY INCOME	HEALTH OPINION
OPINION OF FAMILY INCOME	Pearson Correlation	1	.696*
	Sig. (2-tailed)		.012
	N	12	12
HEALTH OPINION	Pearson Correlation	.696*	1
	Sig. (2-tailed)	.012	
	N	12	12

*. Correlation is significant at the 0.05 level (2-tailed).

Figure 11.22   The SPSS® correlation matrix.

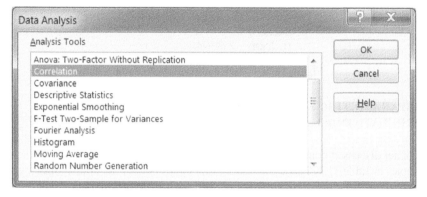

Figure 11.23   The "Correlation" window in the Excel Data – Data Analysis menu.

Correlation Using Excel

Figure 11.23 shows the menu window when you select "Data – Data Analysis" from the main menu in the spreadsheet where the data are located. This should be a familiar menu now that you have used it in past procedures. When you select "Correlation" you are presented with another specification window as shown in Figure 11.24. As you can see, I selected both columns of data at the same time in the "Input Range:" window. Since I included the labels, I made sure to check the "Labels in First Row" box. The default is to create the data in a separate spreadsheet.

When you select "OK" from the button shown in Figure 11.24, you will see the correlation results in a matrix form, even though there is only one correlation pair. Figure 11.25 shows the IncomeOP–HealthOP correlation as 0.696, which matches the manually calculated value.

Note that Excel does not specify the p value of the result. You must consult the correlation table of values to obtain the comparison value for the hypothesis test.

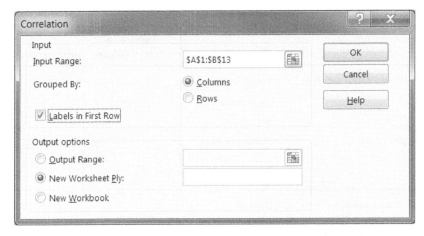

Figure 11.24   The "Correlation" specification window in Excel.

	IncomeOP	HealthOP
IncomeOP	1	
HealthOP	0.695608	1

Figure 11.25   The Excel correlation matrix.

NONPARAMETRIC STATISTICS: SPEARMAN'S RANK ORDER CORRELATION (r_s)

I have not discussed nonparametric correlation procedures thus far, but I listed some examples in Table 11.1. Those listed in the first three columns are nonparametric procedures designed to measure correlations with other than interval data. I will briefly describe one of these in this chapter, Spearman's Rho.

Up to now, I have discussed using two interval-level variables for calculating Pearson's r. However, researchers often do not have access to interval data. For example, researchers might be limited to discussing hospital rankings as a way to discuss quality care. If this is the case, these rank-ordered data are ordinal data, and you can make no assumption that the interval between the rankings is equal.

If you use ordinal data, you can use a variation of correlation called Spearman's r. Also called Spearman's rank order correlation, or Spearman's Rho, this procedure calculates a correlation *using ordinal data* or *interval data that have been ranked*.

Spearman's Rho results vary between −1 and +1 as with Pearson's r. You can obtain a negative value, which is interpreted as it is with Pearson's r. However, since this not a parametric statistic, you cannot square the r_s value to arrive at a "variance explained" figure as in Pearson's r. You can perform the hypothesis test to see whether the value is significant.

The manual calculation for Spearman's Rho is as follows:

$$r_s = 1 - \frac{6 \sum d^2}{N(N^2 - 1)}$$

The formula appears somewhat strange in comparison to the other procedures I have presented. Like some nonparametric tests, the Spearman's Rho formula includes a *constant* in the formula (a constant is a number that does not change). The "6" appears mysterious, but the nonparametric formula is created to yield a value that fits the $-1/+1$ range, and the value of 6 allows the computed values to fall in this range. There is a longer explanation, but this gives you some insight into nonparametric procedures.

The preceding formula is used with two sets of ranks like the hypothetical example of data in Table 11.4.

If you use the formula I included earlier, the following is the calculation for Spearman's Rho:

$$r_s = 1 - \frac{6 \sum d^2}{N(N^2 - 1)}$$

$$= 1 - \frac{6(8)}{5(25 - 1)}$$

$$= 1 - \frac{48}{120}$$

$$= 0.60$$

Spearman's Rho calculations can be part of hypotheses tests using the same process as the hypothesis tests in the parametric procedures. The null and alternative hypotheses state that the correlation will be 0 (or not 0, respectively) in the population the sample data represent. Spearman's Rho is calculated with the previous formula, and the researcher can compare the calculated value to a critical test value.

Spearman's Rho has a special table of comparison values to use for hypothesis tests. In this table, *the researcher does not use degrees of freedom* since no parameters are estimated. However, if a table of values is not available (I do not include such a table in this book), the researcher can use the *T* table of values with the same formula I noted earlier for Pearson's r. *When you use the T distribution table for identifying a comparison value, you can use degrees of freedom as you did with Pearson's r* since

TABLE 11.4   Hypothetical Correlation of Hospital Rankings by Patient Satisfaction Ranking

Hospital Ranking	Patient Satisfaction Ranking	d	d^2
1	2	−1	1
2	1	1	1
3	5	−2	4
4	3	1	1
5	4	1	1
	Totals	0	8

the table is created for a parametric comparison:

$$t = \frac{r_s \sqrt{N - 2}}{\sqrt{1 - r_s^2}}$$

$$= \frac{0.6\sqrt{3}}{\sqrt{0.64}}$$

$$= 1.30$$

Using the T table of values, I note that the critical value of rejection at the 0.05 (two-tailed) level with df $= 3$ (5 − 2) is 3.182. Therefore, since the calculated t value (from Spearman's Rho) is 1.30, you cannot reject the null hypothesis.

The one-tailed 0.05 exclusion value using the Spearman's table of critical values for 5 data pairs is 0.90. (Spearman's table does not provide a two-tailed value with $N = 5$.) You would therefore need a 0.90 correlation or higher to reject the null hypothesis. Using either table would therefore indicate the same result: you cannot reject the null hypothesis with this brief example.

Variations of the Spearman's Rho Formula: Tied Ranks

Researchers oftentimes use rank order procedures when they have data that are interval, but the data are not normally distributed, as I mentioned earlier when I discussed skewed variables. Situations in which this is common involve using financial data, like housing values, physician salaries, or hospital funding. I will provide an extended example of this later.

More commonly, researchers have studies in which they may have *both* ordinal- and interval-level variables. In either case, however, the simple Spearman's Rho formula earlier will most likely not be appropriate as I will discuss later. The reason is that larger studies with more cases or studies that involve ranking of interval variables usually result in *tied ranks*, which are problematic to the "basic" Spearman's Rho formula.

If skewed interval-level variables are used along with ranked variables, *the skewed interval data must first be ranked and then correlated with variables already ranked.* In these cases, the Spearman's Rho formula earlier should not be used.

In the fictitious study earlier, I used hospital ranking as one of the ordinal (ranked) variables. What if I had used the number of positive citations the hospitals had received *instead* of the ranking variable? I would then have an interval-level variable. In such a case, I would need to rank order the interval data so that both of the study variables would be ordinal (remember, the other variable, patient satisfaction ranking was already an ordinal variable). Table 11.5 shows the comparison of these variables and how the interval-level variable can be changed to rankings.

I placed the original ranked variable in the first column. The second column is the interval-level variable used in place of the original ordinal variable (hospital ranking) in the study *instead* of the ranked variable. The problem with these data

TABLE 11.5   Ranking an Interval Variable

Hospital Ranking	Number of Citations	Citations Rankings
1	12	2
2	14	1
3	6	3.5
4	6	3.5
5	1	5

values, however, is that the third and fourth citation listings tied since they received the same number of citations (6). If you wanted to rank this variable, you must *average the tied ranks*.

When you rank the hospitals in the order of the greatest number of citations (you can also rank them the other direction), the top two hospitals are ranked 2 (second) and 1 (first), but the next two hospitals occupy the same rank (third). Therefore, you must *average the rank positions* of the citations (average the <u>rank</u> positions, not the <u>actual values</u>). This means that you would need to average the <u>third and fourth rank positions</u> resulting in two ranks of 3.5 (since $\frac{3+4}{2} = 3.5$). I showed this in Table 11.5 in the third column (shaded).

Once this variable has been changed to a rank order variable from an interval-level variable, you can proceed with the Spearman's Rho calculation with the new ranked variable and the other original variable (patient satisfaction) in Table 11.4.

Remember, however, the basic Spearman's Rho formula I used earlier for this calculation works well with small samples, but it is affected by variables with *tied ranks*. If you have tied ranks, you should use another formula that takes the tied ranks into account. (I do not introduce that formula in this chapter.) Larger data sets, especially those involving skewed interval data that have been ranked, should be analyzed by SPSS or similar statistical software. As you can see, ranking skewed data can be quite difficult manually if the data set is large.

A Spearman's Rho Example

I began this chapter with the example of the relationship between wealth and health using opinion data that I treated as interval data. In this section, I examine the same topic but with at least one variable that might not best be used with Pearson's *r*.

The data are hypothetical but similar to studies using financial revenues and health ratings. One variable "funding" is the dollar amount (in thousands) received by 50 hospitals of the same size and configuration for a new procedure designed to reduce spinal nerve compression after automobile accidents. The "health outcome" variable is a hospital figure measuring the average number of complaints over a 1-month span resulting from the procedures used to treat nerve compression. Is there a relationship between funding and complaints?

The design for such a study is a very simple one. If performed in the real world, a great danger would be to make causal attributions of the positive effects of funding if indeed there were a positive correlation with health outcomes. Correlation,

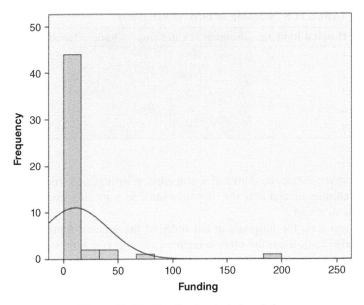

Figure 11.26   Funding for study hospitals.

whether measured by Pearson's *r* or Spearman's Rho, can only establish relationship, not causality. One of the reasons for this potential problem in interpretation is that a great many factors (in addition to funding) might have an impact on health outcomes. More complex associational designs, like the ones discussed in the next two chapters, would help the researcher to speak more precisely about the specific contribution of funding to health outcomes.

As I noted earlier, any variable measuring income, funding, or wealth is always suspect for being normally distributed because in real life funding is not normally distributed across society. This presents a problem for measuring correlation using Pearson's *r*. In such cases, researchers might use Spearman's Rho <u>because this procedure can be used effectively with skewed data</u>. Creating ranks with these kinds of variables would be very tedious, especially with large data sets. Fortunately, SPSS includes Spearman's procedure that can be very helpful.

Figure 11.26 shows the SPSS histogram for funding received by the study hospitals, indicating that this variable is markedly skewed. Under these circumstances, with the example study question, the researcher might seek an alternative to Pearson's correlation despite the fact that the data are interval (even ratio) level data. If the researcher has interval data that depart this far from the assumptions of parametric tests to the extent they cannot be reasonably used, then Spearman's Rho can be used instead of Pearson's *r*.

Figure 11.27 shows the Spearman's r results for this research question. As you can see, the correlation (−0.324) is significant at $p = 0.022$. (Figure 11.21 shows how to obtain this SPSS output. There is simply a box to check for Spearman's correlation in the same specification window in which you call for Pearson's *r*.)

Correlations

			Funding	HealthOutcome
Spearman's Rho	Funding	Correlation Coefficient	1.000	−.324*
		Sig. (2-tailed)	.	.022
		N	50	50
	HealthOutcome	Correlation Coefficient	−.324*	1.000
		Sig. (2-tailed)	.022	.
		N	50	50

*. Correlation is significant at the 0.05 level (2-tailed).

Figure 11.27 The Spearman's Rho correlation between the study variables.

Correlations

		Funding	HealthOutcome
Funding	Pearson Correlation	1	−.135
	Sig. (2-tailed)		.350
	N	50	50
HealthOutcome	Pearson Correlation	−.135	1
	Sig. (2-tailed)	.350	
	N	50	50

Figure 11.28 The Pearson's *r* correlation between the study variables.

Figure 11.28 shows the same correlation using Pearson's *r*. As you see, $r = -0.135$ and is not significant ($p = 0.350$). In this example, a more meaningful outcome may be achieved by using the appropriate statistical procedure (Spearman's Rho). Hospitals with greater funding correlate inversely with the number of complaints about the funded procedures. Again, the researcher cannot make causal attributions from these findings, but the outcome generally speaks to at least one facet of the wealth–health relationship using Spearman's Rho.

TERMS AND CONCEPTS

Aggregate data: Aggregate data are those data gathered on large-scale social units such as states, counties, industries, and the like, which combine data from smaller analytical levels (e.g., individual opinions, individual salaries, etc.).

Coefficient of determination:	The squared value of r, the Pearson correlation coefficient, which represents the proportion of variance in the outcome variable accounted for by the predictor variable of a study.
Dichotomized variables:	Continuous scores that have been transformed into variables with only two values (e.g., high or low). This is related to but not the same as "dichotomous variables" which are those variables that naturally have two categories (e.g., male or female).
Heteroscedasticity:	A violation of the assumption of equal variation. In this condition, the variance of one study variable is not equal at each value of the other study variable.
Homoscedasticity:	The assumption of equal variance in a study in which the variance of one variable is equal at values of the other variable in a study.
Linear relationship:	The relationship among study variables that forms a straight line if plotted on a graph. Violations of linearity might take the form of "curvilinear" relationships in which the graphed line is not straight but curved.
Outliers:	Extreme scores in a distribution that may result in a distortion of values of the total set of scores.
Proportional reduction in error (PRE) measures:	Procedures that measure how much variation is reduced or explained by knowing the relationship among study variables. In correlation, r^2 is such a measure in that it describes the proportion of variance in the outcome variable that is accounted for by the predictor variable.
Restricted range:	A problem in correlation studies in which the entire set of scores are not used in an association, but rather a selected group of the scores is used that that do not represent the total variability.
Scattergram:	A graph that shows the relationship between study variables when they are plotted together. Also called "scatter diagram," "scatterplot," or "scatter graph."

DATA LAB AND EXAMPLES (WITH SOLUTIONS)

Problem 1

A research professor wanted to check the relationship between the score on a quiz and the minutes it took students to complete the quiz. Does time matter to test scores? Table 11.6 presents the data for this problem.

TABLE 11.6   Test Taking Minutes and Test Score Data

Minutes	Test Score
16	19
3	17
6	18
12	19
7	16
16	20
12	19
15	20
8	17
9	19

Problem 2

Earlier in this book I introduced data from a partial housing survey I conducted some years ago that focused on neighborhood characteristics. (Table 3.4 presents partial data from this survey.) In this problem, I present a sample of residents' survey responses to two neighborhood characteristics: job opportunities and community involvement. Are these variables related?

Table 11.7 presents the data for this problem. Conduct a correlation analysis and summarize your responses using SPSS. Be sure to discuss whether the assumptions were met for this procedure.

DATA LAB: SOLUTIONS

Problem 1

Findings

The minutes taking the test and the test score are positively correlated with these data. The longer the time taking the test, the higher the score:

- Pearson's $r = 0.81$
- Critical value $= 0.632$
- Reject H_0, $p < 0.05$

Manual calculations

The SS_{XY}

$$SS_{XY} = \sum XY - \frac{(\sum X)(\sum Y)}{N}$$

$$SS_{\text{Minutes} \times \text{Test Scores}} = 1958 - \frac{(104)(184)}{10}$$

$$SS_{\text{Min.} \times \text{Scores}} = \mathbf{44.4}$$

TABLE 11.7   The Job Opportunity–Community Involvement Study Data

Job Opportunities	Community Involvement
1	1
1	3
1	1
1	1
2	4
2	1
2	1
2	2
2	4
2	3
3	2
3	4
3	5
3	4
4	4
4	3
4	4
4	3
4	4
4	6
5	5
5	5
5	7
6	5
7	7
7	7
7	6
7	7

The SS_X

$$SS_X = \sum X^2 - \frac{\left(\sum X\right)^2}{N}$$

$$SS_{\text{Minutes}} = 1264 - 1081.6$$

$$= 182.4$$

The SS_Y

$$SS_Y = \sum Y^2 - \frac{(\sum Y)^2}{N}$$

$$SS_{Scores} = 3402 - 3385.6$$

$$= \mathbf{16.4}$$

Pearson's r

$$r_{XY} = \frac{SS_{XY}}{\sqrt{(SS_X)(SS_Y)}}$$

$$= \frac{44.4}{\sqrt{(182.4)(16.4)}}$$

$$= \frac{44.4}{54.69}$$

$$= \mathbf{0.81}$$

Problem 2

The elements of the solution for this problem include an examination of assumptions, the hypothesis test, and effect size. The database I used is only to illustrate the correlation procedure and should not be taken to indicate real-world findings.

Assumptions

1. Randomly chosen sample. I chose the respondents from the database (of about $N = 140$) to illustrate the correlation procedure.

2. Variables are interval level. Data are from respondent survey that I treat as interval.

3. Variables are independent of one another. Respondent data were not dependent in this study.

4. Variables are normally distributed.
   The SPSS outcome shown in Figure 11.29 (from "Analyze – Compare Means – Means" menus) indicates that the two variables are normally distributed based on skewness and kurtosis. The histograms in Figure 11.30 (Community Involvement) and Figure 11.31 (Job Opportunities) show some skewness in Job Opportunities but "somewhat" normal distribution in Community Involvement, findings indicated by the Shapiro–Wilk test of normality shown in Figure 11.32. Despite minor irregularities in the normal assumption, Pearson's r is robust and can provide meaningful results.

5. Variances are equal. Pearson's r is robust for these violations unless one or both variables are significantly skewed. Although the results indicate some skewness in

Report

	Job Opportunities	Commnity Involvement
Mean	3.61	3.89
N	28	28
Std. Deviation	1.950	1.969
Kurtosis	−.806	−.912
Std. Error of Kurtosis	.858	.858
Skewness	.439	.035
Std. Error of Skewness	.441	.441

Figure 11.29   Descriptive findings for study variables.

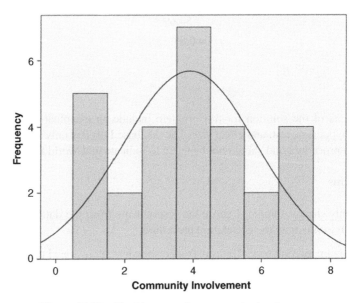

Figure 11.30   The histogram for community involvement.

one variable (Job Opportunities), I will proceed with this study problem. The scattergram shown in Figure 11.33 is partial evidence of bivariate normality, discussed in the next assumption.

6. Linear relationship. The two variables must display a "straight line" when plotting their values. Violations of this assumption might include "curvilinear" relationships in which plotted data appear to be in the form of a "U" pattern. Figure 11.33 shows the scattergram for the study variables, the data of which appear to be uniformly distributed around the regression line. In a later chapter, I show how to detect "curvilinear" and other relationships through SPSS. Using this example, those tests and the visual examination of the scattergram provide evidence of linearity.

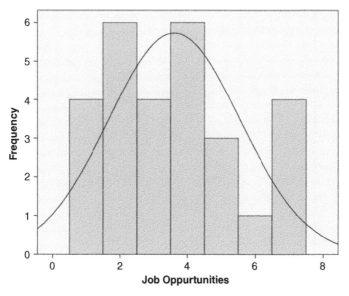

Figure 11.31 The histogram for job opportunities.

Tests of Normality

	Kolmogorov-Smirnov[a]			Shapiro-Wilk		
	Statistic	df	Sig.	Statistic	df	Sig.
Job Opportunities	.152	28	.095	.912	28	.022
Community Involvement	.129	28	.200[*]	.924	28	.042

[*]. This is a lower bound of the true significance.

a. Lilliefors Significance Correction

Figure 11.32 The tests of normality for the study variables.

Hypothesis Test

1. The null hypothesis (H_0): $\rho = 0$.
2. The alternative hypothesis (H_A): $\rho \neq 0$.
3. The critical value $r_{28(0.05)} = 0.374$.
4. The calculated value (0.874) (see Figure 11.34 for the correlation findings).
5. Statistical decision: Reject the null hypothesis. The calculated correlation falls into the exclusion area and is therefore unlikely a chance finding.

Effect Size

The effect size for this result is $r^2 = 0.76$ ($0.847^2 = 0.764$). The predictor variable (job opportunities) accounts for 76.4% of the variance in the outcome variable

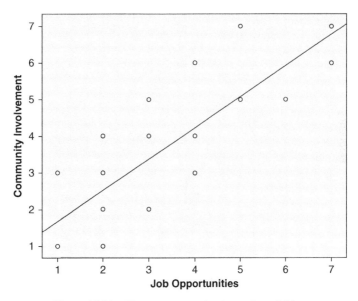

Figure 11.33   The scattergram for the study variables.

Correlations

		Job Opportunities	Community Involvement
Job Opportunities	Pearson Correlation	1	.847**
	Sig. (2-tailed)		.000
	N	28	28
Community Involvement	Pearson Correlation	.847**	1
	Sig. (2-tailed)	.000	
	N	.28	28

**. Correlation is significant at the 0.01 level (2-tailed).

Figure 11.34   The correlation findings for the study variables.

(community involvement). This amount is considered large by the Cohen (1988) criteria.

Discussion

For this example study, respondents indicated that job opportunities in a sub-sidized housing project were positively correlated to community involvement. The high correlation ($r = 0.847$) indicated that respondent's judged community involvement to be higher with increased job opportunities.

12

BIVARIATE REGRESSION

This chapter discusses a very important statistical procedure for researchers. Regression techniques use correlation to help predict the values of an outcome variable knowing values of the predictor variable. If you recall, I mentioned at the outset of Chapter 11 that correlation helps researchers to explain and predict. By extension, regression techniques use correlations between variables to explain variance in outcome variables and predict specific *outcome values* at different values of predictor variables.

I made reference to regression procedures in the scattergrams I created and discussed in Chapter 11. For example, Figure 11.2 showed the scattergram of the correlation between the opinion of family income and the opinion of health. The scattergram used a line to show the pattern of the respondent scores. Correlation is stronger when the dots are close to the line, and the direction of the line indicates whether the relationship is positive or inverse.

The line that "captures" the pattern of the correlation relationship is actually the *regression line of best fit*. You will learn in this chapter to calculate the equation for this line so that you can understand the dimensions of the relationship between the two variables. You can use the line to help predict values of the outcome variable knowing values of the predictor variable, and you can identify the "explained variance" between the two variables knowing the dimensions of the line.

If a researcher created a regression equation for the relationship between respondents' opinions of their income and their health, they could use this information to understand other respondents not in the study. For example, knowing that the correlation between opinions of income and health is 0.699 would help the researcher to

Using Statistics in the Social and Health Sciences with SPSS® and Excel®, First Edition.
Martin Lee Abbott.
© 2017 John Wiley & Sons, Inc. Published 2017 by John Wiley & Sons, Inc.

make better predictions of the income or health of other individuals who were not in the study. For example, if you asked a nonrespondent to give you an opinion of their income, you could use the $r = 0.699$ to calculate a better estimate of their health opinion than if you simply guessed at their health.

The researcher could also understand how much of the variance in health opinions is explained by respondents' income opinions and how much variance is left unexplained. The researcher would in this way create a "model" of explanation that would help them in subsequent studies to add other possible explanations that might help to explain further the "unexplained variance."

THE NATURE OF REGRESSION

Technically, regression refers to the *spread of the values of Y for values of X*. This refers to the fact that at fixed values of the predictor variable (X), there are several values of the outcome variable (Y). This spread of Y values will have a mean at each X value. The path of a line that crosses through all the means is what we refer to as the regression line. It is a "line of best fit" since it passes through the means of the Y points across the values of X.

Consider Figure 12.1, a hypothetical example using the data from problem 2 in Chapter 11 (relationship between job opportunities and community involvement). As you can see, I placed several elements on the chart to explain the nature of the regression line:

- The dots represent the values of job opportunities and community involvement for each respondent in the data set. (Note that each dot may represent more than one respondent if they have the same values.)
- The line passes through the means of both variables ($M_{JO} = 3.61$, $M_{CI} = 3.89$).
- The bracket in Figure 12.1 indicates that at each X value (job opportunities), there may be several values of Y (community involvement). Figure 12.1 shows the Y values in the bracket where $X = 2$.
- The regression line makes it possible to predict values of Y at each value of X. For example, in Figure 12.1, the dashed vertical and horizontal lines represent extending a vertical line from $X = 3$ to the regression line and then extending a horizontal line from the regression line to the Y-axis to indicate a predicted value of Y (3.37). Thus, when $X = 3$, the predicted value of $Y = 3.37$.

In Figure 12.1, you can see that when job opportunities (X) is 2, there are several respondents represented. This means that several respondents indicated a "2" on the survey regarding their opinion of job opportunities, but not all of these respondents had the same opinion of community involvement. I drew a bracket around the dots at $X = 2$ to show that at any value of X there will be a spread of values of Y.

Figure 12.2 shows another dimension of regression analysis. When you create the regression line, the predicted value of Y represents the mean of the distribution of Y predicted values at values of X. However, the *actual* values of Y (which you may not

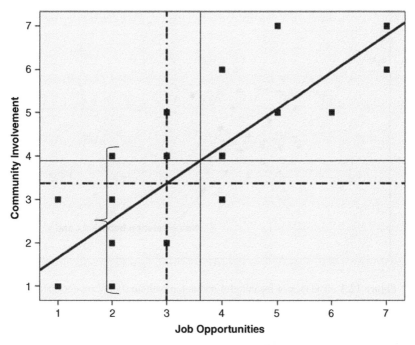

Figure 12.1   The regression line for job opportunities and community involvement.

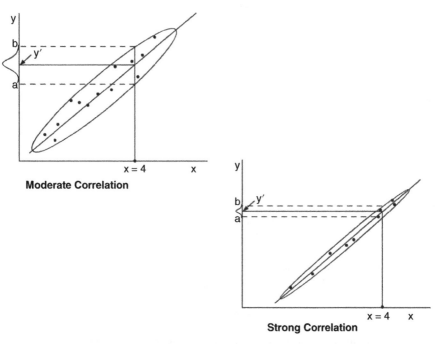

Figure 12.2   The effect of correlation on prediction accuracy.

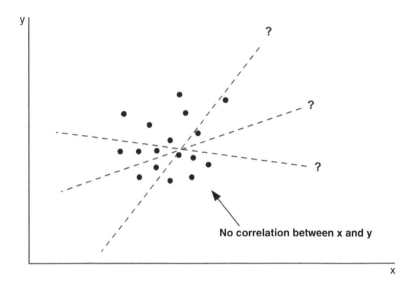

Figure 12.3   The lack of meaningful prediction with no significant correlation.

know) might vary from this predicted value. I represented this variability of prediction with a small distribution around the predicted values on the *Y*-axis. (In these graphs, *y′* indicates the predicted value of *Y*.)

As you can see, when the correlation between the two variables is stronger (bottom panel), the predicted *Y* values have less variability and can be thought to be more accurate. Since in this case there is less variability of *Y* scores at each value of *X*, the "mean of the predicted values of *Y*" is a more precise estimate of the actual value of *Y*.

Figure 12.3 shows yet another dimension of regression. When there is no significant correlation, the predictability of *Y* at values of *X* is very poor. You can see how this is problematic because with very low correlation, you cannot establish a meaningful regression line that will provide good estimates or predicted *Y* values.

THE REGRESSION LINE

Just as there were two methods for calculating Pearson's *r*, there are two methods for calculating the regression line. The first of these methods uses *Z* scores. The logic of this formula is best understood by first looking at the raw score formula which is the second way of creating the equation for the regression line.

Both the *Z* score formula and the raw score formula are variations of the equation for a line that you probably learned in an algebra class:

$$Y = mX + b$$

In this formula, the *m* is the slope of the line (rise over run), and *b* is the *y* intercept. Statisticians use the same formula but with different symbols. In the statistical

TABLE 12.1   The Fictitious Data on Income Class and Healthy Days

Income Class	Healthy Days
5	76
1	58
6	81
8	86
9	90
3	62
0	45

formula, *b* represents the slope of the line and *a* is the *y*-intercept. So, the statistical equation for the straight line (i.e., regression line) we use is

$$\hat{Y} = bX + a$$

You will note that the $\hat{Y}$ is the symbol for "*Y* predicted," which is the predicted value of *Y* at values of *X*. This is often represented as *Y′* as you can see in Figure 14.2, or simply as Y_{pred}. I will use the latter (Y_{pred}) in this chapter.

The "*b*" and "*a*" values in the equation have research meanings beyond "slope" and "intercept." Here is how to use them in research:

- *b* is the slope of the regression line. When you calculate the equation, the *b* is the coefficient for the predictor variable that indicates *the unit change in Y with each unit change in X*. That is, for every 1 unit change in the *X* variable, how many units will the *Y* variable change?
- *a* is the *Y*-intercept. This refers to the value of *Y* when *X* = 0. (You must examine research graphs carefully since some do not show 0 on the *X*-axis. I will discuss this later.)

Table 12.1 shows a fictitious set of data that follows the theme in Chapter 11 of correlating respondents' opinions of their income with opinions of their health. These data represent income by "classifying" income in groups from 0 to 10, with higher groups representing higher incomes. Health is represented by the number of days in a 3-month period a respondent considered themselves healthy.

In regression, you use the correlation to help better predict the values of an outcome variable (*Y* = Healthy Days) using values of a predictor (*X* = Income Class). Thus, you use regression to create a model that will accomplish two things:

1. Explain as much variance as possible in the outcome variable
2. Predict values of the outcome variable with values of the predictor

Figure 12.4 shows the scattergram between the two variables (from SPSS®). As you can see, the regression line ("line of best fit") has been calculated and drawn

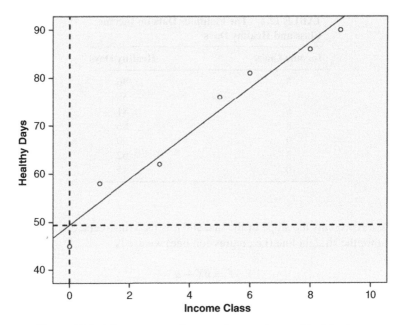

Figure 12.4   The scattergram between income class and healthy days.

through the dots in such a way as to minimize the distance of each dot from the line. As I discussed earlier, you may also think of the line representing the mean of all the predicted Y values that lie at each value of X. Since there are so few observations, this is not visually apparent, but you can see it more clearly with more observations as in a following example.

The task is to calculate the regression line so as to understand better the properties of regression. I will calculate both b and a for this equation.

Note that in Figure 12.4, the Y-intercept is shown (i.e., the regression line is shown crossing the Y-axis), but the intercept value ("a") is the value of Y when $X=0$. *This value lies directly above the "0" on the X axis where the regression line would intersect the Y-axis.* I indicated this with the vertical and horizontal lines in the scattergram. Since the $X=0$ is not directly on the Y-axis, the value of "a" might be deceptive. On the graph, "a" appears to be about 47 (the point of intersection of the regression line and the Y-axis). However, as I will show, the calculated value of $a = 49.41$, which is seen more clearly by the dashed lines extending from the X-axis to the regression line to the Y-axis.

CALCULATING REGRESSION

As I noted earlier, I will begin by calculating the <u>raw score formula</u> for regression. This formula uses the <u>actual values</u> of X and Y as they appear in the raw score data table. Both variables are measured in their own scales. If you look at the data in

Table 12.1 you will see that both X and Y are interval-level variables (at least, that is how I am presenting them in this fictitious example), but the magnitudes of the scale values are different. (Actual) X values range from 0 to 9, whereas Y values range from 45 to 90. The raw score formula uses the values as they exist in the table:

$$Y_{pred} = bX + a$$

If you look carefully at the formula, there are four elements, two of which are dependent upon the calculation of the other two:

- Y_{pred} is the outcome that depends on the values of the other calculations.
- X takes the values from the data the researcher uses as the predictors.

The aforementioned two values are "resident" in the equation; they are there but do not show a value in the equation. The other two elements are calculated:

b, the slope, is calculated by the following equation:

$$b = \frac{r\sqrt{SS_Y}}{\sqrt{SS_X}}$$

a, the intercept, is calculated by the following equation:

$$a = M_Y - b(M_X)$$

The Slope Value b

Note that the slope is simply the r value times the relationship between the variance (standard deviation (SD)) of Y to that of X (in the formula, I use the sum of squares (SS) value that represents the SD when the square root is taken). Here are some observations about the slope:

- When r *is large*, the slope value will be larger, indicating a larger slant to the regression line and a *greater impact of X on Y*.
- When r *is small*, the slope will be flatter. The r value thus modifies the slope by influencing the size of the "rise" (Y) over the size of the "run" (X).
- When $r = 1.0$, a perfect correlation, the slope is the direct relationship between the SD values of Y and X.
- When $r = 0$, or no correlation, the slope will be flat, *indicating no predictive value of X for Y values*.
- Intermediate values of r "weight" the impact of the slope.

The Regression Equation "in Pieces"

The regression equation looks difficult but it is manageable if you think of it in "pieces." Figure 12.5 shows how you might consider the calculation formula.

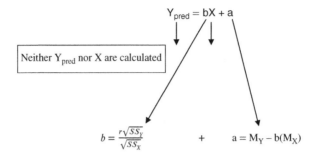

Figure 12.5 The formula in pieces.

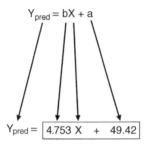

Figure 12.6 The completed regression formula.

The Fictitious Example

Table 12.2 shows the values from Table 12.1 needed for calculating the pieces of the regression equation. Remember you must calculate r as you did in Chapter 11.[1] The value of regression depends upon a significant and meaningful r value:

r value : $r_{XY} = \dfrac{SS_{XY}}{\sqrt{(SS_X)(SS_Y)}} = \dfrac{331.429}{\sqrt{(69.714)(1636.857)}} = 0.981$

b value : $b = \dfrac{r\sqrt{SS_Y}}{\sqrt{SS_X}} = \dfrac{0.981\sqrt{1636.857}}{\sqrt{69.714}} = 4.753$

a value : $a = M_Y - b(M_X) = 71.14 - 4.753(4.57) = 49.42$

You can now place the calculated elements in the regression equation as shown in Figure 12.6. As you can see, the X value simply stays in the equation without a value.[2]

---

[1] See SS formulas in Chapter 11 for calculating Pearson's r.
[2] The beta and intercept values from the hand calculations are slightly different from SPSS which calculates values with several decimal points.

TABLE 12.2   The Calculated Sums of the Fictitious Data

	Income Class (X)	X^2	Healthy Days (Y)	Y^2	X*Y
	5	25	76	5776	380
	1	1	58	3364	58
	6	36	81	6561	486
	8	64	86	7396	688
	9	81	90	8100	810
	3	9	62	3844	186
	0	0	45	2025	0
Σ	32		498		2608
$Σ^2$		216		37066	
Mean	4.57		71.14		372.57
SS	69.714		1636.857		331.429

Interpreting and Using the Regression Equation

Once you arrive at the final regression formula, you can interpret the parts and use it for prediction. The b is a coefficient of X and indicates the unit change in Y with every unit change in X. Thus, when X changes by 1 unit (i.e., when a respondent increases one income class), the Y value increases by 4.753. This means that healthy days increase by almost 5 for each income class advancement.

If you wished to predict a value of Y for a certain value of X, you can simply insert the X value in the equation and solve for the Y_{pred}. For example, if you wanted to predict a healthy days value for a respondent in an income class of 4, the predicted healthy days value would be 68.43:

$$Y_{pred} = 4.753(4) + 49.42$$

$$= 68.43$$

Figure 12.7 shows the predicted healthy days value (68.43) when the respondent's income class is 4.

EFFECT SIZE OF REGRESSION

Regression is based on correlation, so the effect size is r^2 as in correlation. In this instance, you can conclude as you did with correlation that with this sample, the income class accounts for 96.3% of the variance in healthy days. As with correlation,

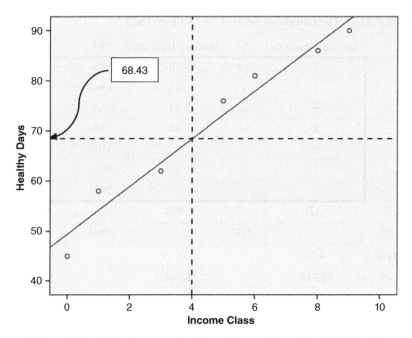

Figure 12.7   Using the regression formula to predict a value of Y at $X = 4$.

you can use the same criteria from Cohen (1988) of r^2 values of 0.01, 0.09, and 0.25 for small, medium, and large effects, respectively.

THE Z SCORE FORMULA FOR REGRESSION

If you recall, I noted earlier that there is another way to calculate the regression formula using Z scores. Like correlation, this would involve creating Z scores for each of the scores in the data table. The resulting formula shows that with bivariate regression, the slope is equal to the correlation (slope $= r$).[3] You can see how this works if you consider that the SD of Z scores $= 1$. Thus, the following would apply:

$$b = \frac{r\sqrt{SS_Y}}{\sqrt{SS_X}} = \frac{r(1)}{(1)} = r$$

If both X and Y were transformed to Z scores, their SDs would $= 1$. Thus, as you can see from the formula for calculating b, this would mean that you would be dividing the Y SD (which equals 1) by the X SD (which also equals 1) to yield 1. (Remember that the $\sqrt{SS}$ value in the equation is a measure of SD.)

---

[3]This is only true for regression studies with one predictor variable (bivariate regression). Multiple regression creates a different value for the slope value with Z score formulas.

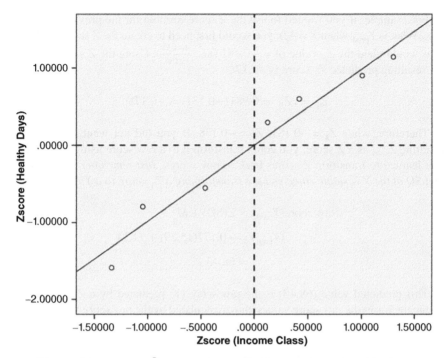

Figure 12.8   The SPSS® Z score scattergram of income class and healthy days.

When both X and Y values are Z scores, the scattergram would show the change in scales for both variables. Since both would be in Z score scales, there would be no Y-intercept; the regression line would cross the "Y-axis" at the origin (where $X = 0$ and $Y = 0$). Figure 12.8 shows this. As you can see, the vertical and horizontal lines create the Y- and X-axes at values of 0 for both. They cross at the origin, which represents $X = 0$ and $Y = 0$. (Note that both the Y and X axes have negative values since Z scores are negative as well as positive.) Since the regression line passes through the origin, the Y-intercept is always 0, unlike the intercept with the raw score formula.

The Z score formula therefore changes due to the revised values for b (i.e., $b = r$) and a ($a = 0$ since there is no Y-intercept). The following shows the raw score formula and the resulting Z score formula that incorporates the changes in values from using Z scores:

$$\text{Raw score formula: } Y_{\text{pred}} = bX + a$$

$$Z \text{ score formula: } Z_Y = rZ_X \text{ which in final form is } Z_Y = \beta Z_X$$

Using the Z Score Formula for Regression

If you use the Z score formula to predict Z_Y values, you need to remember to use Z_X values. Thus, if you wanted to predict a Z_Y value, you would need to obtain Z values for the X scores.

For example, if you wanted to use the Z score formula for the previous problem (i.e., What is Y_{pred} when $X = 4$?), you would first need to create the Z score for $X = 4$. This would yield the Z_X value of $= -0.181$ (i.e., $\frac{4-4.57}{3.156}$). Using the Z score formula, the resulting predicted Z_Y score is -0.178:

$$Z_Y = rZ_X = 0.981(-0.181) = -0.178$$

Therefore, when $Z_X = -0.181$, $Z_Y = -0.178$. If you did not want to report the resulting Z_{pred} as a Z score, you could transform it to a raw score using the formula you learned to transform Z scores back to raw scores. *Just remember to use the M and SD of the Y variable since you are transforming a Z_Y score to a Y raw score*:

$$\text{Raw score}(Y_{pred}) = Z(SD) + M$$

$$(Y_{pred}) = -0.177(15.29) + 71.14$$

$$= 68.43$$

This predicted value (68.43) is the raw score (Y) predicted by a Z_X of -0.181. Compare this to the raw score values above calculated by the raw score formula since these are the Z score values corresponding to predicting Y from an X score of 4.

Unstandardized and Standardized Regression Coefficients

You will notice that the slope values in the raw score formula and in the Z score formula have different symbols. This is because in the raw score formula, you are using *unstandardized* (i.e., raw score) values, that is, values that have not been transformed to Z scores. When you use Z scores, the slope is referred to as "beta" and symbolized by β. You refer to this value as the *standardized* coefficient since Z scores are scores expressed in standard deviation units.

This may seem to be a petty distinction, but I show later that it is an important difference. Statistical software reports regression results in different ways depending on whether standardized values are used, so you need to keep this difference in mind.

TESTING THE REGRESSION HYPOTHESES

When you calculate a regression equation, you can use it to explain variance and to predict values. But the same question remains with regression as with the other procedures we have discussed thus far: Are the results statistically significant?

There are two considerations for statistical significance in bivariate regression:

1. The *omnibus* test is the statistical significance of the *overall regression model*.
2. The *individual predictor test* assesses the statistical significance of each predictor in the model (in bivariate regression there is only one predictor).

I will discuss the results for both of these tests by examining the results from SPSS and Excel. I note here that the *omnibus test is an F test* since the F test assesses the significance by comparing components of variance. The raw score formula uses SS values which allows you to see the relationships among the variables in the analysis. The *individual predictor test is a T test of whether the slope differs from 0* (in effect, a *T* test of a single sample). I discussed both of these tests in past chapters, so you will be prepared to understand the results.

THE STANDARD ERROR OF ESTIMATE

I have discussed several inferential statistical tests that use sampling distributions as comparisons for transformed test values. The regression analysis creates a sampling distribution of sorts, the standard deviation of which is called the standard error of estimate, symbolized by "s_{est}."

When using the regression equation to make predictions, the estimate will infrequently match exactly the "actual" value of Y. Rather, the Y_{pred} value will be somewhat different than an actual value. This difference is called the "error of prediction" or simply "error." The differences between Y_{pred} values and actual *Y* values are also known as *residuals*.

The s_{est} is the standard deviation of the distribution of prediction errors (residuals). You can use this value as a comparison of all individual prediction errors and to create a confidence interval of scores within which the actual value of *Y* will fall a given percentage of time (e.g., 95% of the time).

Calculating the s_{est}

Calculating s_{est} is straightforward and can be performed in two (at least) ways. The first method uses residual scores, as I noted earlier. I will demonstrate this formula in the following when I discuss residual scores. The formula for this approach is

$$s_{est} = \sqrt{\frac{\Sigma(\text{residuals})^2}{N-2}}$$

The second method calculates s_{est} by making reference to the variance measure of Y (rather than residual scores), so you simply adjust the variance measure by using the correlation measure and the degrees of freedom for regression. This will yield the standard deviation of the distribution of prediction errors.

This formula uses SS_Y, the variance measure of *Y*, and uses the degrees of freedom of regression (and correlation), which as you recall is $N-2$ since you estimate two parameters (predictor and outcome variables). This is the same in bivariate regression where there are two variables. When you divide the variance measure by the degrees of freedom, you create an estimate of the SD of the sampling distribution (i.e., the standard error). Taking the square root creates an SD measure from the variance measure (SS_Y) you used to create the estimate

$$s_{est} = \sqrt{\frac{SS_Y}{N-2}(1-r^2)}$$

The s_{est} measure is made more precise by taking into account the correlation between the predictor and outcome variables. Thus, in the formula, you "modify" the estimate by multiplying by $(1 - r^2)$, which is the unexplained variance. As you see, when there is a large correlation (as there is in our fictitious sample), this unexplained variance will be very small and will therefore result in a s_{est} that is small. However, when the original correlation is weak (i.e., approaching 0), there will be a greater amount of unexplained variance. This will result in a larger standard error of estimate.

In the fictitious example, the s_{est} is calculated as follows. Your results may be slightly different depending on whether you round off the elements of the formula before the final calculation or if you complete the formula in one step. SPSS uses values with several decimal places for this calculation so the resulting value of 3.499 is reported. In the following manual calculations, I used more than the typical (for me) three decimal places, so the manual calculations match the SPSS reported s_{est} of 3.499:

$$s_{est} = \sqrt{\frac{SS_Y}{N - 2}(1 - r^2)}$$

$$= \sqrt{\frac{1636.857}{7 - 2}(1 - 0.962)}$$

$$= \sqrt{327.3714\,(0.0374)}$$

$$= 3.499$$

The result is 3.499. What does this mean? *It is the estimated standard deviation of all the prediction errors of the regression equation.*

The original correlation ($r = 0.981$) was very large, so the standard error is not large. If the correlation had been small, for example, $r = 0.10$, look what would happen to the s_{est} calculation:

$$s_{est} = \sqrt{\frac{1636.86}{7 - 2}(1 - 0.01)}$$

$$= \sqrt{327.372(0.99)}$$

$$= 18.00$$

You can see by comparing these s_{est} results that a stronger correlation reduces the prediction error. The range of the s_{est} is therefore:

$s_{est} = 0$, when there is perfect correlation, $r = 1$

$s_{est} =$ the maximum value is equal to SD_Y when the correlation $= 0$

CONFIDENCE INTERVAL

Earlier, I predicted a value of Y (68.43) when X was 4. You can have confidence that this value is *close* to the actual value of Y, but it will likely not be exactly the same. Therefore, you can <u>estimate a range of values that will capture the true value of Y</u> (a parameter estimate) by using the s_{est} value. This is the same process you followed with other statistical procedures using confidence intervals that identified the boundary values within which the true (population) value fell a given percent of the time (e.g., 95%).

You can use the s_{est} to identify the interval within which to expect the true (parameter) value of Y to fall. Recall that in Chapter 7, I used the following formula to establish the confidence interval for the single sample population estimate:

$$\text{Confidence interval} = \pm t(s_M) + M$$

With regression, you use the same approach, but substituting the different elements. The CI for the (estimated) true value of Y is

$$\text{Confidence interval} = \pm t(s_{est}) + Y_{pred}$$

In this formula, use the tabled value of T since the sample size is very small. With larger samples, you can use the Z value (± 1.96 at the 0.05 level, etc.). Please remember, however, that when you identify the exclusion value with the T table for regression, you need to use the df value of $N - 2$ (since the regression procedure estimates two parameters). The s_{est} replaces the standard error of the mean (s_M) in the single sample formula since you estimate values of Y rather than the population mean. You establish boundary values around the predicted value of Y (Y_{pred}), so this value replaces "M" in the single sample CI formula.

Using the CI formula, you can estimate the true value of Y when $X = 4$ as follows:

$$\text{Confidence interval} = \pm t(s_{est}) + Y_{pred}$$

$$CI_{0.95} = \pm 2.571(3.499) + 68.43$$

Lower Boundary = 59.43	Upper Boundary = 77.43
$CI_{0.95} = -2.571(3.499) + 68.43$	$CI_{0.95} = +2.571(3.499) + 68.43$

According to these estimates, you can be confident at the 0.95 level that the true value of Y will fall between 59.43 and 77.43. The s_{est} helps to identify these values which are much more accurate because you use the value of the correlation to help estimate more precisely. Without the knowledge of the correlation, you would estimate the boundaries somewhere between approximately 25.97 and 110.90 using the s_Y (16.52). The high correlation between X and Y helps create a more precise estimate.

EXPLAINING VARIANCE THROUGH REGRESSION

I mentioned earlier that the main functions of regression are prediction and explanation. Correlations greater than 0 (i.e., significant) improve the predictions of the outcome variable at various levels of the predictor variable. You saw this in the figures that showed "tighter" patterns of dots around the line having stronger correlations and, therefore, more precise predictions.

You can also use regression relationships to explain the proportion of variance in the outcome variable resulting from its relationship to the predictor variable. The r^2 value is a numerical expression of this explained variance, as you saw in Chapter 11. Now I can delve a bit more deeply into the relationships to show how this works. You can use sum of square calculations to measure components of variance that will "partition the variance" or break the variance down into recognizable parts.

The following formula expresses these parts of the variance in the relationship between income class and healthy days. The equation has three parts:

$$\Sigma(Y - M_Y)^2 = \Sigma(Y_{pred} - M_Y)^2 + \Sigma(Y - Y_{pred})^2$$

The part of the equation on the left of the = sign is the total variance measure of Y. As the equation shows, there are two parts on the right side of the equation produced by the regression relationship that contributes to the total variance in the outcome variable. Here are the three parts and how they are calculated:

$$\Sigma(Y - M_Y)^2 = \text{the total sum of squares of } Y, \text{ or simply } SS_Y$$

The next component (immediately to the right of the "=" sign) is the portion of variance in the outcome variable that you identify through the predictive power of the correlation with the predictor variable. It is the "known" portion of variance in the outcome variable and is called regression, or simply the sum of squares of regression:

$$\Sigma(Y_{pred} - M_Y)^2 = \text{sum of squares of regression, or } SS_{reg}$$

The last portion represents the part of the variance in the outcome variable that is unknown or that which you cannot identify through the variables in the regression equation. It is called "error" since its origin cannot be determined. This part is measured by creating residual values that exist between the predicted Y values and the actual Y values. This "residual sum of squares" value is a combination of random error and unexplained variance:

$$\Sigma(Y - Y_{pred})^2 = \text{sum of squares of residual, or } SS_{res}$$

In regression, you account for total variance by "partitioning" it, or breaking it down, so that you can understand the contributing parts. The following is a simplification of the larger regression equation shown earlier:

$$SS_Y = SS_{reg} + SS_{res}$$

Stated differently:

Total variation in Y = known variation (SS_{reg}) + unknown variation (SS_{res})

These parts of total Y variation are similar to the sources of variance I discussed in the ANalysis of VAriance (ANOVA) chapter. Recall that you determined the following with respect to the portions of variance in an ANOVA study:

$$SS_T = SS_B + SS_W$$

Like the regression equation, I explained total variance as a combination of between (known) and within (unknown or error) variance. There is a very close relationship between ANOVA and regression that I will discuss further in the following text.

You learned with ANOVA that you can calculate eta square (an effect size measure) as follows:

$$\eta^2 = \frac{SS_{Between}}{SS_{Total}}$$

Like ANOVA, you can create a similar measure, r^2, from the proportions of variation identified in regression. Consider the following formula and compare it to the eta square formula shown earlier:

$$r^2 = \frac{SS_{reg}}{SS_Y}$$

Hopefully, you can see the parallels between these two formulas. Both measure the proportion of known variance (regression) to total variation. Both express the amount of explained variance in an outcome variable accounted for by a predictor variable.

Using Scattergrams to Understand the Partitioning of Variance

The parts of the regression equation are easier to understand through a visual examination of the scattergram. Remember that residuals are the "prediction errors" that result from using the regression equation to predict values of the outcome variable Y. Each prediction yields a value that is a certain distance from the actual value of Y.

Figure 12.9 shows the regression relationship between the two variables in the example I used earlier. The regression line is established between the X variable (Income Class) and the Y variable (Healthy Days).

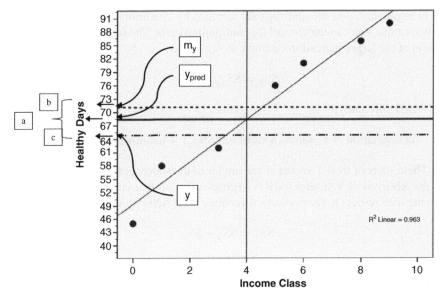

Figure 12.9 The elements of the Y variance.

I included three lines in Figure 12.9 that help to show the parts of variation:

1. The dashed line in the scattergram (the lowest of the three lines) is the *actual value of Y*. (There was no actual value of Y in the study data, so you can assume this to be 65 for illustration purposes. That is, you assume that a respondent has an income class of 4 and has 65 healthy days.)
2. The solid black line just above the (dashed) line is *the predicted value of Y* at a certain value of X. (The value shown in the figure is $X = 4$, which, as calculated in the earlier section of the chapter predicted a value of Y of 68.43. Remember, there was no respondent with an income class of 4 in the study; I simply demonstrated earlier that the regression equation could help predict values of Y at certain values of X.)
3. The dotted line above the predicted value line is the mean of Y (71.14). This is a primary reference point for the analyses since the M_Y is the best guess of the value of Y if you had no other information. That is, without any help from the regression with X, if someone asked to guess a value for healthy days for a respondent, the best guess would be the mean of the healthy days scores since most respondent values would fall there.

I added three "identifiers" to Figure 12.9 to point out the parts of the variation:

- "a" = SS_Y. This is the SS measure for the differences between the mean of Y and the actual value of Y. Remember that variance is a measure of how far from the mean all the scores in a distribution scatter out. Thus, in Figure 12.9, this represents the large distance of the actual Y value from the mean of Y.

- "b" = SS_{reg}. This distance represents the "known" variation. Think of this part as representing the distance that a predicted value moves away from the mean and closer to the actual value as a result of the correlation between X and Y. Thus, the correlation has the effect of identifying the known relationship between X and Y, resulting in the predicted value moving closer to the actual value. The stronger the correlation, the greater this portion of the variance, since the predicted values will fall further from the mean and closer to the actual values.

- "c" = SS_{res}. This part represents the distance between the predicted value of Y and the actual value. It is the "unknown" portion of the variation because there is no information about what might cause it to be as large as it is. The SS_{reg} moved the predicted value closer to the actual value (due to the influence of X), but couldn't get it all the way! The SS_{res} is what remains, or error.

Now, examine the r^2 equation again. As you can see, the equation compares the elements of variation from the regression analysis. The r^2, or effect size, increases as the SS_{reg} increases relative to the overall variation in Y. Another way of saying this is that as the predicted scores move further away from the mean toward the actual values of Y, the more variation explained in the Y variable:

$$r^2 = \frac{SS_{reg}}{SS_Y}$$

A NUMERICAL EXAMPLE OF PARTITIONING THE VARIATION

You can use the actual calculations from the example study to measure the proportions of variation. Table 12.3 shows these calculations. (I show the values from the example study sorted by the X variable.)

Remember the equation for these elements is as discussed earlier. I have shown this equation with the actual values in Table 12.3:

$$SS_Y = SS_{reg} + SS_{res}$$

$$1636.86 = 1575.64 + 61.21$$

TABLE 12.3   The Calculations for the Components of Variance

X	Y	$(Y-M_Y)$	$(Y-M_Y)^2$	Y_{pred}	$(Y_{pred}-M_Y)$	$(Y_{pred}-M_Y^2)$	$(Y-Y_{pred})$	$(Y-Y_{pred})^2$
							Residuals	
0	45	−26.14	683.46	49.41	−21.73	472.33	−4.41	19.45
1	58	−13.14	172.74	54.16	−16.98	288.29	3.84	14.72
3	62	−9.14	83.59	63.67	−7.47	55.81	−1.67	2.80
5	76	4.86	23.59	73.18	2.04	4.15	2.82	7.95
6	81	9.86	97.16	77.93	6.79	46.12	3.07	9.40
8	86	14.86	220.73	87.44	16.30	265.68	−1.44	2.08
9	90	18.86	355.59	92.20	21.05	443.26	−2.20	4.83
$M_Y = 71.14$								
			$SS_Y = 1636.86$			$SS_{reg} = 1575.64$		$SS_{res} = 61.21$

As you can see from the equation, the total variation in Y is a combination of known (SS_{reg}) and unknown (SS_{res}) variation. Comparing these two sources, you can see that the unknown proportion is much smaller than the known proportion because the correlation was so large ($r = 0.98$).

You can calculate r^2 from the variance sources, as I discussed previously. Partitioning the variance is an important avenue for understanding the relationships between an outcome and a predictor variable:

$$r^2 = \frac{SS_{reg}}{SS_Y}$$

$$= \frac{1575.64}{1636.86}$$

$$= 0.96$$

Using Residuals to Calculate s_{est}

I mentioned earlier that you can use residuals to calculate the standard error of estimate. Using the residual data (SS_{res}) value from Table 12.3 (61.21) in this formula will yield the same s_{est} value (3.499) as that yielded by using the second formula (shown earlier) which used the SS_Y:

$$s_{est} = \sqrt{\frac{\sum (\text{residuals})^2}{N - 2}}$$

$$= \sqrt{\frac{61.21}{5}}$$

$$= 3.499$$

USING EXCEL AND SPSS® WITH BIVARIATE REGRESSION

I explored the value of regression for prediction and explanation in the previous sections. I now turn to exploring the regression output to illustrate these procedures. I will use the same fictitious data in this section but then will introduce a more extended example in a later section.

THE SPSS® REGRESSION OUTPUT

In this section I note some unique features from SPSS that are helpful for bivariate regression and that establish a model for interpreting multiple regression results. The SPSS procedure is available through the main "Analyze – Regression" menu. When you select this option, you will be presented with several regression procedures from which to choose. For bivariate regression, select "Linear" since this procedure applies

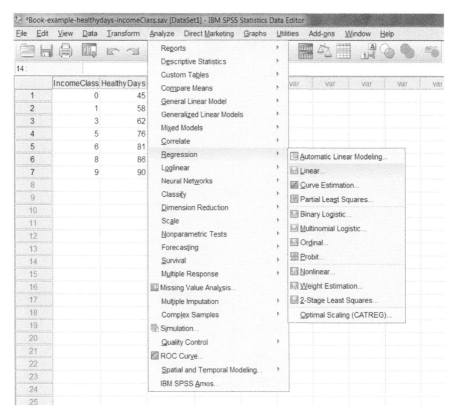

Figure 12.10 The regression options in SPSS®.

to regression equations that manage one (bivariate) or many predictors (multiple). Note that this regression procedure <u>assumes a linear relationship</u> that I discussed earlier. I will review all the regression assumptions in a later section in this chapter.

Figure 12.10 shows several ways to specify the bivariate regression study. The main specification window "Linear Regression" requires that you place the predictor variable in the "Independent(s)" window and the outcome variable in the "Dependent" window. As you see, I specified both variables using the example data.

Once the variables are specified, the user can choose from a number of buttons on the right side of the "Linear Regression" window. All of these are important for different kinds of studies, but the "basic" bivariate regression can be created by including only a few additional specifications from the "Statistics" button. Figure 12.11 shows these specifications.

The "Linear Regression: Statistics" window allows the user to create descriptive information on the study variables ("Descriptives") as well as to produce the ANOVA table ("Model Fit") results and identify changes to the R^2 from predictors added to the analysis ("R squared change"). The "Estimates" and "Confidence intervals" choices produce the a and b coefficients with their confidence intervals.

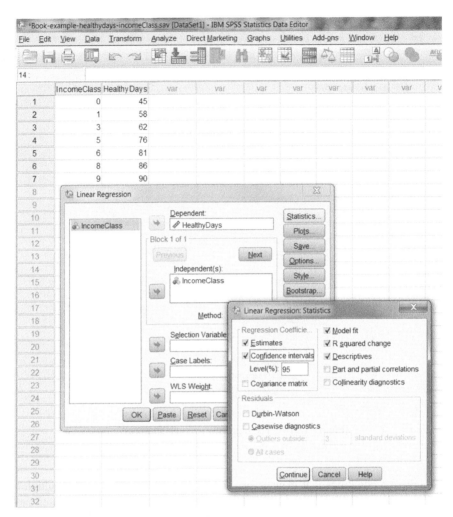

Figure 12.11   The SPSS® regression specification windows.

The Omnibus Test and Model Summary

Making these specification choices results in several SPSS outcome panels. After reports on descriptive statistics for each variable and the correlation matrix, the outcome includes the ANOVA table used to assess the omnibus test for the regression. Figure 12.12 shows the data that allow you to test the null hypothesis for regression. If you recall, I mentioned that there are two kinds of significance tests with regression. One is the *omnibus test* that determines whether the overall results establish a non-chance predictive model between the two study variables. Note that the omnibus test

ANOVA[a]

Model		Sum of Squares	df	Mean Square	F	Sig.
1	Regression	1575.644	1	1575.644	128.702	.000[b]
	Residual	61.213	5	12.243		
	Total	1636.857	6			

[a]Dependent Variable: Healthy Days.
[b]Predictors: (Constant), Income Class.

Figure 12.12 The ANOVA table providing data for the omnibus test.

results are provided in an ANOVA table. I discussed previously the close relationship between ANOVA and regression because both procedures use sum of squares calculations to understand how the components of variation between the study variables relate to each other.

Figure 12.12 shows two important elements of the ANOVA results:

1. The omnibus significance test is provided by the F ratio (128.70, significant beyond $p < 0.000$) which indicates that the proportion of total variance explained by the SS of regression is beyond the value expected by chance (according to the F distribution).
2. The total explained variance, or R^2 (0.96) can be obtained by dividing the SS_{reg} (1575.64) by the total variation, or SS_Y (1636.86).

The results panel in Figure 12.13 ("Model Summary") shows values for R, R square, adjusted R square and s_{est}. There are some additional results reported in this panel, however. I will list these in the following text.

- "R Square Change" shows the impact of the predictor variable on the overall regression model. There is only one predictor, so this is a bit harder to understand, but if there were additional independent variables, there would be separate lines of data and the R Square Change value would show how the addition of each predictor would change the overall R^2 value. Since there is only one predictor in the current study, the R Square Change value is the same as the R Square value in the second column. You might think of this value as the predictor variable (income class) increasing the explained variance in Y (healthy days) from 0% to 96%.
- "F Change" similarly shows the impact of adding the predictor (only one in this study) to the F value.
- "Sig. F Change" registers the change in the significance of the F value from the addition of the predictor variable. Both this and the former will change when additional predictors are included in the model.

Model Summary[b]

Model	R	R Square	Adjusted R Square	Std. Error of the Estimate	Change Statistics				
					R Square Change	F Change	df1	df2	Sig. F Change
1	.981a	.963	.955	3.499	.963	128.702	1	5	.000

[a]Predictors: (Constant), Income Class.

[b]Dependent Variable: Healthy Days.

Figure 12.13   The SPSS® model summary results panel.

Coefficients[a]

Model	Unstandardized Coefficients		Standardized Coefficients	t	Sig.	95.0% Confidence Interval for B	
	B	Std. Error	Beta			Lower Bound	Upper Bound
1 (Constant)	49.410	2.328		21.226	.000	43.426	55.394
IncomeClass	4.754	.419	.981	11.345	.000	3.677	5.831

[a]Dependent Variable: Healthy Days.

Figure 12.14   The SPSS® coefficients panel results for the bivariate regression.

The Regression Coefficients

Figure 12.14 shows the "Coefficients" panel which provides the information necessary to create the regression equation and assess the significance of the individual
predictor. Among the results is the column "Standardized Coefficients" reported just
before the T test results are provided. This column of data includes the beta (β) coefficient which is the *standardized coefficient* for the regression equation.

If you recall at the outset of this chapter, I discussed two ways of creating
the regression equation. The method I used in the calculations of the example study
involved the regression equation that used the actual (raw score) scales of the
variables. This method produces the regression equation that can be derived from
the values from the panel in Figure 12.14. The y-intercept value "a" is listed as the
"(Constant)" value of 49.41, and the slope value "b" is listed adjacent to the name of
the independent variable "Income Class" (4.754). Both of these values are located in
the "Unstandardized Coefficients." Using these coefficients produces the regression
equation[4]

$$Y_{pred} = 4.75X + 49.41$$

The other method I discussed was the Z score method that transform raw score
values of both X and Y variables and then create the regression equation

$$Z_Y = \beta Z_X$$

[4]The SPSS output differs slightly from my hand calculations above due to slight rounding differences.

Recall that with bivariate regression, the slope coefficient is equal to the Pearson's r value using standardized X and Y values. Thus, Figure 12.14 shows the beta (β) coefficient which can be used in the standardized equation. If you check the values in Figure 12.14, you will see that the standardized coefficient is equal to Pearson's r since there is only one predictor variable:

$$Z_Y = \beta Z_X$$
$$= 0.981 \, Z_X$$

You may be curious as to *why* SPSS produces both sets of coefficients. There are several answers to this question, but the most common answer is that researchers often wish to work with both of their variables on the same scale of measurement. In the example study, each variable is expressed in different scales. The y variable "Healthy Days" potentially has values from 0 to 100, whereas the x variable "Income Class" has a range of values from 0 to 9. If you transform the values to standardized (Z) scores, they would be expressed in similar ranges of values (i.e., z score values typically from ranging from -3.00 to 3.00). In this way, SPSS presents raw score values as Z scores and reports the resulting regression formula as a standardized equation.

The Significance Test of Individual Predictors

Figure 12.14 also shows values that allows you to perform the second significance test, the test of the individual predictors. Recall I mentioned that once the omnibus test was performed, you would need to perform a test on the individual predictor(s) to determine whether the slope was significantly different from 0. This test is primarily important for "multiple regression" which has more than one independent (predictor) variable. In such a study you would need to perform individual significance tests on the separate predictors to see which added most to the overall prediction.

Figure 12.14 shows the "t Stat" for the predictor variable X (Income Class) as 11.345 and is determined to be significant (shown in the "P-value" column as $p < 0.000$). This test uses the single sample t ratio to determine whether the derived slope coefficient (4.754) is significantly different than a population value of 0. With these results, you can conclude that the individual predictor Income Class is a significant predictor of the Healthy Days for this sample of respondents.

Note also the confidence interval values provided in the output (lower bound: 3.667 and upper bound: 5.831).[5] These values indicate a 95% confidence that the population value for the sample slope of 4.754 will be between 3.667 and 5.831. In addition to the t test of the slope, you can determine that the slope is significant (i.e., nonzero) if the confidence limits do not include the possibility of "0."

---

[5] Do not confuse these values with the confidence limits I calculated for a predicted value of y for a given value of x, as I showed above. The SPSS output lists the confidence limits for the slope value in order to provide an estimate of the population value for the slope.

THE EXCEL REGRESSION OUTPUT

I will again use the data in Table 12.1 to demonstrate the Excel regression procedure. At the "Data Analysis" window that results from using the main menu options "Data – Data Analysis," you can choose "Regression" which will produce the window in Figure 12.15.

As you can see, I entered the spreadsheet locations of the Y (Healthy Days) and X (Income Class) data. I checked the "Labels" box since I included the variable labels to identify the variable data in the output. I asked for "Confidence Level 95%" that applies to the regression coefficients ("b" and "a") as I showed in the SPSS results. I also asked for "Residuals" so you can see how these values appear. Recall that I used these values earlier when I discussed partitioning the variance.

When you run this specification, Excel returns four panels of results. I show these below in Figures 12.16–12.19.

Figure 12.16 confirms the values that I produced in the manual calculations. Note that Pearson's r is called "multiple R" when it is used in regression. The "adjusted R

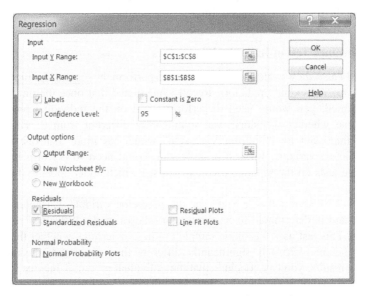

Figure 12.15 The Excel regression specification window.

Regression Statistics	
Multiple R	0.98
R Square	0.96
Adjusted R Square	0.96
Standard Error	3.50
Observations	7

Figure 12.16 The Excel regression Statistics output.

ANOVA	df	SS	MS	F	Significance F
Regression	1	1575.64	1575.64	128.70	0.00
Residual	5	61.21	12.24		
Total	6	1636.86			

Figure 12.17   The Excel Regression Model output.

	Coefficients	Standard Error	t Stat	P-value	Lower 95%	Upper 95%
Intercept	49.41	2.33	21.23	0.00	43.43	55.39
Income Class (X)	4.75	0.42	11.34	0.00	3.68	5.83

Figure 12.18   The Excel regression output showing the regression coefficients.

	RESIDUAL OUTPUT	
Observation	Predicted Healthy Days (Y)	Residuals
1	49.41	–4.41
2	54.16	3.84
3	63.67	–1.67
4	73.18	2.82
5	77.93	3.07
6	87.44	–1.44
7	92.20	–2.20

Figure 12.19   The Excel predicted values and residuals for the study data.

square" measure is affected by the sample size among other considerations. You can see that the "standard error" is the same value $s_{est} = 3.499$ from the manual calculations and the SPSS output (with rounding).

As in the SPSS results, Figure 12.17 shows the data that will help test the null hypothesis for regression. The F value (128.70) shows that the *omnibus test* is significant ($p < 0.00$) and determines that the overall results establish a nonchance predictive model between the two study variables. The total explained variance, or R^2 (0.96), can be obtained by dividing the SS_{reg} (1575.64) by the SS_Y (1636.86) as I discussed in the SPSS results shown earlier.

Figure 12.18 shows the table of values for second significance test, the test of the individual predictors. As you can see, the t test for the slope of the predictor variable X (Income Class) is 11.34 and is determined to be significant (in the "P-value" column at $p < 0.00$). This test uses the single sample t ratio to determine whether the derived slope coefficient (4.75) is significantly different than a population value of 0. With these results, you can conclude that respondents' income class can significantly predict their healthy days.

Figure 12.18 also provides the calculated value of the slope (b) and intercept (a) values used to create the regression equation (49.41 and 4.75, respectively).

The "standard error" values reported for the intercept and X variable (2.33 and 0.42) in Figure 12.18 are not s_{est} which is shown in Figure 12.16. These standard errors are those connected to both the a and b coefficients (i.e., the standard deviation of the sampling distributions of estimates for intercept and slope to create CI values for each). The confidence intervals shown in the last two columns ("Lower 95%" and "Upper 95%") reference population estimates of the coefficients as I discussed in above in the SPSS results.

The last Excel panel is shown in Figure 12.19 and lists the predicted and residual values for each case in the data set. (You can compare these values with those in Table 12.3). Remember the s_{est} is the estimated standard error of these residuals. Excel has an option for "standardized residuals" (that I did not request) which transforms the residual values to standardized values (i.e., Z values) so you can see at a glance which exceed 2 or 3 and might therefore be considered "extreme" or "outlier" values. In our example database, we would expect no such outliers, but you can use this feature with actual data in your studies.

COMPLETE EXAMPLE OF BIVARIATE LINEAR REGRESSION

In this section, I provide an example of bivariate regression using data from my community survey I introduced in past chapters. This example uses adjusted data ($N = 24$) from the survey in order to demonstrate the issues in the following sections of this chapter. This part of the study concerned the possibility that the presence of Recreational Opportunities (RO) in the neighborhood might affect community involvement positively.[6] Thus, the study question might be posed as: Can RO significantly predict community involvement values and be helpful in accounting for variance in respondent opinions about community involvement?

I do not provide data analysis using manual calculations, but I do provide the SPSS and Excel findings used to interpret the results. First, I will address whether the assumptions of the data are met before I proceed with the regression analysis.

ASSUMPTIONS OF BIVARIATE REGRESSION

As in the case of the other statistical procedures in this book, there are assumptions for linear regression that, when met, will likely yield the best predictions and explanation of variance. Different authorities look at these assumptions differently, so I will list the common assumptions here.

---

[6] Since I adjusted the values for the demonstration, the outcomes should not be taken as a reflection of the outcomes of the overall (actual) study. However, despite the changes I made to demonstrate the procedures that follow, the findings using the entire data set are generally the same as those with the sample set. The predictor variable (Recreational Opportunities) significantly predicts the outcome variable (community involvement). In fact, the results of the overall study show stronger results!

When proceeding with a regression study, the first step is to check the assumptions since using data that meet the assumptions promise a more accurate result. In what follows, I address each of the assumptions with the example database:

1. <u>Variables are interval level</u>. Regression procedures can use ordinal and even nominal data *as the predictor variable* but not the outcome variable. In advanced courses, you will learn how to create and use categories of data to predict interval-level outcomes. I treat this in detail in other publications (see Abbott, 2010). There are other regression procedures for studies with categorical outcomes (e.g., logistic regression), but I will use interval-level variables for the bivariate regression examples.

2. <u>Variables are normally distributed</u>. This assumption is primarily for the outcome variable, but using normally distributed predictors will help with the other assumptions.

3. <u>Variances are equal</u>. As with Pearson's *r*, regression is robust for these violations unless one or both variables are significantly skewed. You can use scattergrams to detect patterns that may indicate violations of this assumption. If the pattern of dots is not generally evenly distributed around the regression line, the variances may not be equal, for example. Technically, this assumption means that *the variance of one variable should be generally the same at different levels of the other variable*.

4. <u>Linear relationship</u>. With the linear regression procedure I am discussing in this book, the two variables must display a "straight line" when plotting their values. Thus, for example, if you correlated the age of a car with the value of a car, the correlation would probably be a straight line (in a downward direction, indicating an inverse relationship), but at some point the line would likely change in an upward direction since really old cars increase in value. Formally, you can detect these "curvilinear" relationships through SPSS as I will show.

5. <u>Cases are independent of one another</u>. As I mentioned with correlation, this assumption is somewhat difficult to understand, but it deals primarily with not using variables in which there are linkages among the participants. The pairs of data from each participant must not be connected to others.

In the next two sections, I will expand on the assumptions that warrant an extended view: normality, equal variance, and linearity. The sections below examine these assumptions using SPSS and Excel procedures.

Normal Distribution and Equal Variance Assumptions

Figures 12.20 and 12.21 show the descriptive data from SPSS and Excel with respect to these study variables. As you can see from both figures, the study variables are

Report

	Recreational Opportunities	Community Involvement
Mean	3.391	3.619
N	23	21
Std. Deviation	1.6717	1.4310
Kurtosis	−.428	−.302
Std. Error of Kurtosis	.935	.972
Skewness	.463	−.604
Std. Error of Skewness	.481	.501

Figure 12.20   The SPSS® descriptive summaries of the study variables.

	Recreational Opportunities	*Community Involvement*
Mean	3.39	3.62
Standard Error	0.35	0.31
Standard Deviation	1.67	1.43
Sample Variance	2.79	2.05
Kurtosis	−0.43	−0.30
Skewness	0.46	−0.60
Range	6	5
Minimum	1	1
Maximum	7	6
Sum	78	76
Count	23	21

Figure 12.21   The Excel descriptive summaries for the study variables.

normally distributed as indicated by skewness and kurtosis values that are within acceptable boundaries.[7]

Since neither study variable is extremely skewed, the scattergram should show an even distribution of dots around the regression line. Figure 12.22 shows this to be the case, with a wider bit of scatter around the origin of the graph. This would be something to keep in mind for our later procedures (especially linearity), but for this small data set, you can proceed with the assumption of equal variance.

Linear Assumption: Curvilinear Relationships

Thus far, I have discussed bivariate *linear* relationships. As you check the assumptions for a study, however, you might find that the variables are not related to one

---

[7]The Kolmogorov–Smirnov and Shapiro–Wilk tests of normality obtained through the "Explore" procedure in SPSS also confirm that the two study variables are within normal bounds.

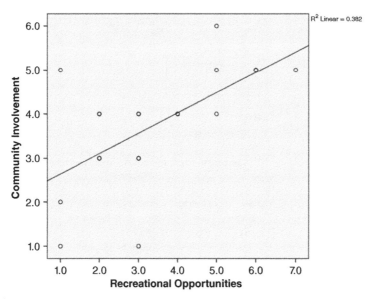

Figure 12.22 The scattergram between recreational opportunities and community involvement.

another in linear fashion. Scattergrams are always helpful to detect these possible violations of assumptions, but SPSS has a procedure that provides a numerical analysis.

In what follows, I demonstrate procedures for checking curvilinearity in the community survey sample data I described earlier. This procedure tests the assumption that the predictor (Recreational Opportunities) is related in linear fashion to the outcome (community involvement).

In order to test the assumption of linearity, use the "analyze – regression – curve estimation" menu to get the screen shown in Figure 12.23.

As you can see, I placed the community involvement variable in the "Dependent" window and Recreational Opportunities (RO) in the "Independent" window. In the "Models" box, there are several choices for curve fitting that might be applicable to the data. I have chosen two of these ("Linear" and "Quadratic") to show how each method fits the data to the regression line. In essence, these methods (and the others listed) are attempts to provide the best fit of the line to the dots. As you can see, there are several different models that might provide a better regression equation than a linear fit. Also check the "Display ANOVA table" box in the lower left part of the box for additional diagnostic information.

Figure 12.24 shows the scattergram that is created when you proceed with the Curve Estimation procedure. As you can see, the graph includes two lines placed on the data. The linear (solid) line is shown along with the quadratic (dashed) line. The pattern of the dots *appear* almost to overlap, indicating that the data indicate the same fit model. The two lines appear to be very close to one another, but you must rely on the numerical analysis to decide the better fit.

The curve estimation procedure provides a numerical analysis of the two fit lines so you can compare their fit to the data. Figure 12.25 shows the results of this analysis.

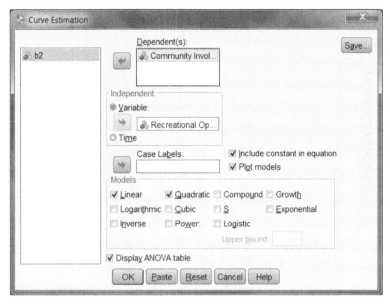

Figure 12.23   The Curve Estimation procedure in SPSS®.

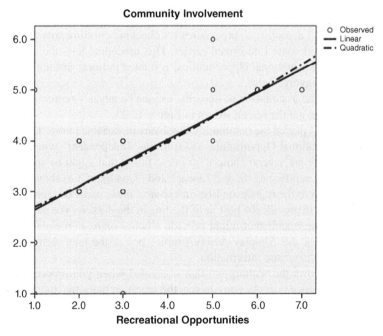

Figure 12.24   The Curve Estimation procedure for recreational opportunities and community involvement.

Model Summary and Parameter Estimates

Dependent Variable: Community Involvement

Equation	Model Summary					Parameter Estimates		
	R Square	F	df1	df2	Sig.	Constant	b1	b2
Linear	.382	11.129	1	18	.004	2.184	.461	
Quadratic	.383	5.276	2	17	.017	2.326	.362	.013

The independent variable is Recreational Opportunities.

Figure 12.25 The curve estimation model summary.

You interpret this output as you would a given linear regression output such as the example shown with the Income Class–Healthy Days (example) data. Figure 12.25 output shows two equations that correspond to two different statistical models. The first equation ("Linear") shows that the regression equation between RO and community involvement would result in an R^2 of 0.382 and the following linear equation:

$$Y_{pred} = 0.461X + 2.184$$

The second equation ("Quadratic") shows the regression equation with an R^2 of 0.383 and the following result:

$$Y_{pred} = 0.362X_1 + 0.013X_1^2 + 2.326$$

These equations look different because the quadratic equation adds a predictor with a b_2 of 0.013. This b_2 consists of a separate predictor variable that is comprised of the squared values of the original predictor (RO), or $X_1{}^2$, according to the requirements for the quadratic formula. The quadratic model adds the squared values of RO to the linear regression equation in order to see whether a curvilinear pattern presents a better fitting line. This process shows whether squared values *add information to estimating the curve.* Predicted *Y* values are created by *combining* two estimated coefficients: the coefficient for the values of the *X* variable and the coefficient for the squared values of the *X* variable. *The resulting equation would therefore represent a line that curves or contains two different trajectories.*

The quadratic model (curvilinear) and the linear model explain virtually the same amount of total variance in the dependent variable (0.383 and 0.382, respectively). Along with the visual evidence from the scattergram, you might therefore conclude that both models are equal in their ability to explain variance in the dependent variable. The Curve Estimation procedure provides an additional bit of information to help understand the nature of the line.

Figure 12.26 shows the output coefficient analysis for the quadratic formula. As you can see, neither of the predictor variables in this equation is significant. Therefore, the quadratic formula does not add sufficient information to warrant its use over the linear formula, which does show a significant b_1 for the single predictor RO.

Coefficients

	Unstandardized Coefficients		Standardized Coefficients		
	B	Std. Error	Beta	t	Sig.
Recreational Opportunities	.362	.632	.486	.573	.574
Recreational Opportunities ** 2	.013	.082	.135	.159	.875
(Constant)	2.326	1.045		2.226	.040

Figure 12.26 The quadratic coefficients analysis for Curve Estimation.

THE OMNIBUS TEST RESULTS

Recall that the omnibus test assesses the statistical significance of the overall regression model. You can use both SPSS and Excel to examine the omnibus test results through the ANOVA table. I show the SPSS results in Figure 12.27 (Excel provides identical results). As you can see, the F (11.129) is significant ($p = 0.004$) which indicates that the overall model significantly predicts opinions about community involvement from opinions about Recreational Opportunities.

EFFECT SIZE

You can calculate the effect size by using the SS values reported in Figure 15.26. As you can see, the calculated value of r^2 is 0.382, which is considered a large effect according to the guidelines I discussed earlier:

$$r^2 = \frac{SS_{reg}}{SS_Y}$$
$$= \frac{12.895}{33.750}$$
$$= 0.382$$

ANOVA[a]

Model		Sum of Squares	df	Mean Square	F	Sig.
1	Regression	12.895	1	12.895	11.129	.004[b]
	Residual	20.855	18	1.159		
	Total	33.750	19			

[a]Dependent Variable: Community Involvement.

[b]Predictors: (Constant), Recreational Opportunities.

Figure 12.27 The SPSS® omnibus test results.

Model Summary[b]

Model	R	R Square	Adjusted R Square	Std. Error of the Estimate	Change Statistics				
					R Square Change	F Change	df1	df2	Sig. F Change
1	.618a	.382	.348	1.0764	.382	11.129	1	18	.004

[a]Predictors: (Constant), Recreational Opportunities.

[b]Dependent Variable: Community Involvement.

Figure 12.28   The SPSS® model summary results for recreational opportunities–community involvement study.

THE MODEL SUMMARY

Both SPSS and Excel provide overall model summary data which provide further information for the omnibus test and effect size. I show the SPSS results in Figure 12.28 because of the additional information contained in the output as I described earlier in this chapter. As you can see, the effect size is as I calculated it earlier, and both the F Change and R Square Change values are significant. The $s_{est} = 1.0764$ will be helpful for predicting specific values of community involvement given values of RO.

THE REGRESSION EQUATION AND INDIVIDUAL PREDICTOR TEST OF SIGNIFICANCE

I will show the individual coefficient results from both SPSS and Excel in order to point out the unique results of the outputs. Both report identical findings for the test of the predictor slope and for the coefficient values.

Both Figures 12.29 (SPSS) and 12.30 (Excel) show that the t value (3.336) for RO is significant ($p < 0.004$). This indicates that the slope for RO is significantly

Coefficients[a]

Model		Unstandardized Coefficients		Standardized Coefficients	t	Sig.	95.0% Confidence Interval for B	
		B	Std. Error	Beta			Lower Bound	Upper Bound
1	(Constant)	2.184	.527		4.141	.001	1.076	3.292
	Recreational Opportunities	.461	.138	.618	3.336	.004	.171	.751

[a]Dependent Variable: Community Involvement.

Figure 12.29   The SPSS® coefficients output for the recreational opportunities–community involvement study.

	Coefficients	Standard Error	t Stat	P-value	Lower 95%	Upper 95%	Lower 95.0%	Upper 95.0%
Intercept	2.184	0.527	4.141	0.001	1.076	3.292	1.076	3.292
RO	0.461	0.138	3.336	0.004	0.171	0.751	0.171	0.751

Figure 12.30   The Excel regression output for the reading assessment – FR study.

different from 0, or nonzero. The confidence intervals for the coefficients indicate that the estimated population slope fall between 0.171 and 0.751 at the 95% level. If this interval had included 0, you would have to conclude that a 0 population slope was possible and therefore that the slope is not significant. However, the values do not include 0, so you can be confident (at the 0.95 level) that the slope is significantly different from 0.

Figures 12.29 and 12.30 show the coefficients that create the regression equation:

$$Y_{pred} = 0.461X_{RO} + 2.184$$

Thus, you can identify that with a change of one value in RO, the community involvement value increases by 0.461.

Figure 12.29 also includes the standardized regression coefficient (β) of 0.618, which is also r in this analysis. If you wanted to create the standardized regression equation, it would be as follows:

$$Z_{CI} = 0.618Z_{RO}$$

Either of these regression formulas can be used for prediction. However, you must remember to use the Z score formula to transform the outcomes if you wish to create raw score values using the standardized (Z) formula.

ADVANCED REGRESSION PROCEDURES

Correlation and regression are very useful statistical techniques. However, they are somewhat limited in that only one predictor variable accounts for the variance in an outcome variable. Real-life research is much more complex. In the example, 38.2% of the variance in the opinion of community involvement among a small group of respondents is accounted for by the opinion of Recreational Opportunities. There is still a great deal of variance in community involvement opinions unexplained. Fortunately, there are several statistical procedures that help to account for more of the unexplained variance by adding predictors to the study.

Multiple Correlation

If you recall, I discussed a fictitios study in which I predicted healthy days from respondents' income class. You know that no one variable by itself will explain all of the variance of another; life is not that simple. Therefore, you might use several predictor variables, analyzed at the same time, to explain more of the variance of a dependent variable. *Multiple correlation is a technique that correlates several predictors with a dependent variable.* Will the combined influence of the set of independent variables explain more of the variance in a dependent variable than a single predictor?

You can extend this fictitious example to understand multiple correlation. If you look at Figure 11.11, you will see a Venn diagram illustrating how a correlation results

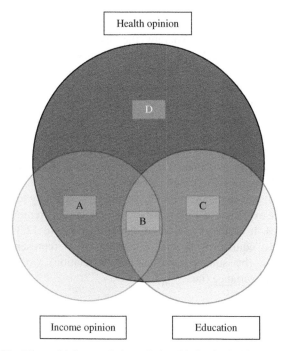

Figure 12.31 The multiple correlation relationship in the fictitious study example.

in explained variance (i.e., through r^2). Recognizing the complexity of the research situation, you might add education level to the original correlation to see what *additional* explanation of health opinion it provides. Figure 12.31 shows how this might appear through Venn diagrams.

As you can see, the addition of the second predictor, Education, results in additional overlap with the dependent variable health opinion. Therefore, the amount of overlap by both predictors shows that this multiple correlation explains more of the variance in Health Opinion than using a single predictor as shown in Figure 11.11.

You may never be able to explain all of the variation in health opinion in this manner, because there are probably an infinite number of potential explanations. However, adding predictors helps to get closer to understanding the variance in the distribution of dependent variable scores.

You will not calculate multiple correlation in this book. I wanted to introduce you to the procedure so you can understand how correlation and regression are used in research. You add (and subtract) variables from the models you build so that you can increase understanding of a study (i.e., outcome) variable.

With a single predictor, r^2 is the effect size indicator. With multiple correlation, the effect size (the "multiple coefficient of determination") is indicated by the capital r as R^2. You will note that the regression summaries presented in both SPSS and Excel show the multiple R^2 since they are designed to describe the effects of multiple predictors.

Partial Correlation

Partial correlation is a process whereby the researcher assesses the correlation between an outcome variable Y and one independent variable (X_1) while holding a second independent variable (X_2) constant. What this means in practice is that you take into account all of the various pieces of the overall set of correlations.

Recall the Venn diagram in Figure 12.31. As you can see I labeled the various overlapping sections of the circles with A through D. The partial correlation of income opinion and health opinion is like saying you are going to correlate these two variables *after you remove the influence of education from both of the other variables*. This is like saying that among respondents of the same education, the correlation of income opinion and health opinion is a certain calculated value.

In this situation, you can understand the partial correlation by looking at the pro-portion of variance explained in Y after the second predictor is removed from both of the other variables. In terms of the Venn diagram in Figure 12.31, the explained variance would be equivalent to the proportion of D represented by A. Cal-culating this value (by squaring the partial correlation) would represent the percent of explained variance (i.e., $\frac{A}{A+D}$).

Multiple Regression

If multiple correlation can explain additional variance in Y as a result of adding more predictors, multiple regression can use the additional variables in a formula measur-ing the influence of all the predictors on the outcome variable. The incremental gain of each predictor in explaining more of the variance in Y is identified in a multi-ple regression formula. The slope values of each independent variable measure the effects of that particular predictor on Y *when the influence of the other predictors is controlled*. These regression coefficients can be tested for significance to provide a view of how important each of the independent variables are in predicting Y.

I will cover multiple regression in greater depth in Chapter 13. I encourage you to pursue an understanding of this procedure, which I believe is one of the most valuable statistical techniques for researchers. I explore the topic in depth in Abbott (2010).

Additional Considerations

In advanced books and courses, you will learn about several statistical techniques that are built on correlation and regression procedures. Path analysis, structural equation modeling, canonical correlation, discriminant analysis and hierarchical linear mod-eling are just a few of many such powerful techniques.

DETECTING PROBLEMS IN BIVARIATE LINEAR REGRESSION

I mentioned earlier that I have dealt with detecting problems with statistical assump-tions in other publications (see Abbott (2010) in particular about regression proce-dures). You can see that performing a regression study can be quite complex but that *your results can be improved if you meet the assumptions of the procedure*. This is a general rule in statistics: the power of a study is improved by using the proper procedure and meeting the assumptions for each.

SPSS provides several diagnostic procedures to assist researchers with their attempts to meet the assumptions of their chosen statistical measures. You may want to explore these further as you advance in the use of statistics for problem solving. I discussed some of these procedures in this chapter on bivariate regression (e.g., using residual analyses and curve fitting). I encourage you to seek other diagnostic techniques to help with your real-world studies.

TERMS AND CONCEPTS

Beta: The *standardized* regression coefficient. Sometimes called "beta weight" and "beta coefficient."

Confidence interval: In regression, the confidence interval is the range of y values within which the "true" population value of a predicted y value is likely to fall.

Line of best fit: This is the term for the regression line calculated from the slope and y-intercept values. It is called the line of best fit since a line is drawn through the bivariate scatter of values in such a way that distances from the line are minimized.

Multiple correlation: A statistical procedure that measures the association of several predictors with a single outcome variable.

Multiple regression: A statistical procedure assessing the influence on an outcome variable of more than one predictor variable.

Partial correlation: *Generally*, the process of assessing the correlation between an outcome and predictor variable when holding a second predictor constant. Technically, it represents the correlation of two variables *after you remove the influence of a third variable from both of the other two variables.*

Slope: In a regression equation, the slope is the "angle" of the line which is measured by comparing "rise over run." In regression analyses, the slope helps to indicate how the values of a dependent variable change with unit changes in the independent variable.

Standard error of estimate: The standard deviation of the distribution of estimates in a regression study (i.e., the distribution of prediction errors).

Y-intercept: In a regression equation, this value refers to the y value when $X = 0$. This value falls at the intersection of the regression line and the y axis.

DATA LAB AND EXAMPLES (WITH SOLUTIONS)

Problem 1

Predict the number of absences from work (absence) from knowing the stress score (stress) of a small group of hospital intake workers. Answer the questions listed in Table 12.4 by using manual calculations.

TABLE 12.4   The Stress-Absence Data

Stress	Absence
9	5
2	3
12	10
11	9
4	6
1	3

1. Is there a significant correlation between Stress and Absence?

2. What is the effect size?

3. What is the regression equation?

4. Predict the number of absences of a new worker not in the original study who has a Stress value of 7.

5. Identify the $CI_{0.95}$ values for the prediction in #4.

Problem 2

Table 12.5 shows data from my community study in which respondents indicated their opinions on the extent of job opportunities in their community and their view of community involvement.[8] For this problem, use SPSS and Excel to analyze the data and report the following:

- Assumptions met?
- Correlation – is it significant?
- Effect size and interpretation
- Omnibus test results
- Individual predictor test of significance

---

[8] As with the sample above using community involvement and RO, this is a sample of the total data set, but I adapted some values for space consideration and demonstration purposes. Data from the total data set show the same (significant) trend shown in the sample data set, albeit not as strong.

TABLE 12.5 The Job Opportunity
and Community Involvement Data

Job Opportunities	Community Involvement
1	1
1	1
1	2
2	2
2	2
3	2
2	3
3	3
3	3
4	3
4	3
3	4
3	4
3	4
3	4
4	4
5	4
3	5
4	5
4	5
4	5
5	5
5	5
4	6
5	6
5	6
7	6
5	7
6	7
7	7

DATA LAB: SOLUTIONS

Problem 1

1. Is there a significant correlation between stress and absence? (Table 12.6)
   - Yes: $r = 0.89149$, $p < 0.05$ ($r_{0.05, 4df} = 0.811$)

2. What is the effect size?
   - $r^2 = 0.795$
   - 79.5 of the variance in absence is accounted for by stress.

TABLE 12.6   Manual Calculations for Problem 1

	Stress (X)	X^2	Absence (Y)	Y^2	X*Y
	9	81	5	25	45
	2	4	3	9	6
	12	144	10	100	120
	11	121	9	81	99
	4	16	6	36	24
	1	1	3	9	3
Σ	39		36		297
Σ^2		367		260	
Mean	6.50		6.00		49.50
SS					
SS	113.5		44		63

3. What is the regression equation?
   - Slope b: $b = \dfrac{r\sqrt{SS_Y}}{\sqrt{SS_X}} = \dfrac{0.891\sqrt{44}}{\sqrt{113.5}} = 0.555$
   - Intercept a: $a = M_Y - b(M_X) = 6 - 0.555(6.5) = 2.392$
   - $Y_{pred} = 0.555X + 2.392$

4. Predict the number of absences of a new worker not in the original study who has a stress value of 7.
   - $Y_{pred} = 0.555(7) + 2.392$
   - $Y_{pred} = 6.277$: A worker with a stress value of 7 will have a predicted absence value of 6.277.

5. Identify the $CI_{0.95}$ values for the prediction in #4.

$$s_{est} = \sqrt{\frac{SS_Y}{N-2}(1-r^2)}$$

$$= \sqrt{\frac{44}{4}(1-0.795)}$$

$$= \sqrt{11(0.205)}$$

$$= 1.502$$

$CI_{0.95}$ values for the prediction: $= \pm t(s_{est}) + Y_{pred}$

- Lower bound: $-2.776(1.502) + 6.277 = 2.11$
- Upper bound: $2.776(1.502) + 6.277 = 10.45$

Problem 2

1. Assumptions met? Yes

Normality: Yes. According to Figure 12.32, Sk and Ku values indicate no departure from normal for either variable (using SPSS Compare Means – Means). Also, Figure 12.33 shows nonsignificant tests of normality (using SPSS Explore).

Report

	Job Opportunities	Community Involvement
Mean	3.700	4.133
N	30	30
Std. Deviation	1.5790	1.7367
Kurtosis	−.138	−.827
Std. Error of Kurtosis	.833	.833
Skewness	.196	−.050
Std. Error of Skewness	.427	.427

Figure 12.32 Sk and Ku data for the two study variables.

Tests of Normality

	Kolmogorov-Smirnov[a]			Shapiro-Wilk		
	Statistic	df	Sig.	Statistic	df	Sig.
Job Opportunities	.138	30	.151	.947	30	.145
Community Involvement	.124	30	.200[*]	.952	30	.187

[*]. This is a lower bound of the true significance.

[a]Lilliefors Significance Correction.

Figure 12.33 Tests of normality are nonsignificant for the study variables.

Equal variance: Yes. The scattergram in Figure 12.34 shows a fairly even distribution of dots around the regression line. Along with the normality test, you can assume this assumption is met.

Linearity: Yes

The model summary in Figure 12.35 shows relatively similar R square values,[9] as is the scattergram comparison of the linear and quadratic models coefficients (Figure 12.36).

---

[9]The quadratic coefficient for Job opportunity is significant, but the JO^2 variable is not.

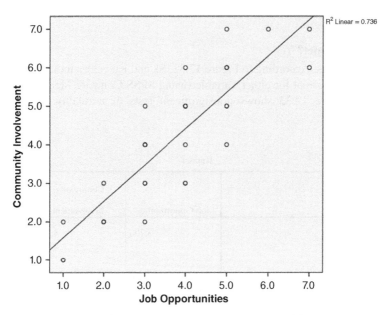

Figure 12.34   The scattergram of the study variables.

Model Summary and Parameter Estimates

Dependent Variable: Community Involvement

Equation	Model Summary					Parameter Estimates		
	R Square	F	df1	df2	Sig.	Constant	b1	b2
Linear	.736	77.864	1	28	.000	.643	.943	
Quadratic	.748	40.078	2	27	.000	−.118	1.417	−.062

The independent variable is Job Opportunities .

Figure 12.35   Model summary comparisons for linear and quadratic equations.

2. Correlation

The correlation is significant as indicated by the correlation matrix shown in Figure 12.37.

3. Effect size and interpretation

Figure 12.38 shows an R square of 0.736. This indicates that 73.6% of the variance in community involvement is accounted for by JO in this set of data.

4. Omnibus Test results

Figure 12.39 shows the ANOVA result ($F = 77.864, p < 0.000$), indicating that the model specifies JO as a significant predictor of CI in this one predictor model.

5. Individual Predictor test of significance

The regression formula: $Y_{pred} = 0.943X + 0.643$ (CI values increase by 0.943 with unit increases in JO.)

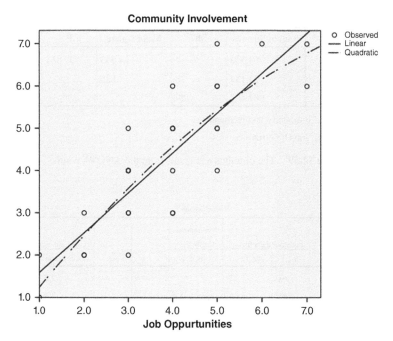

Figure 12.36   The scattergram of linear and quadratic regression equations.

Correlations

		Community Involvement	Job Opportunities
Pearson Correlation	Community Involvement	1.000	.858
	Job Opportunities	.858	1.000
Sig. (1-tailed)	Community Involvement	.	.000
	Job Opportunities	.000	.
N	Community Involvement	30	30
	Job Opportunities	30	30

Figure 12.37   Correlation matrix indicating a significant correlation.

Model Summary

Model	R	R Square	Adjusted R Square	Std. Error of the Estimate	Change Statistics				
					R Square Change	F Change	df1	df2	Sig. F Change
1	.858[a]	.736	.726	.9090	.736	77.864	1	28	.000

[a]Predictors: (Constant), Job Opportunities.

Figure 12.38   The model summary indicating the correlation and squared correlation (effect size).

ANOVA[a]

Model		Sum of Squares	df	Mean Square	F	Sig.
1	Regression	64.333	1	64.333	77.864	.000b
	Residual	23.134	28	.826		
	Total	87.467	29			

[a]Dependent Variable: Community Involvement.
[b]Predictors: (Constant), Job Opportunities.

Figure 12.39   The omnibus test result from the ANOVA result.

Coefficients[a]

		Unstandardized Coefficients		Standardized Coefficients			95.0% Confidence Interval for B	
Model		B	Std. Error	Beta	t	Sig.	Lower Bound	Upper Bound
1	(Constant)	.643	.429		1.499	.145	−.235	1.522
	Job Opportunities	.943	.107	.858	8.824	.000	.724	1.162

[a]Dependent Variable: Community Involvement.

Figure 12.40   The coefficients findings summary.

Figure 12.40 shows the following results pertinent to the significance of the predictor:

- The T test of the slope ($t = 8.824$) is significant ($p < 0.000$).
- The confidence interval for the slope does not include 0.

13

INTRODUCTION TO MULTIPLE LINEAR REGRESSION

I return to a topic in this chapter that I introduced in several earlier chapters, the connection between health and income. There is a common assumption that the greater the income, the better the health in the United States. Although this assumption is widely held, it is not strictly accurate among all indicators. A well-known example of this discrepancy is that the United States is among the wealthiest nations, but it is not the top in terms of life expectancy, among other indexes of health.

If wealth does not produce good health, what does? This is a question explored by many social science and health researchers. One such researcher, Marmot (2004) suggests that social standing might be a variable primarily responsible for health status, beyond income. Since social status consists of a number of elements (e.g., extent of education, nature of work, achievements, etc.), income or wealth may not be the best predictor of health. In the example that follows, I explore the impact of work and status on health, along with income.

THE ELEMENTS OF MULTIPLE LINEAR REGRESSION

At the end of Chapter 12, I mentioned that multiple linear regression (MLR) is an extension of bivariate linear regression in which more than one predictor variable is added to an equation that predicts values of an outcome variable. MLR is a complex procedure and well beyond the scope of this book. However, I believe it is important, and necessary, for all researchers to understand at least the basics of the procedure.

Using Statistics in the Social and Health Sciences with SPSS® and Excel®, First Edition.
Martin Lee Abbott.
© 2017 John Wiley & Sons, Inc. Published 2017 by John Wiley & Sons, Inc.

I will identify some of the primary elements of MLR and provide a simple example to highlight how to analyze and interpret MLR findings. I will not discuss the hand calculations but will instead examine the SPSS® and Excel output for the research example.

You will need to explore more advanced treatments of MLR in order to gain a depth of understanding of this versatile process. I encourage you to explore my more comprehensive treatment of MLR in Abbott (2010) as a starting point.

SAME PROCESS AS BIVARIATE REGRESSION

MLR like bivariate regression is a process that creates a model for *predicting* values of an outcome variable from predictor variables and a way of *explaining* the variance in an outcome variable. Although the hand calculations are more complex, the overall procedure is the same. *I discuss the linear relationship among variables (predictors and outcome) that will improve on the prediction of an outcome variable knowing the correlation between the outcome and predictors.*

Statistical Significance

Like bivariate regression, MLR can be examined for statistical significance by examining the *omnibus* test and the *individual predictor* test(s). Both procedures make use of the analysis of variance (ANOVA) table since both examine how the various components of variance relate to one another. Bivariate regression has only one individual predictor test, while MLR has several but the statistical significance of each individual predictor can be tested with an individual T test.

Effect Size

Effect size is measured the same way in MLR as in bivariate with the omnibus test of the model. In both cases, R^2 is an indicator of how much variance is explained in the outcome variable as a result of the predictor(s). Effect size in MLR measures the contribution of a set of predictors upon the explained variance of the outcome variable. There are more specific effect size indicators for individual predictors in MLR, but they are based on the same principle.

Coefficients

Like bivariate regression, there is a regression equation with coefficients that explain the relationship among the study variables. In MLR, of course, there are additional coefficients because there are additional predictors. The beta coefficient(s) express the same thing: the changes in Y_{pred} when the beta for a specific predictor changes one unit. Since MLR has multiple beta coefficients, this interpretation changes to "the changes in Y_{pred} when the beta changes one unit and the effects of the other predictors are controlled." This last restriction allows the researcher to understand how a particular predictor affects the outcome *at similar levels of all the other predictors*. This is the way in which the other predictors are understood as being <u>controlled</u>.

Scatter Diagrams

I have shown how scattergrams visually express the relationship between a predictor and an outcome. MLR can use scattergrams for models that include a second predictor by creating a 3D graph that includes a "Z" axis as well as X and Y axes. More complex MLR designs use graphical methods that capture the additional influences of other variables, but these are beyond the scope of this book.

Fixed- versus Random-Effects Modeling

Many statisticians make a distinction between "fixed effects" and "random effects" modeling, which can have an impact on the findings of a study and in particular on the generalizability of the findings. Fixed-effects modeling uses the same categories of variables across studies. The predictor variable (x) has a set number of categories, like gender or experimental method, where the same categories are used in all situations. In this situation, generalizability of findings is limited to the fixed category values.

On the other hand, random-effects modeling is most common in non-experimental social science research analyses; it is used in situations where the evaluator takes a random set of observations from a larger population of values, with the categories or levels of the predictor variable (x) "emerging" from and determined by the data sampled. The categories and values of x are thus random.

According to many authorities, when the main assumptions for regression are met, fixed-effects and random-effects models are interchangeable. This is particularly the case when errors are not correlated to predicted values.

SOME DIFFERENCES BETWEEN BIVARIATE LINEAR REGRESSION AND MULTIPLE LINEAR REGRESSION

There are some differences between bivariate and multiple regression due to the added complexity of additional predictors. These differences are not related to the structure of the process but are due to the added complexity.

Multiple Coefficients

I mentioned this difference earlier. Added predictors do not change the essential nature of regression but rather call for additional methods for interpretation of output.

Explanation of R^2

The explanation of components of explained variance in the outcome is related to the complexity of multiple coefficients and multicollinearity. MLR can be used to pinpoint the contribution to the R^2 of individual predictors. This is one of the chief contributions of MLR to research.

Although I cannot pursue this matter very far in this book, I will mention that interpretation of the components of R^2 rests with some procedural elements ("order of entry schemes") as well as with the very important correlation procedures of *partial* correlation and *semipartial* (or "part") correlation. I will demonstrate how to use semipartial correlation for interpreting MLR results.

Entry Schemes

MLR results can be affected by the order in which predictors are "added" to the equation by statistical software. Some software procedures allow the user to add (and remove) the predictors to the overall model in "stepwise" fashion using a set of predetermined statistical guidelines that judge whether the predictors meet certain numerical thresholds. Other schemes allow the researcher to add predictors to an MLR model in the order they determine based on a priori theoretical considerations.

The researcher can use several approaches to identify the influence of predictors on an outcome variable. (I will show a couple of these in the example in the following.) "Hierarchical" regression is simply an MLR study in which the researcher adds predictors according to an indication of importance to the study and observes the changes to the overall R^2 as a result of adding the predictors.

STUFF NOT COVERED

Because of the complexity of MLR, I cannot hope to discuss all the dimensions in this book. I mentioned some of these areas earlier (e.g., partial and semipartial correlation). Here are some other areas of MLR I cannot cover here. You might consult another of my works (Abbott, 2010) for further consideration of MLR processes.

Using MLR with Categorical Data

MLR is quite versatile and allows the researcher to use categorical as well as continuous predictors. It can even be used in experimental studies; there is a statistical connection between MLR and ANOVA, the latter of which is typically used for experimental study.

MLR uses categorical predictors through procedures in which the researcher "transforms" each of the categories of a predictor into separate "vectors" (or "subvariables") which together comprise the predictor. Each of these vectors can then be understood in their relationship to the outcome variable. (An example might be creating four vectors from a treatment variable "noise" in predicting human learning in the fictitious study I introduced in an earlier chapter.) Transforming predictors to "sets" of vectors can be done using "dummy," "effect," or "contrast" coding according to the needs of the researcher.

MLR also uses categorical outcome variables (e.g., where values are "0" or "1") in a process called "logistic regression." In this procedure, predictor variables can be either or both continuous or/and categorical. The overall attempt is to identify the likelihood of an outcome taking place or not. An example might be to determine the likelihood of contracting a certain disease given inputs of certain enzyme levels, age, diet, etc.

Curvilinear Regression

Like bivariate regression, the relationship of the predictors to the outcome variable in MLR may be nonlinear as well as linear. Statistical software like SPSS have ways of identifying these trends, so the researcher can express the most efficient model for predicting the outcome variable.

Multilevel Analysis

Multilevel analyses are procedures that recognize different "levels of data" in a regression study. For example, I might want to understand the relationship between patient survival rates of a certain illness and treatment protocols for treating the illnesses. Typically, researchers simply want to see if one variable (i.e., protocols) can predict outcomes (i.e., survival rates). This approach "understands" the relationship between two variables that are measured at the same (individual) level of analysis. However, might the hospitals within which the treatments are applied also affect the outcomes? Viewed thus, individual protocols used are "nested" within hospitals which aggregate the incidents in which the protocols were used. This is a different level from the individual level of analysis.

Viewing hospitals as a different variable in such a study suggests several questions: Are all hospitals equal, with respect to this research question? Would the unequal funding levels for newer technology, newer understandings of the disease process, more and easier analytical processes available, and other such considerations likely affect the relationship between given individual treatments and survival rates for this particular disease?

Multilevel analysis is a way of understanding what the relationships are at one level of analysis (treatment) by recognizing the influence of another level of analysis (hospital). These are very powerful tools for a researcher, but they are not easy to learn. You might explore hierarchical linear modeling approaches if you are interested in this topic.

ASSUMPTIONS OF MULTIPLE LINEAR REGRESSION

Generally speaking, MLR shares the assumptions of Bivariate regression, but I added several later due to the complexity of the data where there is more than one predictor.

Normal Distribution

The values of the variables are normally distributed by themselves and are normally distributed at each combination of levels of the other variables. This is multivariate normal distribution, and is very difficult to achieve in practice. You can use a scattergram to view the normal distribution of each variable (especially the outcome variable), but you will rely on the tests for the other assumptions that I describe later. Multivariate normality results in a linear relationship.

Homoscedasticity

As I discussed with correlation, homoscedasticity refers to equal variance among the variables in an MLR analysis. Since more than one predictor defines MLR, you cannot rely on scattergrams to test this assumption. You still need to examine visual patterns of relationships, but in MLR you rely on the analysis of residuals since these are an index of the set of predictor variables in relationship to the outcome variable. I discuss these procedures in the following.

Linear

Linearity is an important assumption to meet for most research uses of MLR. I discussed the procedure for checking linearity with bivariate regression in Chapter 12; MLR assumptions can be checked with a similar process in addition to using residual analysis discussed later.

Multicollinearity

Multicollinearity is a facet of MLR that relates to the *relationship among the predictors* as well as the relationship between predictors and outcome. MLR takes into account that predictors probably have some relationship *to one another* as well as to the outcome variable. For example, if I explain health as a combination of inputs like education, income, and work, each of these predicators probably is at least somewhat related to the others. This overlap among predictors makes it difficult to determine the extent of the relationship of each predictor with the outcome variable when the other predictors are controlled. If the overlap is too great, the set of relationships is too murky to make useful conclusions.

The MLR output can be examined to understand the size and nature of the components of variance produced in a model with several predictors. Statisticians have devised guidelines for detecting problems in which "too much" of the predictor-to-predictor variance clouds the understanding of explained variance in the outcome variable and makes it difficult to understand the contribution of individual predictors. I will show in the following example how SPSS reports information that is helpful for understanding the interrelationship among the predictors.

ANALYZING RESIDUALS TO CHECK MLR ASSUMPTIONS

Residual analyses can help to determine whether assumptions are met for normality, equal variance, and linearity in an MLR analysis. Recall that residuals are errors in predicting true values of an outcome variable in a regression procedure. In an analysis in which the variables are multivariate normal, have equal variance, and are related in linear fashion, the residuals will display certain patterns that can be assessed visually and by other tests.

Standardized Residuals Normally Distributed

When the assumptions are met, the residuals in an MLR analysis should be normally distributed. This would indicate no "biases" among the data, especially in relationship to the outcome variable. SPSS provides a residual analysis program that includes a histogram of the residuals to determine whether the residuals fit a normal distribution. The "*P–P* Plot" is also produced that allows the researcher to determine the extent to which residuals adhere to a straight line representing expected cumulative probabilities of the normal distribution.

Random Relationship Between Residuals and Predicted Values

When residuals are plotted with predicted values in a scattergram, the dispersion of the residual values can reveal nonlinear relationships and heteroscedasticity. When assumptions are met for normality, linearity and equal variance, <u>there should be no pattern in the residuals when plotted with predicted values</u>.

- Residuals should show a zero slope and even distribution of values when plotted with predicted values. This would indicate the assumptions are met and there is no additional predictability of the outcome by the errors, or randomness.
- When the pattern of residuals around the zero slope line is curved, there is likely a nonlinear relationship among the variables. This might appear like the bottom left panel of Figure 11.3 which showed a curvilinear pattern between two variables. When the residuals appear thus, the assumption for linearity is violated.
- When the pattern of residuals gets increasingly wider along the zero slope line (i.e., outward like a shotgun pattern), homogeneity of variance may be compromised. This pattern would look similar to the scattergram shown in the bottom panel of Figure 11.14, although this figure explained the general condition of heteroscedasticity.

DIAGNOSTICS FOR MLR: CLEANING AND CHECKING DATA

For an extended discussion of regression diagnostics, see Abbott (2010). In this section, I present some of the most important considerations for understanding the nature of the data you use in an MLR analysis. Diagnostic procedures such as these are used to detect problematic patterns within an MLR analysis that may have great influence on the outcome. I discuss the primary diagnostic categories here, and then I discuss the diagnostics of the MLR example later.

In the following, I will use a small and brief example to demonstrate the steps for the diagnostic procedures. Table 12.2 shows the data for the fictitious study relating Healthy Days to Income Class. Table 13.1 shows the same data except I changed one value, case #7, from (0, 45) to (0, 80), to help illustrate the diagnostic procedures.

TABLE 13.1   The Diagnostic Study Values

Income Class (X)	Healthy Days (Y)
5	76
1	58
6	81
8	86
9	90
3	62
0	80

IncomeClass	HealthyDays	ZHealthyDays	ZIncomeClass	ZRE_1	COO_1	LEV_1	DFB0_1	DFB1_1
5	76	−0.012	0.126	−0.128	0.002	0.003	−0.161	−0.009
1	58	−1.518	−1.048	−1.003	0.361	0.183	−5.235	0.711
6	81	0.406	0.419	0.144	0.003	0.029	0.080	0.033
8	86	0.825	1.006	0.153	0.008	0.169	−0.170	0.102
9	90	1.160	1.299	0.318	0.065	0.281	−0.760	0.327
3	62	−1.183	−0.461	−1.102	0.160	0.035	−3.076	0.282
0	80	0.323	−1.341	1.618	1.865	0.300	11.990	−1.776

Figure 13.1   The SPSS® report of diagnostic values for the study data.

Figure 13.1 shows the results of several diagnostic procedures that I will use as a reference in the following sections.

These diagnostic measures result from choosing the "Regression – Linear" menus in SPSS as shown in Figure 12.10. When you use this menu, the specification menu shown in Figure 13.2 results.

You can specify the regression analysis using the submenu selections (top right buttons) as I demonstrated in Chapter 12 (see Figures 12.11 and following). I did not discuss diagnostics in those examples, so I introduce them here. Choosing the "Save" button in the Regression menu in Figure 13.2 results in the further specification window shown in Figure 13.3.

As you can see in this menu, I checked some of the boxes in the "Distances," "Residuals," and "Influence Statistics" sections to obtain the diagnostic values I reported in Figure 13.1. I will discuss these in the following sections as I encounter each of the values.

EXTREME SCORES

I have alluded several times thus far that "outlier" scores, or those scores that fall outside the group of other scores in a correlation or regression analysis, can dramatically affect results. Extreme scores can be a matter of examining the study variables

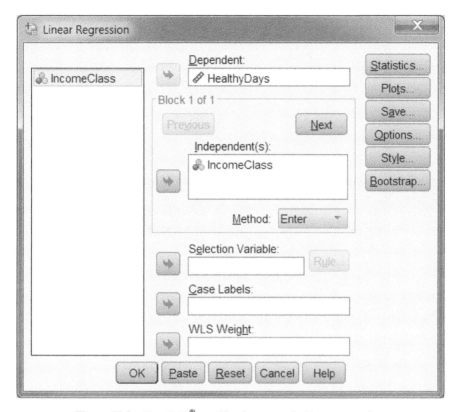

Figure 13.2 The SPSS® specification menu for linear regression.

individually ("univariate extreme scores") or taken together in a regression study ("multivariate extreme scores"). Therefore, the first diagnostic tool for understanding potential problems with study data is to find any such scores.

Univariate Extreme Scores

One of the ways to detect extreme scores of the study variables is simply by running a descriptives program such as I have described for analyzing skewness and kurtosis. These measures may identify values of a variable that might inflate one or the other of these measures.

Another way to detect possible extreme scores of individual variables is to examine standard scores (z scores) for each of the values. SPSS creates these by you simply checking the box that requests saving standard scores when you use the "Descriptives" command ("Save standardized values as variables"). You can examine the standard scores (at both positive and negative ends) and look at scores of ±3.00 as extreme scores.

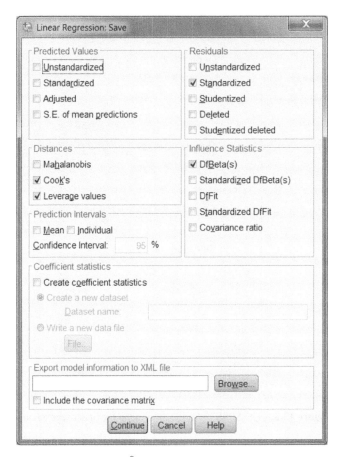

Figure 13.3   The SPSS® specification menu for diagnostic values.

Standard scores for both variables are listed in columns 3 and 4 of Figure 13.1 as "ZIncomeClass" and "ZHealthyDays." As you can see, there are no z scores listed above 2.0, so it appears that none of the values are extreme within their own value distributions.

A scattergram of the bivariate relationship might provide additional visual clues of possible extreme values. Figure 13.4 shows the scattergram of these variables. I highlighted the value I changed for this demonstration (0, 80). Compare this graph to the scattergram in Figure 12.4 that shows the unchanged case (0, 45). The scattergram for the unchanged data shows the study values deviating closely to the regression line. The scattergram in Figure 13.4 shows the changed values separated from the other values and the regression line by quite a distance. Remember, this is a change in value of only one study variable (Healthy Days).

The impact of this change is quite large on the study findings. The effect size changes from 0.96 in the original analysis to 0.492 in the study that includes the one

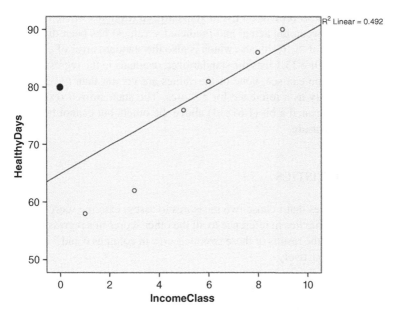

Figure 13.4   The scattergram of the study variables.

changed value. This is a reduction in the effect size of 0.47 (0.96 − 0.49), a very large impact from one extreme value.

When you encounter extreme values using this procedure, you need to think about how to manage the data and how to account for the extreme values: How many extreme scores are there? Are these "real" scores (e.g., are the extreme values accurate representations of respondent attitudes, or are they clerical errors)? How would it impact the analysis to delete or change them? These are considerations researchers must face as they model the data from the study.

Multivariate Extreme Scores

Often, extreme scores are identified by examining the analyses of the variables taken together rather than individually. The procedures I demonstrate are available for regression problems with more than one independent variable, but I am using an example from a bivariate regression procedure to illustrate how they work.

As you recall, residual scores (the difference between actual and predicted scores) provide a way of understanding how scores disperse around the regression line. Residual scores can be an excellent way of looking for extreme scores since large residual values indicate large distances between predictions from a regression equation and the actual value used to create it. Obviously, this has a great deal to do with the size of the correlation between the variables, but residuals can indicate extreme values and whether these might be problematic to an analysis.

You can view the residuals as <u>unstandardized values</u> that retain the scale of the study variables, but it is important to remember that each may have different variances. Thus, SPSS provides a list of <u>standardized residuals</u> where each residual (the difference between the actual and predicted y values) has been divided by the standard deviation of the residuals (which is also the standard error of estimate).

Column 5 in Figure 13.1 lists the standardized residuals in the regression analysis as "ZRE_1." As you can see, none of the values are greater than ($\pm$) 3.00 which I discussed previously as a reference for z scores. The standardized residual for the changed case is elevated a bit (1.61813) above the others but cannot be considered extreme by this measure.

DISTANCE STATISTICS

Figure 13.3 indicates that I chose two measures to assess extreme scores. These calculate how each score lies in reference to all the other scores in a regression analysis. Figure 13.1 shows the results of these two measures in columns 6 and 7 as "COO_1" and "LEV_1," respectively.

- "COO_1" are Cook's distance values (CDV).
- "LEV_1" are centered leverage values (CLV).

Centered Leverage Values (CVL)

These values indicate distances for the independent variable. The greater the distance between each x value and the mean of x, the larger the CLV, whereas values closer to the mean of x are increasingly smaller. The maximum leverage score is 1.0. Statisticians differ in their opinions of cutoff criteria based on these values, and some suggest that cutoff values may be misleading and somewhat artificial.[1] It may be helpful first to look for extreme values by sorting the CLV and then examining the scores for the highest values.

In this example, the highest values are 0.28 and 0.299 for cases 5 and 7, respectively. The mean CLV (reported in the SPSS output) for these data is 0.143 (SD = 0.123). Taking a broad view, these values are near but do not approach high values (e.g., mean + 2SD) of the reported residual statistics for CLV scores (i.e., 0.143 + 0.246 = 0.389). Remember, the CLV measures extreme <u>independent variable values</u>, so you can examine the IV values in the data and find that these two cases represent the lowest and highest IV values but do not appear from the scattergram to be inordinately removed from the other values.

Cook's Distance Values (CDV)

These values measure the effect on all the residuals if a particular case were dropped from the analysis. It therefore is <u>a measure of both independent and dependent</u>

---

[1]Pedhazur (1997) discusses high leverage values noting $(k + 1)/N$ as average leverage: multiplying $(k + 1)$ by 2 or 3 might generally identify a high value. Thus, in this case, 3(2)/15 = 0.40, compared to the 0.389 calculated above.

<u>variables</u> acting in concert in the analysis, with large values indicating more impact on the regression coefficients. Here again, cutoff criteria are debated by various researchers. One way to examine CDV visually is to sort the database by the values and to identify how extreme they become. They typically range from small values of "0" to larger values where the extreme scores may be several times larger than the immediately preceding scores.

Using this method, you can identify one CDV score that appears to be quite distant from the others in the regression analysis. Case 7 (the case I changed) shows a CDV of 1.865. With the database sorted according to these values, the next nearest high CDV is 0.36073 (case 2) and then 0.16020 (case 6). Given these range of values, Case 7 appears to be extreme.

The scattergram provides a helpful visual clue to whether this value might be extreme and therefore problematic to the analysis. As you can see in Figure 13.4, the highlighted case (0, 80) is clearly "outside the pack" of the other values. Since the CDV measures the joint influence of independent and dependent variables in the analysis, this case may be one to flag for further investigation. Recall that this case produced a larger but no inordinately large residual value.

INFLUENCE STATISTICS

As I noted, it is important to examine the data for extreme scores since they may have a large impact on the regression equation. Examining the residuals and distance statistics is helpful in locating potential extreme scores, but SPSS provides other measures that identify the impact on regression coefficients <u>if individual scores are deleted from the analysis.</u>

The last two columns (8 and 9) of Figure 13.1 show values for two measures that represent the change in the regression coefficients when a particular score is deleted from the analysis. These are "DfBeta(s)" that indicate changes on the intercept value (DFB0_1) and slope value (DFB1_1) of a regression equation when a specific case value is dropped from the database.

Thus, for example, if I dropped the changed case 7, what would be the impact on the regression equation? Essentially, these measures represent the amount of change in the intercept and slope of the regression line if you were to run the regression, delete the scores, and then rerun the regression line. If you subtract the values from the original regression, you will observe the change is equal to the DfBeta measures.

To take the example from my discussion earlier, I can show how the original regression equation is changed by dropping case 7. The overall (unstandardized) regression equation based on the regression analysis (including case 7) is

$$\text{Healthy Days} = 2.459 \text{ Income Class} + 64.902$$

<u>Adjusted intercept value</u>: Subtracting the DFB0 value (11.98987) score from the intercept in the original equation (64.902) yields the value of the intercept that would result if the extreme score (case 7) were deleted:

$$(64.902)-(11.990) = \mathbf{52.912}$$

Adjusted slope value: Subtracting the DFB1 score (-1.776) from the slope value in the original equation (2.459) yields a value of the slope value that would result if the extreme score (case 7) were deleted:

$$(2.459)\text{--}(-1.77628) = \mathbf{4.235}$$

The resulting (unstandardized) regression equation with case 7 deleted is

$$\text{Healthy Days} = 4.235\text{Income Class} + 52.912$$

The impact of deleting an extreme score (in this example case #7) is registered in the regression equation as shown before. But you can also measure these changes by the change in effect size:

$$\text{Initial database(including extreme case \#7)} : \; R^2 = 0.492$$
$$\text{Revised database(deleting extreme case \#7)} : \; R^2 = 0.969$$

The overall impact of deleting the extreme case is therefore increasing the effect size by 0.477 (0.969 − 0.492).

MLR EXTENDED EXAMPLE DATA

In the introduction to this chapter, I noted the questions that have arisen among social science researchers about the connections between income and health. As I noted there, a common assumption states that the greater the income, the better the health in the United States, although this is not so simple a relationship as one might expect.

If wealth does not always produce good health, what other factors may help to elaborate an understanding of this relationship? In the example that follows, I explore the impact of social status and work factors that might help to shed light on the relationship between health and income.

Table 11.2 shows the data I used to explain correlation procedures. Although hypothetical, these are the kinds of data that researchers might use to explore the "income–health" relationship. In this chapter, I extend those considerations by adding two predictors of health in addition to income. In this section, I use an MLR procedure to show some of the ways to interpret the findings from SPSS and Excel. Both perform MLR analyses, but the Excel capacity is more limited than SPSS. In addition, because SPSS is specifically designed for these kinds of complex analytical procedures, there are more custom features provided in the menus.

In the study database, I use variables modeled after those in GSS as I did in the correlation study. I took a small random sample from the overall (GSS, 2014) database to demonstrate the procedures a researcher might use in a larger, more complete, MLR analysis. My primary concern in this example is to demonstrate the MLR procedures used in any study, not to produce a primary research finding. Therefore, as in the correlation study, the conclusions I reach in this demonstration cannot be taken as representative of larger, more comprehensive studies.

Ordinarily, larger samples produce more representative findings. I use a small sample in this demonstration ($N = 78$) that is lower than most researchers would use in actual studies.[2] The data do illustrate the MLR procedures, however, and the findings help to illustrate how the study variables might be understood in terms of the income–health question.

The following are the variables I use. These are survey-based questions that record respondent opinions on each of the following:

- HeathOP – Opinion of health ($1 =$ poor, $2 =$ fair, $3 =$ good, $4 =$ very good, $5 =$ excellent)
- IncomeOP – Opinion of family income ($1 =$ far below average, $2 =$ below average, $3 =$ average, $4 =$ above average, $5 =$ far above average)
- RankOP – Opinion of social position ($1 =$ bottom rank through $10 =$ top rank)
- StressOP – How often the respondent finds work stressful ($1 =$ always, $2 =$ often, $3 =$ sometimes, $4 =$ hardly ever, $5 =$ never)

Before I proceed to the MLR procedure, I address whether the assumptions are met for the study. Analyzing the residuals requires that I run the procedure, so I will look at this section independently of the primary MLR findings.

ASSUMPTIONS MET?

Normal Distribution

As I noted earlier, the study variables can be examined individually as well as through residual analyses that incorporate all the study variables taken together. Visually, according to Figure 13.5, the outcome variable (HealthOP) appears to be slightly skewed negatively (indicating that slightly more of the respondent sample rated their health positively).

Using the Compare Means procedure, I gain additional numerical indications of normality for the other study variables. Figure 13.6 shows the descriptives report for all the study variables showing skewness and kurtosis figures that are in bounds of a normal distribution.

The optimal way to assess normality for the MLR with multiple predictors is to examine the residuals. This analysis will help to assess several assumptions, so I provide these findings in the following.

---

[2]There are numerous suggestions among researchers about the number of cases per number of predictors used in MLR studies. For smaller studies, less than 100 cases with three predictors would typically not be viewed as acceptable.

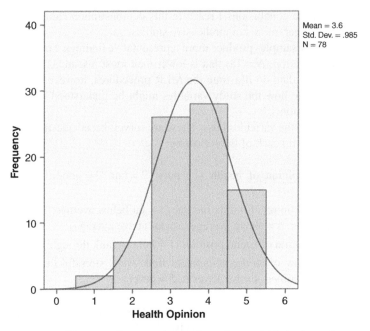

Figure 13.5   The histogram for the dependent variable in the study.

Report

	OPINION OF FAMILY INCOME	HOW OFTEN DOES R FIND WORK STRESSFUL	Health Opinion	Rank Opinion
Mean	2.91	3.00	3.60	6.04
N	78	78	78	78
Std. Deviation	.871	1.162	.985	1.848
Kurtosis	.223	-.565	-.146	.754
Std. Error of Kurtosis	.538	.538	.538	.538
Skewness	-.186	-.051	-.378	-.058
Std. Error of Skewness	.272	.272	.272	.272

Figure 13.6   The SPSS® descriptives report showing skewness and kurtosis findings.

Homoscedasticity

As I discussed with correlation, homoscedasticity refers to equal variance among the variables in an MLR analysis. Since more than one predictor defines MLR, you cannot rely on scattergrams to test this assumption. You still need to examine visual patterns of relationships, but in MLR you rely on the analysis of residuals since these are an index of the set of predictor variables in relationship to the outcome variable. I discuss these procedures and findings later.

Linear

Linearity is an important assumption to meet for most research uses of MLR. I discussed the procedure for checking linearity with bivariate regression in Chapter 12. MLR assumptions can be checked with a similar process, but a straightforward procedure is to examine the residuals which I discuss later.

Multicollinearity

Multicollinearity is a facet of MLR that relates to the *relationship among the predictors* as well as the relationship between predictors and outcome. MLR takes into account that <u>predictors</u> probably have some relationship *to one another* as well as to the outcome variable. For example, if I explain health as a combination of inputs like education, income, and work, each of these predicators probably is at least somewhat related to the others. This <u>overlap</u> among predictors makes it difficult to determine the extent of the relationship of each predictor with the outcome variable when the other predictors are controlled. If the overlap is too great, the set of relationships is too murky to make useful conclusions.

The MLR output can be examined to understand the size and nature of the components of variance produced in a model with several predictors. Statisticians have devised guidelines for detecting problems in which "too much" of the predictor-to-predictor variance clouds the understanding of explained variance in the outcome variable and makes it difficult to understand the contribution of individual predictors. I will show in the example later how SPSS reports information that is helpful for understanding the interrelationship among the predictors.

ANALYZING RESIDUALS: ARE ASSUMPTIONS MET?

As I noted previously, residual analyses can help to determine whether assumptions are met for normality, equal variance, and linearity in an MLR analysis. Recall that residuals are errors in predicting true values of an outcome variable in a regression procedure. In an analysis in which the variables are multivariate normal, have equal variance, and are related in linear fashion, the residuals will display certain patterns that can be assessed visually and by other tests.

Standardized Residuals Normally Distributed

When the assumptions are met, the residuals in an MLR analysis should be normally distributed. This would indicate no "biases" among the data, especially in relationship to the outcome variable. SPSS provides a residual analysis program that includes a histogram of the residuals to determine whether the residuals fit a normal distribution.

I will demonstrate how to produce the residual findings when I explain the SPSS procedure in the following. For now, examine Figure 13.7 showing a histogram of the (standardized) residual values from the study. As you can see, the residuals appear to be normally distributed, which is an indication the primary assumptions for the data are met.

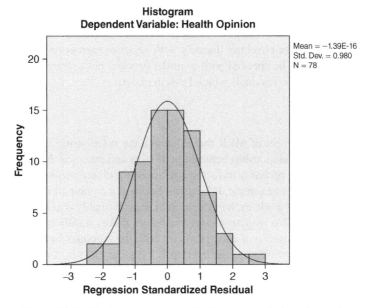

Figure 13.7 The histogram of standardized residuals from the study.

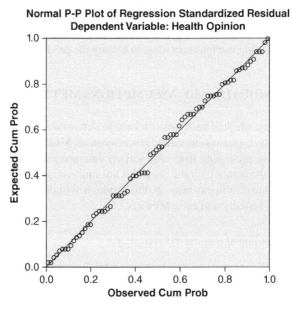

Figure 13.8 The *P–P* plot of standardized residuals from the study.

Figure 13.8 demonstrates a "*P–P* Plot of Regression Standardized Residual" values that also indicate assumptions are met. As you can see, the residual values conform to expected probabilities of a normal distribution by closely "hugging" the straight line.

Random Relationship between Residuals and Predicted Values

When residuals are plotted with predicted values in a scattergram, the dispersion of the residual values can reveal nonlinear relationships and heteroscedasticity. When assumptions are met for normality, linearity, and equal variance, there should be no pattern in the residuals when plotted with predicted values. Examine Figure 13.9 as a reference to the following elements of the assumptions:

- Residuals should show a zero slope and even distribution of values when plotted with predicted values. This would indicate the assumptions are met and there is no additional predictability of the outcome by the errors, or randomness. As you can see in Figure 13.9, the slope is "0" and the cases are evenly distributed around the regression line. There are a few extreme values that you might examine, but overall, the figure shows the pattern of residuals indicating assumptions are met.

- When the pattern of residuals around the zero slope line is curved, there is likely a nonlinear relationship among the variables. This might appear like the bottom left panel of Figure 11.3 which showed a curvilinear pattern between to variables. When the residuals appear thus, the assumption for linearity is violated. The curved pattern of residuals is not present in the study report as indicated in Figure 13.9.

- When the pattern of residuals gets increasingly wider along the zero slope line (i.e., outward like a shotgun pattern), homogeneity of variance may be compromised. This pattern would look similar to the scattergram shown in the bottom panel of Figure 11.14, although this figure explained the general condition of heteroscedasticity. No such pattern is shown in Figure 13.9.

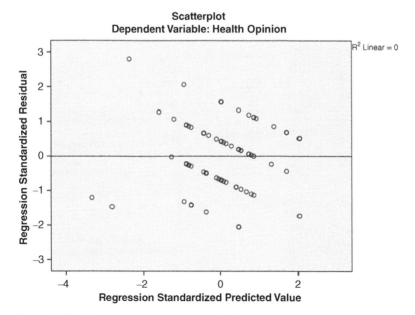

Figure 13.9   The scatterplot between standardized residuals and predicted values.

INTERPRETING THE SPSS® FINDINGS FOR MLR

In what follows, I present the SPSS findings for the study. The Excel program also produces a summary of findings for MLR, but the SPSS program produces a great deal more detail for this type of study. In what follows, I will point out some of the unique features of SPSS that help to explain some of the nuances of the model.

I will discuss several ways to analyze the impact of a set of predictors upon an outcome variable. Although this topic goes far beyond the space I have in this chapter to explain, I will cover the most important procedures and discuss the merits of each. I start with adding the predictors as a set (or block) together so that I can determine the overall impact on the outcome variable. The second method is to add predictors to the model sequentially so that the user can see what happens to the MLR model as each predictor is added (which I refer to as "hierarchical regression"). I will mention further methods that some researchers use to add predictors to the model.

Figure 13.10 shows the result of specifying linear regression through the "Analyze – Regression – Linear" instruction. I presented similar procedures for bivariate regression in Chapter 12 in Figures 12.10 and 12.11. Recall that this series of menus is available through the same Analyze menus. This selection yields the option window in Figure 13.10. I reproduce it here because I want to point out a couple of very important specifications for MLR analyses that go beyond bivariate regression.

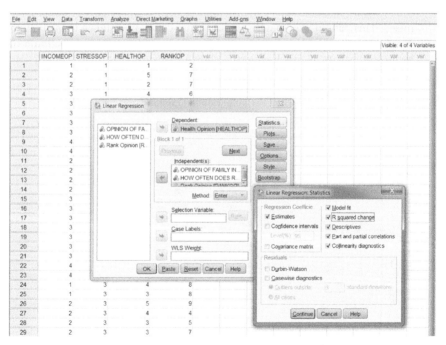

Figure 13.10   The specification menus for SPSS® MLR.

ENTERING PREDICTORS TOGETHER AS A BLOCK

In Figure 13.10, you see that I placed Health Opinion in the "Dependent" window, and the three predictor variables (IncomeOP, StressOP, and RankOP) in the "Independent(s)" window. This allows the researcher to determine the impact of <u>all the predictors together on the outcome variable</u>. The "Statistics" menu button produces the further specification menu in Figure 13.10 and allows me to call for a range of procedures.

- The "Model fit" provides the omnibus test result.
- The "R squared change" provides information relevant to effect size and to further analysis of the impact of each predictor (under a different model for adding predictors to the model, discussed later).
- "Part and partial correlations" are procedures critical for interpreting MLR findings. One very helpful use is to identify and <u>square the part correlation</u> for each variable in the analysis to show the contribution to R^2 for each variable added to the model. I will demonstrate this in my further explanation as follows.
- "Collinearity diagnostics" show the extent to which the predictors correlate to one another as well as to the outcome variable. This "intercorrelation" among the predictors can present difficulties for the MLR analysis. Choosing collinearity diagnostics helps to ensure that the study avoids serious violations of this assumption.

Figure 13.11 shows the further specification of the MLR by calling for several outputs helpful for understanding individual outcomes as well as for checking whether the assumptions have been met. Making these selections results in the output shown in Figures 13.7–13.9.

Partial Regression Plots

This specification also provides scatterplots for each predictor ("partial plots") with the outcome variable, when the remaining predictors are "held constant." Holding predictors constant is like saying that the model is assessing the relationship between a single predictor and the outcome variable at *all the different levels of the other predictors*. Thus, the model does not allow the values of the other predictors to interfere with the understanding of how the single predictor uniquely relates to the outcome. Figure 13.12 shows the "Partial Regression Plot" of Rank Opinion with the outcome Health Opinion while the other predictors are held constant.

As you can see in Figure 13.12, there is a positive relationship between rank and health opinion when the other predictors are held constant. In the upper right corner of the figure, you will see that "R^2 linear = 0.124" which indicates the effect size of this single variable. The further output for the model (which I present later) shows that this effect size is the <u>squared partial correlation</u> for this predictor. (Refer to the "Partial Correlation" section of Chapter 12 to understand this concept.)

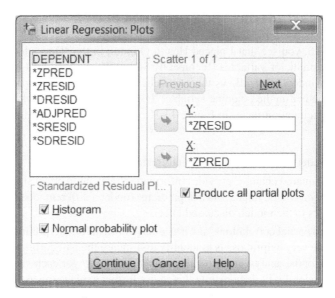

Figure 13.11   The SPSS® MLR specification for assumptions and individual predictors.

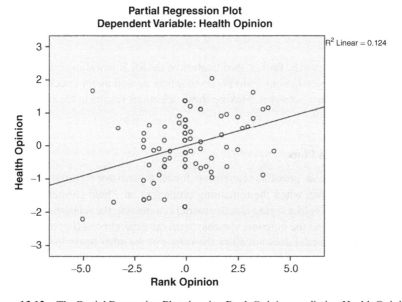

Figure 13.12   The Partial Regression Plot showing Rank Opinion predicting Health Opinion.

Assessing the MLR Findings

When you run the regression analysis (by hitting "OK" on the Linear Regression menu), you will be able to assess the primary elements of the MLR analysis: overall model significance, effect size, and significance of individual predictors. I will address these in the sections that follow.

Overall Model Significance

Figure 13.13 shows the ANOVA table that indicates the three predictors significantly predict values of Health Opinion. The F value (6.884) indicates the significance of the entire model, or omnibus test.

Effect Size

Figure 13.14 shows the overall effect size of this model. The adjusted R Square (0.186) indicates that about 18.6% of the variance in Health Opinion is due to the predictors in this model, for this sample group. As I noted in Chapter 12, the Adjusted R Square values take into account sample size (where smaller samples produce greater adjustment typically) and the number of predictors.[3]

Figure 13.14 also reports "R Square Change." (I discussed this value in Chapter 12 with "Bivariate Regression.") With this method of entry (i.e., entering all predictors as a block), the R Square Change value is equal to the R Square since the model does not highlight the impact of adding predictors separately, as I will show in the section in the following section for the hierarchical regression method of adding predictors. The "F Change" and "Sig. F Change" values likewise report global figures, while the hierarchical regression method will show these values for each variable added to the regression model.

ANOVA^a

Model		Sum of Squares	df	Mean Square	F	Sig.
1	Regression	16.294	3	5.431	6.884	.000^b
	Residual	58.385	74	.789		
	Total	74.679	77			

a. Dependent Variable: Health Opinion
b. Predictors: (Constant), Rank Opinion, HOW OFTEN DOES R FIND WORK STRESSFUL, OPINION OF FAMILY INCOME

Figure 13.13 The MLR omnibus test result.

Model Summary^b

Model	R	R Square	Adjusted R Square	Std. Error of the Estimate	Change Statistics				
					R Square Change	F Change	df1	df2	Sig. F Change
1	.467^a	.218	.186	.888	.218	6.884	3	74	.000

a. Predictors: (Constant), Rank Opinion, HOW OFTEN DOES R FIND WORK STRESSFUL, OPINION OF FAMILY INCOME
b. Dependent Variable: Health Opinion

Figure 13.14 The effect size summary for the MLR procedure.

[3] You can reproduce R^2 (0.218) by calculating the proportion of total variance explained as reported in the ANOVA table (Figure 13.13) by calculating the proportion of regression to total variance ($\frac{16.294}{74.679}$) as I discussed in Chapter 9.

Significance of Individual Predictors

The next output shown in Figure 13.15 reports information about each single predictor in the analysis, among other findings. The regression coefficients are reported as "Unstandardized" and "Standardized" according to whether the researcher seeks to use values in their own raw scales or standardized (Z) scale values.

The researcher uses these coefficients to show the <u>regression equation</u> as I discussed in Chapter 12. The following is the MLR equation using the unstandardized coefficients:

$$Y_{\text{HealthOP}} = 0.207X_{\text{IncomeOP}} + 0.208X_{\text{StressOP}} + 0.179_{\text{RankOP}} + 1.295_{\text{Constant}}$$

Each of the unstandardized "B" coefficients for the predictor variables represents the individual impact on the outcome with the other predictors held constant. The constant is the value of Y when the predictors $= 0$. Researchers can use this equation to predict values of HealthOP using values of the predictor variables, much as I discussed with a single predictor (see Chapter 12). (You would follow the same process of substituting values and then constructing confidence intervals around the predictions using the (multiple) standard error of estimate shown in Figure 13.14.)

Figure 13.15 shows the significance of individual predictors using the t tests for the various predictors. As you can see, the StressOP ($t = 2.385$, $p < 0.02$) and RankOP ($t = 3.240$, $p < 0.002$) are significant predictors of HealthOP, while IncomeOP ($t = 1.770$, $p < 0.08$) is not.

Collinearity Statistics

The "Collinearity Statistics" columns (last two columns on the right side of Figure 13.15) show the results researchers can use to determine if the intercorrelation among the predictors is too high. "Tolerance" represents the extent of the

Coefficients[a]

Model		Unstandardized Coefficients		Standardized Coefficients			Correlations			Collinearity Statistics	
		B	Std. Error	Beta	t	Sig.	Zero-order	Partial	Part	Tolerance	VIF
1	(Constant)	1.295	.533		2.430	.018					
	OPINION OF FAMILY INCOME	.207	.117	.183	1.770	.081	.215	.201	.182	.983	1.017
	HOW OFTEN DOES R FIND WORK STRESSFUL	.208	.087	.245	2.385	.020	.238	.267	.245	.998	1.002
	Rank Opinion	.179	.055	.336	3.240	.002	.358	.352	.333	.985	1.015

a. Dependent Variable: Health Opinion

Figure 13.15   The SPSS® output for individual predictors.

intercorrelation of the predictors.[4] Generally, <u>the lower the Tolerance value the greater the intercorrelation complications</u>. Thus, if the Tolerance value is too low (e.g., <0.10), there is not much variance left to explain in the outcome variable once the intercorrelation of the predictors is accounted for.

The "VIF" (variance inflation factor) values are derived from the Tolerance values, so <u>higher numbers are problematic</u> (e.g., VIF > 10 may indicate problems of multi-collinearity).

The Squared Part Correlation

Part (or Semipartial) correlations are very important values for understanding the impact of individual predictors upon the outcome variable. The Part correlation is not to be confused with the Partial correlation that I discussed in Chapter 12. As you recall, I defined the Partial correlation as the correlation of a predictor variable with the outcome *after you remove the influence of the remaining predictors from both of the other variables* (*target predictor with the outcome variable*).

<u>Part correlations show the relationship of a predictor to an outcome when the effects of the remaining predictors are taken out of the predictor variable but not the outcome variable</u>. Consider Figure 13.16 (this is a reproduction of Figure 12.31) that shows these relationships in the study with two predictors (see the discussion of this figure and "Partial Correlation" in Chapter 12).

The Part or Semipartial correlation is shown as the relationship of the "A" section to the entire variance of the outcome variable (i.e., $\frac{A}{A+B+C+D}$).[5] Thus, in this example, the Part correlation of IncomeOP with HealthOP is represented by the unique correlation between IncomeOP and HealthOP (i.e., section A) as a proportion of the <u>entire variance of HealthOP</u> (i.e., sections $A + B + C + D$).

The importance of this measure is that, <u>when squared</u>, it represents the <u>unique</u> contribution to the outcome variable by one single predictor (when the other predictors are held constant). In the current study with three predictors, you can use the SPSS output for individual predictors to determine the unique impact of each predictor on the outcome variable.

Thus, if you look at Figure 13.15 you can see that squaring the part correlation for RankOP ($0.333^2 = 0.11$) results in the percent of variance in HealthOP contributed uniquely by RankOP, (i.e., 11% of the variance in HealthOP is contributed uniquely by RankOP.) In similar fashion, you can square the part correlations for the remaining predictors to show their unique contributions to the variance in HealthOP. Thus StressOP accounts for 6% (or 0.245^2) unique variance in HealthOP while IncomeOP accounts for 3% (0.182^2). Comparing all the predictors, it appears that RankOP is a better predictor of HealthOP than either StressOP or IncomeOP for this set of data.

---

[4]Tolerance is calculated by subtracting the squared multiple correlation of the <u>additional predictors</u> with the predictor in question from 1.

[5]This is similar to the Partial correlation as referenced in Chapter 12, but that correlation is represented by the relationship of the "A" section to the $(A + D)$ sections.

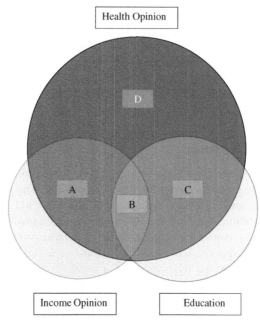

Figure 13.16   Isolating the effects of a predictor variable on an outcome variable through part or semipartial correlation.

ENTERING PREDICTORS SEPARATELY

This second method of entering predictors to an MLR analysis allows the researcher to specify changes in model values when successive predictors are added to the analysis. This constitutes hierarchical regression analysis since each predictor contribution is added sequentially to the others in "building block" fashion. The other facet of this method that sets it apart from other entry methods is that the predictor variables are added to the model according to the researcher's theoretical understanding of the relationships among the variables, or some other a priori rationale.

Figure 13.17 shows the beginning SPSS specification menu for MLR as we discussed with the entry method earlier (i.e., "Entering Predictors Together as a Block" section). As you can see, I entered the IncomeOP as the first predictor because of the theoretical notions I described earlier in the chapter about the widespread assumptions between income and health.

I can add the other predictors separately, as separate "Blocks" by choosing the "Next" button after I add each predictor. Thus, in Figure 13.17, I entered IncomeOP first, and then can hit the Next button to add work stress (StressOP) as a predictor because of the emphasis in some research literature on the importance of work to health. Last, I can hit the Next button again to add the RankOP predictor given the potential importance of social status to health (as I noted in the research reported by Marmot, 2004).

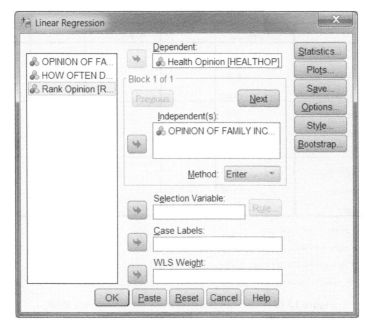

Figure 13.17 The MLR entry method for the first predictor.

The resulting MLR output enables the researcher to determine omnibus test finding, effect size, and individual predictor significance as in the former entry scheme. However, when I enter the predictors in separate blocks, the MLR results produce the results in hierarchical fashion created by adding predictors.

Notice that in Figure 13.18 Model 3 results will be the same as the results for the omnibus results in the first entry method (combined entry) <u>since it includes all the variables specified in the study.</u> This will be the same for the following output, which shows that results for Model 3 are the same in both entry schemes for effect size and individual predictor analyses.

Overall Model Significance

Figure 13.18 shows that the model with only the first predictor (HealthOP) as not being significant ($F = 3.696, p > 0.05$) but nearly so (see "Model 1" results). When the second predictor (StressOP) is added, the model is significant ($F = 4.506, p < 0.014$) (Model 2 results). When RankOP is added, the model is also significant ($F = 6.884, p < .000$) (Model 3 results).

Effect Size (Multiple R^2)

The R Square is likewise reported for each model representing the sequential addition of predictors. As you can see in Figure 13.19, the R Square value changes from 0.046 in Model 1 to 0.107 in Model 2, and to 0.218 in Model 3. <u>Taken together</u> (Model 3),

ANOVA[a]

Model		Sum of Squares	df	Mean Square	F	Sig.
1	Regression	3.463	1	3.463	3.696	.058[b]
	Residual	71.216	76	.937		
	Total	74.679	77			
2	Regression	8.011	2	4.005	4.506	.014[c]
	Residual	66.669	75	.889		
	Total	74.679	77			
3	Regression	16.294	3	5.431	6.884	.000[d]
	Residual	58.385	74	.789		
	Total	74.679	77			

a. Dependent Variable: Health Opinion

b. Predictors: (Constant), OPINION OF FAMILY INCOME

c. Predictors: (Constant), OPINION OF FAMILY INCOME, HOW OFTEN DOES R FIND WORK STRESSFUL

d. Predictors: (Constant), OPINION OF FAMILY INCOME, HOW OFTEN DOES R FIND WORK STRESSFUL, Rank Opinion

Figure 13.18   The omnibus test results for hierarchical MLR.

Model Summary[d]

					Change Statistics				
Model	R	R Square	Adjusted R Square	Std. Error of the Estimate	R Square Change	F Change	df1	df2	Sig. F Change
1	.215[a]	.046	.034	.968	.046	3.696	1	76	.058
2	.328[b]	.107	.083	.943	.061	5.116	1	75	.027
3	.467[c]	.218	.186	.888	.111	10.499	1	74	.002

a. Predictors: (Constant), OPINION OF FAMILY INCOME

b. Predictors: (Constant), OPINION OF FAMILY INCOME, HOW OFTEN DOES R FIND WORK STRESSFUL

c. Predictors: (Constant), OPINION OF FAMILY INCOME, HOW OFTEN DOES R FIND WORK STRESSFUL, Rank Opinion

d. Dependent Variable: Health Opinion

Figure 13.19   The hierarchical results for effect size.

the three predictors account for 21.8% of the variance in HealthOP (or 18.6% using the Adjusted R Square) which agrees with the combined entry method as shown in Figure 13.14.

By using separate entry, you can see how the model results change when you add predictors sequentially. Thus, Model 2 shows that adding StressOP to IncomeOP creates a significant omnibus model, and it adds a significant "amount" of R Square. This addition to R Square is represented in the "Change Statistics" columns as the "R Square Change (0.061)" which shows that StressOP adds 0.061 to the previous overall R^2 (.046) to yield an accumulated value of 0.107.

This change also registers in the "Sig. F Change" column where F Change (5.116) is considered significant ($p < 0.027$). The F Change references the change in the omnibus test, but it is a referent for the R Square Change as well.

Individual Predictors analyses

Adding predictors separately is also very helpful because it allows the researcher to see how the effect sizes change as each is added. Figure 13.20 shows the significance tests and effect size values (i.e., part correlations) for each predictor as they are introduced. You interpret these values similarly to the interpretations produced by the separate entry method. The difference is that you can see the changes to significance and effect sizes as predictors are separately entered.

Note, for instance, that IncomeOP changes in significance depending on the variables in the equation. In Model 1, it is close to significance ($p = 0.058$), in Model 2 it is significant ($p = 0.043$), while in Model 3 it is not significant ($p = 0.081$). The changes are small, but they show that adding predictors changes the interpretation of the findings.

This dynamic is similar for examining part correlations. As with significance numbers, the output shows part correlations for each variable within the block it is introduced. For example, the part correlation for IncomeOP is 0.215 in Model 1 where it is the only predictor. By Model 3, the part correlation has dropped to 0.182 when the two other predictors have been added. Apparently this variable shares variance with variables that are added, as can be understood by squaring the part correlations.[6] (In this particular case, it is understandable since income and social status are quite related variables.)

I mentioned previously that squaring the part correlations yields the unique contribution to understanding the variance in the outcome variable of each predictor.

		Coefficients^a							
		Unstandardized Coefficients		Standardized Coefficients			Correlations		
Model		B	Std. Error	Beta	t	Sig.	Zero-order	Partial	Part
1	(Constant)	2.894	.385		7.522	.000			
	OPINION OF FAMILY INCOME	.244	.127	.215	1.922	.058	.215	.215	.215
2	(Constant)	2.235	.475		4.708	.000			
	OPINION OF FAMILY INCOME	.254	.123	.225	2.059	.043	.215	.231	.225
	HOW OFTEN DOES R FIND WORK STRESSFUL	.209	.093	.247	2.262	.027	.238	.253	.247
3	(Constant)	1.295	.533		2.430	.018			
	OPINION OF FAMILY INCOME	.207	.117	.183	1.770	.081	.215	.201	.182
	HOW OFTEN DOES R FIND WORK STRESSFUL	.208	.087	.245	2.385	.020	.238	.267	.245
	Rank Opinion	.179	.055	.336	3.240	.002	.358	.352	.333

a. Dependent Variable: Health Opinion

Figure 13.20 The individual predictor summary for separate entry.

[6]This feature of separate entry is helpful for determining spuriousness. If, for example, bivariate correlations are high but drop considerably when a separate predictor is added, the bivariate relationship may be spurious to the last predictor added.

TABLE 13.2   The Change Values Resulting from Adding Predictors

		R Square	R Square Change	Part Corr.	Part Corr. Squared for last variable added
Model 1	IncomeOP	0.046	0.046	0.215	0.046
Model 2	ADD StressOP	0.107	0.061	0.247	0.061

Another feature of the output for separate entry is that the R Square Change values (noted in Figure 13.19) correspond to squared part correlations. The R Square Change value reflects the changes represented by the last variable entered into the analysis. These changes are mirrored by the squared part correlations. Table 13.2 shows an example of this.

In Table 13.2, IncomeOP is the first variable entered. Therefore, the R Square and R Square Change for IncomeOP will be the same values since the model changes from "no R Square" to an R Square that results from adding one predictor to the equation. In this example, the Part Correlation Squared is also the same value (0.046) since it is the last variable entered into the equation. Thus, the R Square changes from 0 to 0.046.

Table 13.2 shows the changes to the initial results when a second variable (StressOP) is added to the equation. In this case, the R Square Change (0.061) and "Part Corr. Squared for Last Variable Added" value (0.061) for StressOP are the same. The overall R Square value increases by a value of 0.061 (0.107 − 0.046) as a result of adding StressOP to the equation.

You can see similar results for adding the third predictor, RankOP. The R Square Change value (0.111) reported in Figure 13.20 is equal to its squared part correlation ($0.111 = 0.333^2$) when it is the last variable entered. Thus, the "R Square Change" and squared part correlation of a variable represent the increase in variance of the outcome variable (HealthOP) explained by adding the predictor.

In order to observe the "final" accounting of variance by the individual predictors, you can square the part correlations shown in the final model. Despite how they were entered, the final squared part correlations indicate the unique magnitude of impact of each predictor on the outcome variable.

One important point to remember is that *no matter how the variables are entered into the regression equation, the squared part correlation will indicate the unique contribution of a predictor to the variance of the outcome variable.* If, for example, we reran the MLR analysis but added RankOP in the first model and added IncomeOP in the third model, the R Square and R Square Change reported values would change (along with many others). However, the part correlations in the final model will be the same as in the first MLR analysis. This is a very important feature for interpretation since there are other ways to enter predictors to a model that are contentious among researchers.

ADDITIONAL ENTRY METHODS FOR MLR ANALYSES

I presented two methods for entering predictors in an MLR analysis (adding predictors together and adding predictors separately). Other choices for entry include
"Stepwise" which allows SPSS pre-set entry and removal criteria to enter and retain
each variable in the analysis. For example, if I had a study with five predictors, the
stepwise procedure would add and retain (or delete) predictors depending on the size
of their impact on the model. It might be the case that only two predictors would
be retained and the others excluded even though the researcher has good reason to
include them.

The stepwise procedure can be useful at times, but most researchers avoid
the method since it <u>takes the choice for building the model out of the researcher's
control</u>. If the researcher is including each predictor on some a priori grounds for
inclusion, then it is important to see the impact on the results despite the variable not
"making the cut" established by the program.

If you would like to examine the stepwise (or other) method for entry, you can
specify it by choosing the "Entry" button on the main MLR specification window (see
Figure 13.10). Figure 13.21 shows this window in which I chose "Stepwise" under
"Method" which produces a separate menu of methods to enter predictors other than

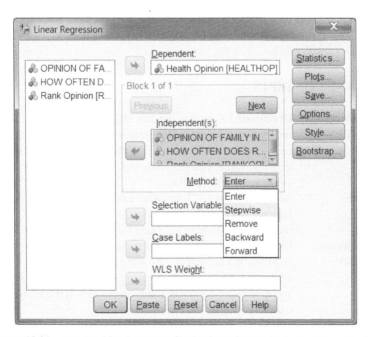

Figure 13.21   The specification menu for the Stepwise (and other) entry method(s).

"Enter". If you were to rerun the MLR I have discussed before, the result would be that two variables would be retained in rank order of their contribution to the outcome (RankOP and then StressOP) according to the criteria used in the program to include and/or exclude variables.[7] In practice, this means that IncomeOP would not be retained despite its theoretical importance and its near significance ($p = 0.081$) in the previous models.

The complete menu of entry schemes includes other methods that exceed the boundaries of this treatment of MLR. However, most researchers can profitably use hierarchical regression ("Enter" method) for their analyses.

EXAMPLE STUDY CONCLUSION

The example study concludes that the two predictors, RankOP and StressOP are significant predictors of HealthOP, while IncomeOP is nearly significant. According to the squared part correlations, RankOP is the best predictor among these variables accounting for 11% of the variance in HealthOP. The other predictors also contribute to an understanding of the variance in HealthOP, but by lesser values (StressOP = 6% and IncomeOP = 3%).

If this were an actual study, we might suggest that social status may be more important than income or work stress for explaining health outcomes. Those with higher social statuses enjoy better health despite the levels of their work stress and/or incomes. These findings would support Marmot's (2004) notions as I discussed above.

TERMS AND CONCEPTS

Centered leverage values (CVL):	Diagnostic values that indicate distances for the independent variable. The greater the distance between each x value and the mean of x, the larger the centered leverage value, whereas values closer to the mean of x are increasingly smaller.
Collinearity statistics:	Statistical values ("Tolerance" and "VIF") reported that indicate whether the intercorrelation among the predictors is too high to obtain meaningful MLR results.
Cook's distance values (CDV):	Diagnostic values that measure the effect on all the residuals if a particular case were dropped from the analysis. It therefore is a measure of both independent and dependent variables acting in concert in the analysis, with large values indicating more impact on the regression coefficients.

---

[7] You can find these criteria under the Options button of the Linear Regression specification menu like that shown in Figure 13.21.

Distance statistics:	A diagnostic measurement that assesses how each score lies in reference to all the other scores in a regression analysis. (See Centered leverage values and Cook's distance values.)
Fixed-effects modeling:	An MLR analysis that uses the same categories of variables across studies. The predictor variable has a set number of categories, like gender or experimental method, where the same categories are used in all situations. In this situation, generalizability of findings is limited to the fixed category values.
Hierarchical regression:	An interpretive technique in multiple regression studies in which the sequential impact of predictor variables on the outcome variable is measured.
Influence statistics:	Diagnostic values that identify the impact on regression coefficients if individual scores are deleted from the analysis.
Multicollinearity:	A measure of the "overlap" (or intercorrelation) among predictors in a multiple regression study. This overlap can obfuscate the overall relationship of the set of predictors to the outcome variable.
Part Correlation:	Part correlations show the relationship of a predictor to an outcome when the effects of the remaining predictors are taken out of the predictor variable but not the outcome variable. (Also called Semipartial correlations.)
Partial Regression Plots:	These are scatterplots for each predictor ("partial plots") with the outcome variable, when the remaining predictors are "held constant."
Random effects modeling:	The most common MLR analysis used primarily in non-experimental social science research analyses; it is used in situations where the evaluator takes a random set of observations from a larger population of values, with the categories or levels of the predictor variable "emerging" from and determined by the data sampled. The categories and values of x are thus random.
Residuals:	Residuals are errors in predicting true values of an outcome variable in a regression procedure
Semipartial correlations:	(See Part correlation.)
Squared part correlation:	Values that indicate the percent of variance in the outcome variable uniquely explained by each individual predictor (when other predictors are held constant).
Stepwise entry method:	This method allows statistical programs to enter/remove and retain predictors in an MLR analysis according to pre-set entry and removal criteria.

TABLE 13.3   The Study Variables and Labels

SPSS Variable	Full Variable Label	Values
JobOpp	Job Opportunities	Low (1) -- High (7)
HlthServices	Health Services	Low (1) -- High (7)
RecOpp	Recreational Opportunities	Low (1) -- High (7)
CommInvolv	Community Involvement	Low (1) -- High (7)
FearCrime	Fear of Crime	Low (1) -- High (7)

DATA LAB AND EXAMPLE (WITH SOLUTION)

In this lab, I present several cases of the community survey I have used in past chapters as an example for MLR.[8] For this example study, investigate the data to determine whether, and to what extent, Community Involvement is predicted by the other four (predictor) variables. Thus, to what extent is community involvement predicted by respondent perceptions of job opportunities, recreational opportunities, health services, and fear of crime? Table 13.3 shows the study variables, their labels, and their values and Table 13.4 shows the study data.

Lab questions: (Enter predictors together as a single block.)

1. Are assumptions met for MLR?
2. What are the findings: omnibus test, omnibus effect size, and individual predictor significance?
3. What are the unique explanations of variance in community involvement by each of the predictor variables?
4. What conclusions can you draw about the research question from the findings of this example study?
5. Briefly examine diagnostics (standardized residuals, Cook's, CLV). Observations?

DATA LAB: SOLUTION

1. Are assumptions met for MLR?

Normal distribution According to Figure 13.22, the outcome variable (community involvement) appears to be fairly balanced with a very slight positive skew. Figure 13.23 shows the Sk/Ku findings that indicate the study variables are within the boundaries of a normal distribution.

---

[8]Once again, due to the small sample size and other features of the data, no conclusions should be drawn from the analyses. The data are shown here for illustration of MLR procedures only.

TABLE 13.4   Problem 1 MLR Data

JobOpp	HlthServices	RecOpp	CommInvolv	FearCrime
2	4	2	2	4
1	1	1	1	1
7	6	6	6	1
4	4	5	4	3
6	5	6	5	5
1	3	1	1	4
7	6	6	6	2
4	5	4	4	3
5	7	7	5	7
5	6	5	5	2
2	5	5	3	2
4	3	4	3	3
4	6	6	5	1
3	2	6	3	5
4	4	7	4	4
4	4	4	4	5
4	5	4	3	7
4	5	5	5	4
3	4	4	2	4
2	2	4	3	2
4	7	6	4	6
3	5	2	2	4
2	5	4	2	4
6	5	6	6	1
4	4	4	3	1
4	4	5	5	4
3	5	4	4	6
1	1	1	1	7
2	5	4	4	3
2	4	2	1	3
6	6	6	4	3
3	5	7	3	4
3	3	3	1	5
4	6	4	2	4
4	4	7	6	3
2	2	6	4	4
1	7	6	4	2
5	2	7	6	1
7	7	5	7	1
3	3	7	2	1
1	6	1	3	7

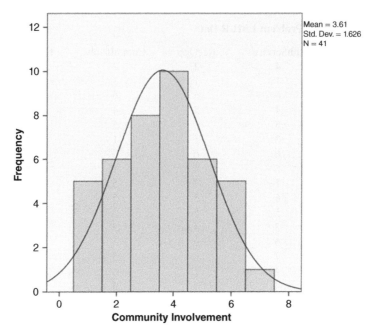

Figure 13.22 The histogram for the outcome variable.

	Community Involvement	Job Opportunities	Recreational Opportunities	Health Services	Fear of Crime
Mean	3.61	3.56	4.61	4.46	3.49
N	41	41	41	41	41
Std. Deviation	1.626	1.689	1.829	1.614	1.846
Kurtosis	−.782	−.395	−.485	−.416	−.632
Std. Error of Kurtosis	.724	.724	.724	.724	.724
Skewness	.050	.348	-.597	-.400	.334
Std. Error of Skewness	.369	.369	.369	.369	.369

Figure 13.23 The findings indicating all study variables are normally distributed.

Multicollinearity Multicollinearity is controlled for this set of data according to Tolerance and VIF values.

Multivariate normality, linearity, and equal variance (using residual analysis)

Standardized residuals normally distributed. Figure 13.24 shows the residuals are fairly normally distributed for the study variables.

Random relationship between residuals and predicted values. Figure 13.25 shows a random array of residuals plotted with predicted values.

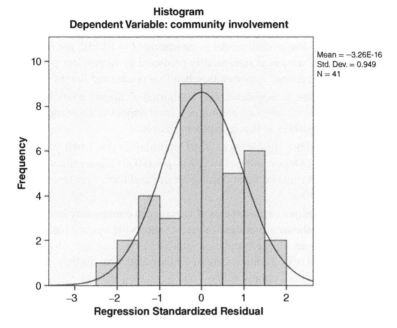

Figure 13.24   The residuals plot for normality assessment.

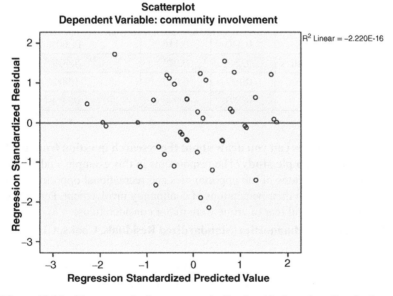

Figure 13.25   The scatterplot between standardized residuals and predicted values.

2. What are the findings (omnibus test, omnibus effect size, individual predictor significance)? (Predictors entered together as a single block.)

Omnibus test – The overall model is significant ($F = 19.610$, $p < 0.000$). Community involvement is significantly predicted by respondent perceptions of job and recreational opportunities, health services, and fear of crime.

Effect size – The R Square $= 0.685$ (Adjusted R Square $= 0.650$) indicating 68.5% of the variance in community involvement is accounted for by the predictor variables in this respondent sample.

Individual predictor significance – Job Opportunities ($t = 3.640$, $p = 0.001$) and Recreational Opportunities ($t = 3.004$, $p = 0.005$) are significant predictors of community involvement. Health service and fear of crime are not significant predictors.

3. What are the unique explanations of variance in community involvement by each of the predictor variables? Table 13.5 shows the squared part correlations and interpretations for each predictor variable. As you can see, job opportunities and recreational opportunities account for the greatest proportion of community involvement in this example study.

TABLE 13.5   The Unique Contribution to Outcome Variance by Predictor Variables

Predictor	Part Correlation	Squared Part Correlation	% of unique variance in Community Involvement accounted for by the Predictor
Job Opportunities	0.340	0.116	11.60%
Recreational Opportunities	0.281	0.079	7.90%
Health Services	0.139	0.019	1.90%
Fear of Crime	−0.080	0.006	0.60%

4. What conclusions can you draw about the research question from the findings of this example study? The respondents in this example study indicated that their perceptions of job opportunities and recreational opportunities were most important in their perceptions of community involvement. Perceptions of health services and fear of crime were minor considerations.

5. Briefly examine diagnostics (Standardized Residuals, Cooks, CLV). Observations?

- One ZResidual value (−2.14) is a bit extreme, but not excessive.
- One Cook's value (0.25883) is high and may be problematic; a second value (0.21808) may also bear investigation.
- One CLV value (0.35911) appears to be high, but not inordinately so.

14

CHI-SQUARE AND CONTINGENCY TABLE ANALYSIS

Up to now, I have explored statistical procedures that use continuous data that are interval level. These are the procedures you will encounter the most often in evaluation reports, newspaper articles, and scholarly articles. However, you cannot conclude a study of statistics without discussing one of the most versatile and useful procedures that can be used with any level of data.

Chi-square is a statistical procedure that primarily uses nominal, or categorical, data. It works by examining "frequency counts" or simply the number (frequency) of people or observations that fit into different categories. An example of such a procedure might be the analysis of soccer injuries as I presented in Chapter 5 (e.g., see Figure 5.1) or comparing the numbers of men and women who choose flexible work schedules in various industries.

The chi-square procedure is used in at least two ways. It is used in a "goodness of fit" test and in hypothesis "tests of independence." I will discuss both of these uses in this chapter. Even though chi-square uses nominal data, there is a chi-square distribution of values with which to determine exclusion values for hypothesis tests. I will therefore treat the chi-square procedures in the same fashion I did with other procedures in this book for hypothesis testing.

CONTINGENCY TABLES

Chi-square data are presented in spreadsheet form in rows and columns. The researcher easily can see how the data are arrayed across the categories of the

Using Statistics in the Social and Health Sciences with SPSS® and Excel®, First Edition.
Martin Lee Abbott.
© 2017 John Wiley & Sons, Inc. Published 2017 by John Wiley & Sons, Inc.

variables. The tables of data containing the frequencies are called "contingency tables" because the data in the row cells are *contingent upon or are connected to* the data in the column cells. Statisticians and researchers often refer to the analysis of contingency tables as "cross-tabulation," or simply "crosstabs."

Having the data displayed in rows and columns according to the categories of the variables making up the contingency table is helpful to the researcher. Simple visual inspection may help to detect patterns not ordinarily apparent when the data are not placed in tables. The question that I have posed with other procedures in this book however is, *how different do the data (in row and column cells) have to be before one could conclude that the data patterns are "statistically significantly different?"*

The answer to the previous question is the reason researchers use chi-square. The chi-square procedure statistically analyzes the differences among the data in contingency tables to determine whether the patterns of difference are different enough to be considered statistically significant.

When researchers wish to present the results of their analyses for interpretation, or to simply list the data in the tables, they use percentages instead of frequencies. This is because the frequencies in cells are often different across rows and columns. Therefore, percentages are a way to present the frequency data "on a level playing field." Raw frequency differences are transformed to a common expression across the entire contingency table. I will examine these facets of contingency table analyses in this chapter and discuss some traditional "rules" on how to present the data in the tables.

One convention some researchers use when presenting data in contingency tables is to present the independent variable categories in columns and the dependent variable categories in rows.[1] In this way, the column data percentages are created to a total of 100%, and the researcher can *compare values of the independent variable categories within rows of the dependent variable categories.* This enables a common way of interpreting the data from visual inspection and from chi-square analyses. I will show how this works in this chapter by using some examples.

THE CHI-SQUARE PROCEDURE AND RESEARCH DESIGN

The chi-square procedure is very important because it is so versatile. Often, researchers are limited as to what data they can gather and may only be able to use simple frequency counts. Chi-square can be used with any kind of data. In some cases, researchers can use chi-square with existing reports of some variable of interest.

Here are some examples of how researchers might use chi-square in *post facto designs*:

- Comparing treatment methods assigned to patients based on sex and age
- Determining whether frequency counts of crimes reported by neighborhood represent statistically significant differences

---

[1] Other researchers organize contingency tables in the opposite fashion, with the independent variable categories in rows. As you will see in the analyses to follow, it does not matter which convention you use as long as you remember how to create the interpretation.

- Comparing attitudes, choices, or behaviors among groups of schoolchildren
- "Windshield surveys" of schools, businesses, or neighborhoods by classifying observed frequencies of human traffic patterns or the physical appearance of buildings
- Comparing the popularity of cafeteria food by classifying amount of waste

You might recognize some of these as studies in which the researcher uses "secondary data" (data that already exist) or "unobtrusive" measures (data that are gathered in natural settings without the researcher intruding into the research context).

Chi-square can also be used with *experimental* data, but the procedures are a bit different than those for post facto designs. These often use designs that include "repeated measures" procedures to control for pre–post differences. An example of this procedure is a study (Trzyna and Abbott, 1991) in which a colleague and I used chi-square to determine if there were pre–post differences in grieving among a group of students in an ethnic literature classroom.

CHI-SQUARE DESIGN ONE: GOODNESS OF FIT

I mentioned earlier that there are two primary uses of chi-square to determine statistical significance. The first of these is the *"goodness of fit" tests used to compare actual data to expected data distributions*. This use of chi-square involves one variable with several categories. The researcher may wish to determine whether the data that are "seen" (*observed frequencies*) are statistically different from the expectations of how the data *should* behave (*expected frequencies*).

As an example, let us suppose that a researcher is interested in whether there is a difference among the number of treatment modalities used in a given hospital over a 1-year period for those experiencing herniated discs. Does the hospital indicate a "favorite" method for dealing with these problems?

If there are four treatments available for these patients, the expected distribution of choices is that there will be the same number of patients who are given each treatment type assuming all patients exhibit the same conditions, and so on.[2] The chi-square procedure compares the actual treatment choices for these patients to see how closely these "actual" treatment numbers compare to what one might expect.

Expected Frequencies: Equal Probability

One of the complexities of this kind of study is how to determine what is expected. Often, expectation is simply a matter of *equal probability*, as inherent to the hospital treatment choices I introduced earlier. In the absence of any other information, the researcher might simply expect equal numbers of treatments in each category. Thus,

---

[2]Obviously, this hypothetical example does not take into account such factors as the differences among patients or the expertise of various medical personnel, among other considerations. This example is used only to demonstrate the chi-square procedure .

if there were 160 patients and four treatment choices, the expected number of patients for each treatment would be 40. This is determined as follows:

$$f_e = \frac{N}{k}$$

I use f_e to represent <u>expected frequency</u>. In this formula, expected frequency is a matter of dividing the total number of subjects (N) by the number of categories (k) in the variable of interest. Therefore

$$f_e = \frac{N}{k}$$
$$= \frac{160}{4}$$
$$= 40$$

If there are 160 patients and four treatment choices, the researcher would expect equal numbers of the patients (40) in each of the treatments.

Expected Frequencies: A Priori Assumptions

Another way to determine expected frequency is to use prior knowledge or theoretical assumptions about what *should* happen. Thus, a researcher may have knowledge (from other studies or on the basis of past observation) that one of the treatment choices is much more popular in hospitals across the country. In this case, the researcher can determine the proportion or probability of each treatment choice and then see how many patients in the study *actually* end up in each of the treatments. It might look like this <u>hypothetical</u> finding:

Treatment A: 0.35 probability, resulting in an expected frequency (f_e) of 56 (0.35 × 160)
Treatment B: 0.25 probability, $f_e = 40$
Treatment C: 0.25 probability, $f_e = 40$
Treatment D: 0.15 probability, $f_e = 24$

A HYPOTHETICAL EXAMPLE: GOODNESS OF FIT

Perhaps the easiest way to explore the nuances of chi-square is to use examples. Since I introduced treatment types earlier, I can use this to show how to proceed with a goodness of fit test using chi-square. This is also referred to as a "one-way chi-square." The "one" represents the fact that there is only one row of data (i.e., one variable with several categories). Thus, this example would be a 1 × 4 chi-square, or a study with one row and four columns.

Let us suppose that a researcher conducts a brief study with 160 herniated disc patients at a large urban hospital. The research question is whether the patients are

TABLE 14.1   The Hypothetical Treatment Differences Data

	Medication	Acupuncture	Manipulation	Surgery
f_o	56	30	34	40
f_e	40	40	40	40
$f_o - f_e$	16	-10	-6	0
$(f_o \text{-} f_e)^2$	256	100	36	0
$\dfrac{(f_o \text{-} f_e)^2}{f_e}$	6.4	2.5	.9	0
$\chi^2 = \sum \dfrac{(f_o - f_e)^2}{f_e} = (6.4 + 2.5 + .9 + 0) = 9.80$				

assigned differently to the different treatment types: medication, acupuncture, manipulation, or surgery. Using what is expect to happen by chance, you can determine that the expected frequency is 40 for each treatment, as I showed earlier:

$$f_e = \frac{160}{4}$$

$$= 40$$

The question is, how do the *actual* treatment choices (observed frequency, f_o) compared to the *expected* choices (expected frequencies, f_e)? For this, the researcher uses the general chi-square (represented by χ^2) formula that compares f_o to f_e as follows:

$$\chi^2 = \sum \frac{(f_o - f_e)^2}{f_e}$$

As you can see, the formula sums up the squared differences between observed and expected frequencies which are divided by the expected frequencies. While this formula sums all the differences up, think of the process as the summing up of the statistical calculations *in each cell*. Table 14.1 shows how you might arrange the data in order to make the required calculations.

Using the Chi-Square Formula

Table 14.1 shows the (actual) data for the study in the top row (f_o) that I shaded. The remainder of the table shows rows that correspond to each of the elements of the formula for chi-square (shown earlier). In essence, these steps "take the formula apart" and calculate the elements separately. The last row shows that the results of the separate calculations are summed for the final chi-square result.

As you can see from Table 14.1, the chi-square results are $\chi^2 = 9.80$. As I described earlier, this is a general measure of how the differences between expected and observed frequencies are arrayed in the data table. The researcher must now decide if 9.8 is a large enough chi-square value to conclude that the treatments are statistically different. To do this, the researcher must conduct a hypothesis test.

The Hypothesis Test for the Goodness of Fit Chi-Square Test

The hypothesis test includes the same steps as those I introduced for the other procedures in this book. The following are the primary elements of the hypothesis test:

1. *Null hypothesis:* $f_o = f_e$ (There is no difference between what I expect to happen and what I observe to happen.)

2. *Alternative hypothesis:* $f_o \neq f_e$ (There is a difference between what I expect to see and what I actually see.)

3. *Critical value of exclusion:* For this value, the researcher uses the chi-square table of values in the appendix. As you have seen with other statistical procedures, you need to establish a value of exclusion on the chi-square distribution to compare with the actual calculated value. If the calculated value exceeds this exclusion value, you would conclude that the results of the study are too large to be considered a chance finding.

   You must use degrees of freedom with the goodness of fit test to identify the appropriate comparison value from the chi-square table of values. For the one-way chi-square, the degrees of freedom are $df = k - 1$, where k is the number of categories. Thus, $df = 3$ in a table with one row and four categories. For the example study I introduced earlier, the 0.05 critical value of exclusion is 7.82. This is represented as $\chi^2_{0.05,3} = 7.82$.

   Like the T distribution, the chi-square distribution is actually several distributions that vary with the size of the sample. Thus, the degrees of freedom identify a "separate" chi-square distribution used as a comparison distribution to establish the critical values of exclusion. *Chi-square is a "directional" test because of the shape of the distribution(s).* The exclusion value is located on the right side of the distribution. Figure 14.1 shows sketches of the general shapes of the chi-square distribution at selected df values. As you can see, the shape of the distribution is quite different depending on the degrees of freedom.

4. *Calculated chi-square:* This is the chi-square value I calculated earlier, $\chi^2 = 9.80$.

5. *Decision:* Since the calculated value (9.80) exceeds the critical value (7.82), I conclude that there is a statistically significant difference among the treatment types for the herniated disc patients at the 0.05 level, $p < 0.05$.

6. *Interpretation:* The patients in the study group were placed in treatment types in statistically different numbers. The question for the researcher is how to report the findings of this study in the words of the study question. For this, I refer back to my earlier statement that researchers need to use percentages to report findings since categories may have unequal raw number values. Table 14.2 shows the hypothetical data with appropriate percentages. Based on these percentages, I would conclude that most patients are assigned "medication" for treatment type by the hospital.

Table 14.2 shows that 35% of the patients were placed in "medication" versus lower percentages in the other treatment categories. This represents almost double the treatment choice of acupuncture, for example (35% vs. 18.75%).

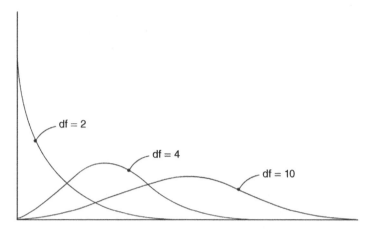

Figure 14.1   The chi-square series of distributions.

TABLE 14.2   The Reporting Data for the Hypothetical Study

	Medication	**Acupuncture**	**Manipulation**	**Surgery**	
f_o	56	30	34	40	$= 160$
%	$35\% \,(\dfrac{56}{160})$	$18.75\% \,(\dfrac{30}{160})$	$21.25\% \,(\dfrac{34}{160})$	$25\% \,(\dfrac{40}{160})$	$= 100\%$

Frequencies versus Proportions

There is a technical point to be made about chi-square and the kind of data used. Most researchers use frequencies or raw counts and numbers in the cells (e.g., the number of patients placed in different treatment categories). In this case, you are actually comparing two different distributions: an actual distribution of occurrences and an expected distribution of occurrences. Statisticians refer to this as a *nonparametric* test because you are not comparing a *sample* set of data to a (known or unknown) *population*. A case in which you compare a sample to a population would be known as a *parametric* test because you refer to population values.

You can use chi-square as a parametric test when you view the distributions as representing populations. This is seen most clearly where you express both expected and observed values as *proportions*, which can express population values. In the herniated disc example mentioned earlier, I showed how to create frequencies from expected probabilities or proportions. Treating the test as comparing sample proportions to population proportions would be considered a parametric test.

There is a relationship between these uses of the data, however. Calculating a chi-square using proportions is equivalent to chi-square calculated from frequencies through the following:

$$\chi^2_{\text{frequencies}} = (\chi^2_{\text{proportions}}) \times N$$

In practice, you can treat the data as parametric and perform hypothesis tests as I have with other statistical procedures. Most critical comparison tables for chi-square use raw score frequencies (as does the one in this book). It is important to understand the difference between these two approaches and to understand that the data can be expressed in different ways.

EFFECT SIZE: GOODNESS OF FIT

Effect size for chi-square is very basic since the procedure uses categorical data. Essentially, *measures of association* determine the impact of the relationship among the study variables. Association measures include the correlation measures I used to show how changes in one variable were linked to changes in another.

In goodness of fit tests, there is only one variable with at least two categories. While there are a number of effect size measures for chi-square, especially for the test of independence that I will discuss next, I will introduce the most common measure called <u>contingency coefficient</u> here, symbolized by "C." The formula for C is

$$C = \sqrt{\frac{\chi^2}{\chi^2 + N}}$$

The contingency coefficient is essentially a correlation measure for nominal data. The chi-square test compares observed and expected frequencies in an attempt to understand if there is a statistically significant difference between the two. Contingency coefficient is a correlation measure of the overall association between the two study variables.

Although this is a measure of association, you cannot interpret it as I discussed for r^2 (i.e., the proportion of variance in one variable explained by the other). Due to the nature of the data, you must refer to a set of values that provide a criteria for judging effect size, as I used with other effect size measures. Because C does not reach the maximum value of 1.00, the effect size values for small, medium, and large vary with the conditions of the study (e.g., number of categories). Cohen's (1988) suggestions are generally 0.10 (small), 0.30 (medium), and 0.50 (large), depending on the factors affecting C.

Using the hypothetical data earlier, we can calculate C:

$$C = \sqrt{\frac{\chi^2}{\chi^2 + N}}$$

$$= \sqrt{\frac{9.80}{9.80 + 160}}$$

$$= 0.24$$

Using the previous criteria, I can suggest a small effect size for the herniated disc treatment study.

CHI-SQUARE DESIGN TWO: THE TEST OF INDEPENDENCE

The second primary use of chi-square is in research studies in which there are two or more variables involved. For example, the researcher may wish to determine whether the treatment choices were equal, as in the previous description, but also may question whether the age of the patient might have an impact on their treatment types. Thus, there are now two variables, treatment types and age, which create a contingency table of data. The question is <u>whether the values of the categories of one variable are in any way linked to the category values of the other variable</u>. Do the cell frequencies of one variable influence the cell frequencies of the other?

The general expectation of chance in which one variable is <u>not linked to another</u> results in what researchers call "independence." That is, the categories of one variable are in no way connected or linked in a pattern to the categories of the other. An example would be that patients of different ages might be placed in treatments equally.

If the categories of data do show a pattern whereby the frequencies of some cells are much greater than the frequencies of other cells, you might speak of the variables being "dependent" on one another. Thus, for example, if younger patients most often are placed in Treatment A and older patients are placed in Treatment C much more frequently, you might say that the choice of treatment is *dependent* on the patient's age. A different way of thinking about this is asking whether <u>knowing the values of one variable helps you to know anything about the values of the other</u>.

Researchers use chi-square to determine whether there are statistically significant differences among the cell frequencies. In this way, they can detect patterns that might indicate relatedness between the study variables. This is the meaning of conducting a <u>test of independence</u>. If a researcher were to reject the null hypothesis (complete independence or no relationship among the cells), then they could conclude that the data are not independent; rather there is a dependent relationship between the study variables.

The goodness of fit test (chi-square one, described earlier) is a very basic assessment of the difference among categories of <u>one variable</u>. With the test of independence, you can add the categories of a <u>second variable</u>, which recognizes additional complexity in a study question and thereby creates a contingency analysis. With two variables, you can express the category data in rows and columns.

Recall my earlier description of the test of independence as concerning whether the values of the categories of one variable are in any way linked to the values of the other variable's categories. That is, do the cell frequencies of one variable influence the cell frequencies of the other?

You can use the same formula for chi-square that I described for the goodness of fit test:

$$\chi^2 = \sum \frac{(f_o - f_e)^2}{f_e}$$

Two-Way Chi-Square

Because you use contingency tables with rows and columns for the test of independence, both of which may have multiple categories, the test is often referred to as the "two-way chi-square." Thus, if you added age categories to the herniated disc treatment study earlier, this chi-square test would be a 2×4 chi-square since it would consist of two age rows and four treatment choice columns.

Assumptions

For this test, I need to note a couple of assumptions. As I have noted with other statistical procedures, the power of a test increases to the extent that the assumptions are met. For the chi-square test of independence, note the following:

1. The categories of both variables should be "independent" of one another. This sounds like a redundancy in a "test of independence," but the idea here is that the cases of the two variables are not related or structurally linked. If I add age to the previous study, for example, I might be concerned if many of the patients were siblings, or related by blood, and so on. Siblings may be perceived differently from others when being assigned treatment.

2. The chi-square test of independence works best if there is no expected cell frequency less than 5. This small value tends to distort the value of the calculation. I will discuss the "Yates correction factor" as a possible remedy in a 2×2 table, but one solution is to "collapse" adjacent cells to avoid the problem. Of course, with sample sizes low enough to cause this problem, you might consider restructuring the study or getting additional cases.

A HYPOTHETICAL EXAMPLE: TEST OF INDEPENDENCE

As I mentioned earlier, the test of independence can recognize additional complexity. Assume the previous research was interested in whether age affected the treatment choice assigned to patients suffering from herniated discs in the hospital. This would yield the contingency table of frequencies shown in Table 14.3.

Creating Expected Frequencies

Please note that the data in Table 14.3 are *observed frequencies*. In order to conduct a chi-square analysis, you need to know the expected frequencies for each of the cells. In the absence of a priori expected frequencies, you can calculate them from the following formula:

$$f_e = \frac{(M_r)\,(M_c)}{GT}$$

The language of this formula is quickly understood if you see that the "M" stands for "marginal total." Thus

M_r is the marginal total for rows.
M_c is the marginal total for columns.
GT is the grand total.

TABLE 14.3   Observed Frequencies for the Test of Independence

	Medication	Acupuncture	Manipulation	Surgery	Totals (M_r)
<45	20	18	22	35	95
GE 45	36	12	12	5	65
Totals (M_c)	56	30	34	40	(Grand Total) GT = 160

Here is an example using the observed frequency cell for patients less than 45 who were treated by medication (see top left cell of Table 14.3):

$$f_e = \frac{(M_r)\,(M_c)}{GT}$$
$$= \frac{(95)\,(56)}{160}$$
$$= 33.25$$

Therefore, the expected frequency for this cell (patients <45 treated with medication) is 33.25, which, as you can see, is different from the observed frequency of 20.

The reason you need to use this method is that there are different numbers of patients <45 ($N = 95$) and patients GE 45 ($N = 65$) in the study. Also, the treatment types are not even (i.e., 56, 30, 34, 40). *Because of the differences of category sizes in both variables, the expected frequencies cannot be equal in all cells.* If you had the same number of patients with ages <45 and patients at least age 45 and the treatment assignments were all the same, you could simply divide the total (160) by the number of cells (8) to get the same expected frequency (20) for all cells, as I showed in the goodness of fit test. However, the unequal sizes mean that the "weighting" of each cell size is different.

I use the previous formula to help create appropriate cell sizes since using the marginal totals. *By multiplying the marginal totals associated with a given cell and dividing by the grand total, you can get a more precise (weighted) expected frequency for each cell.*

Table 14.4 shows the expected frequencies calculated for each cell (in parentheses) along with the observed frequencies. If you calculate these expected frequencies, they should total the marginal totals just the same as the observed frequencies. All the expected frequencies together should be equal to 160.

If you calculate the expected frequencies as I did for the table, you should notice that you actually would only have to calculate three of the row cells to derive all the rest of the expected frequencies. Look at Table 14.4 to see how this works. I bolded the cell values (first three cells of <45) to show that if you create these expected frequencies only, all the other expected frequencies in the other cells can be obtained by simply subtracting the sum of these calculated expected frequencies from the marginal total (M_r) of 95. Here is how you could calculate the expected frequency

TABLE 14.4   The Expected Frequencies for the Study

	Medication	Acupuncture	Manipulation	Surgery	Totals (M_r)
<45	*20 (33.25)*	*18 (17.81)*	*22 (20.19)*	35 (23.75)	95
GE 45	36 (22.75)	12 (12.19)	12 (13.81)	5 (16.25)	65
Totals (M_c)	56	30	34	40	(Grand Total) GT = 160

for the last cell in the first row (<45, surgery):

$$33.25 + 17.81 + 20.19 = 71.25$$

$$\text{Then}, 95(M_r)\text{--}71.25 = 23.75$$

You can use the same logic with the <u>column</u> expected frequencies, but here it is even simpler since there are only two cells per column. Thus, to calculate the expected frequency for GE 45, medication cell,

$$56\ (M_c)\text{--}33.25(\text{the already calculated expected frequency}) = 22.75$$

Degrees of Freedom for the Test of Independence

These calculations express the meaning of degrees of freedom. Only one of the <45 (row) cells cannot change its value when the other three row cells are known. Thus all the row cells (4) are free to vary except for one (thus, $4 - 1 = 3$). The same logic applies to <u>column</u> cells (treatments). Since there are only two cell values making up each column, one is free to change its value, but the other one is not (thus, $2 - 1 = 1$) since it must equal the marginal total number for that column.

The degrees of freedom are therefore calculated as follows:

$$df = (\text{rows--}1)(k\text{--}1)$$

$$\text{In this study}, df = (2 - 1)(4 - 1) = 3$$

Table 14.5 shows the calculated chi-square based on the formula I used earlier in the goodness of fit test:

$$\chi^2 = \sum \frac{(f_o - f_e)^2}{f_e}$$

As you can see, the calculated χ^2 for this study is 26.52. The assumptions were met because there were no expected frequencies less than 5 and the study description of subjects did not specify that the subjects were connected to each other (i.e., dependent). You could therefore proceed to the hypothesis test to determine whether the categories of the two variables show a *pattern of connection* or whether they are "independent" (i.e., do not demonstrate a connection of relationship).

TABLE 14.5 The Calculated Chi-Square for the Test of Independence

| | < 45 | | | | GE 45 | | | |
	Medication	Acupuncture	Manipulation	Surgery	Medication	Acupuncture	Manipulation	Surgery
f_o	20	18	22	35	36	12	12	5
f_e	33.25	17.81	20.19	23.75	22.75	12.19	13.81	16.25
$f_o - f_e$	−13.25	0.19	1.81	11.25	13.25	−0.19	−1.81	−11.25
$(f_o - f_e)^2$	175.56	0.04	3.29	126.56	175.56	0.04	3.29	126.56
$\dfrac{(f_o - f_e)^2}{f_e}$	5.28	0.00	0.16	5.33	7.72	0.00	0.24	7.79
$\chi^2 = 26.52$	(5.28 + 0.00 + 0.16 + 5.33 + 7.72 + 0.00 + 0.24 + 7.79 = 26.52)							

Using the same hypothesis testing steps as with the goodness of fit test, you can determine whether the calculated chi-square of 26.52 falls into the exclusion region of the comparison distribution:

1. *Null hypothesis:* $f_o = f_e$. (There is no difference between what you expect to happen and what you observe to happen.)
2. *Alternative hypothesis:* $f_o \neq f_e$. (There is a difference between what you expect to see and what you actually see.)
3. *Critical value of exclusion:*
   df = 3 (see previous text for calculation):

$$\chi^2_{0.05,3} = 7.815$$

4. *Calculated chi-square:* $\chi^2 = 26.52$.
5. *Decision:* Since the calculated value (26.52) exceeds the critical value (7.815), I conclude that there is a statistically significant difference among the categories of treatments among those patients <45 and those GE 45 at the 0.05 level, $p < 0.05$.
6. *Interpretation:* The patients in this study were assigned different treatments by age in statistically different numbers. The specific interpretation of the direction of the findings is shown in Table 14.6. As you can see, I presented the table with percentages in the cells along with the frequency in the cell in parentheses.

TABLE 14.6 The Percentages of the Study Data for Interpretation of Findings

	< 45	GE 45
Medication	(20) 21.05%	(36) 55.38%
Acupuncture	(18) 18.95%	(12) 18.46%
Manipulation	(22) 23.16%	(12) 18.46%
Surgery	(35) 36.84%	(5) 7.69%
Totals	(95) 100.00%	(65) 100.00%

I changed the nature of the table according to the protocol I noted earlier. That is, the independent variable should be placed in columns, and the dependent variable should be placed in rows. *This way, you can create column percentages (equaling 100%) and interpret across the rows of the dependent variable categories.*

Using the table protocol allows you to frame the results in terms of independent and dependent variables that might be featured in the research design. Thus, you might interpret the findings as "over twice the percentage of patients aged 45 and older were assigned to a treatment of medication" (55.38–21.05%). Also, "over four times the percentage of those less than 45 were treated with surgery than those 45 or over (36.84–7.69%)."

I presented the table in this fashion (with IV categories in columns and DV categories in rows) because it is more meaningful for interpretation. I will also use it this way in SPSS®.

SPECIAL 2 × 2 CHI-SQUARE

There are special formulas for the 2×2 chi-square tests of independence that allow you to calculate values directly from the frequencies in the contingency table rather than calculate f_e. Table 14.7 shows the layout of the 2×2 table with the cells labeled "a"–"d" for clarification. As you can see, the marginal totals simply add the cells across the rows and down the columns.

I present the alternate formula (without a calculated example) for four reasons:

1. The 2×2 table is fairly common in research, so you should be aware of alternate means for manual calculations.
2. There are special effect size calculations for this design that form the basis for effect size calculations that can be used with other types of tables.
3. The 2×2 table illustrates the use of a correction process for tables with low sample size.
4. This design is used with repeated measures studies.

The Alternate 2 × 2 Formula

The formula for the 2×2 table, utilizing the cell identification letters (a–d, as shown in Table 17.7), is as follows:

$$\chi^2 = \frac{N(ad - bc)^2}{(a + b)(c + d)(a + c)(b + d)}$$

TABLE 14.7 The 2 × 2 Chi-Square Contingency Table

a	b	a + b
c	d	c + d
a + c	b + d	N

TABLE 14.8   **The Example Data in a 2 × 2 Table**

	Medication	Acupuncture	Totals (M_r)
< 45	a = 20	b = 18	38
GE 45	c = 36	d = 12	48
Totals (M_c)	56	30	(Grand Total) GT = 86

If you look closely at the formula, it generally expresses the "*ad*" to "*bc*" cell totals as a proportion of all the marginal totals. Thus, as the differences grow between the *ad* and *bc* "axes," the chi-square value increases.

To take an example of this special formula, consider Table 14.8 which is adapted from Table 14.3. The data in the table are simply the patients <45 and those GE 45 between only the first two treatments ("medication" and "acupuncture"). Following the convention shown in Table 14.7, I labeled each cell as "*a, b, c,* or *d.*"

If you calculate chi-square using the special formula, you will find that the result is the same had you used the general formula I introduced earlier in the chapter. The following analyses compare the two approaches showing the same calculated chi-square result (with slight rounding differences):

$$\chi^2 = \frac{N(ad - bc)^2}{(a + b)(c + d)(a + c)(b + d)}$$

$$= \frac{86(240 - 648)^2}{(38)(48)(56)(30)}$$

$$= \frac{14{,}315{,}904}{3{,}064{,}320}$$

$$= 4.67$$

Now, using the general formula on the same data to calculate chi-square, consider the data in Table 14.9. As you can see, the layout is similar to the general formula examples I introduced in earlier sections.

Correction for 2 × 2 Tables: Yates' Correction for Continuity

Some researchers point out that it is important to "correct" 2 × 2 tables, especially those that have small sample sizes because they may not provide the best estimates. The Yates correction for continuity formula allows the researcher to adjust the calculations to make it more difficult to reject the null hypothesis and therefore provide a more conservative chi-square result.

Researchers are divided about whether to use the correction at all because it may be too conservative. If you use chi-square with small samples, especially the special 2 × 2 table, be aware of this issue and investigate the use of the corrected formula.

TABLE 14.9   Using the General Chi-Square Formula on the 2 × 2 Table

	< 45		GE 45	
	Medication	Acupuncture	Medication	Acupuncture
(cell)	a	b	c	d
f_o	20	18	36	12
f_e	24.74	13.26	31.26	16.74
$f_o - f_e$	−4.74	4.74	4.74	−4.74
$(f_o - f_e)^2$	22.468	22.468	22.468	22.468
$\frac{(f_o - f_e)^2}{f_e}$	0.908	1.694	0.719	1.342
$\chi^2 =$	(.908 + 1.694 + .719 + 1.342) = 4.663			

I present the formula here, but do not provide a calculated example. (The previous example from Table 14.8 is inappropriate because the sample size is large.)

$$\chi^2 = \frac{N\left(|ad - bc| - \frac{N}{2}\right)^2}{(a + b)(c + d)(a + c)(b + d)}$$

As you can see, this is simply the special chi-square formula for a 2 × 2 table with the adjustment of subtracting $\frac{N}{2}$ from the $|ad - bc|$ difference before it is squared. (Note that the $\frac{N}{2}$ adjustment is subtracted from the absolute value of the $(ac - bc)$ difference since this value can be a negative value.) In practical terms, it adds one step to the overall set of steps in calculating chi-square.

EFFECT SIZE IN 2 × 2 TABLES: PHI

In a 2 × 2 table under the circumstances I described earlier, the perfect relationship between the categories of two variables equals unity or a proportion of "1." These special properties allow the researcher to express the relationships among the values in terms of a special effect size measure known as phi ("φ"). Phi varies between values of 0 and 1 and when squared can be expressed in terms of explained variance (i.e., the same as r^2). Thus, φ^2 is the proportion of variance in one variable explained by the other.

The formula for phi is very simple. As you can see, it is based on chi-square and can be calculated simply by dividing χ^2 by N and taking the square root of the result

$$\varphi = \sqrt{\frac{\chi^2}{N}}$$

The same criteria for judging C apply also to phi. Cohen's (1988) suggestions are generally 0.10 (small), 0.30 (medium), and 0.50 (large).

CRAMER'S *V*: EFFECT SIZE FOR THE CHI-SQUARE TEST OF INDEPENDENCE

I return now to the question of effect size for the chi-square test of independence. In earlier sections, I discussed C, the general effect size measure for chi-square, especially appropriate for the goodness of fit test, and φ, the effect size measure especially appropriate for the 2×2 test of independence.

Tests of independence that are more complex than the 2×2 table (i.e., that have more than two rows and/or two categories) typically use another measure of effect size, Cramer's V. The φ value calculated from the 2×2 arrangement allows the researcher to express effect size as variance explained, but you cannot do this with larger tables.

Cramer's V calculates effect size values that range between 0 and 1. Since it takes into account tables with different numbers of rows and column categories, the formula includes an adjustable feature:

$$\text{Cramer's } V = \sqrt{\frac{\chi^2}{N(df_{\text{Smallest of } r \text{ or } c})}}$$

As you can see, the formula looks very much like the φ formula except it is modified by the number of rows and columns in the table. The following element of the formula captures the shape of the table and uses it to modify the φ formula:

$$df_{\text{Smallest of } r \text{ or } c}$$

This value refers to the degrees of freedom calculation for the test of independence that I introduced earlier:

$$df = (r{-}1)(k{-}1)$$

Cramer's V uses the smaller of either $(r - 1)$ or $(k - 1)$ in the formula. Thus, in the hypothetical example, I used a 2×4 table. For calculating Cramer's V, I would use $(r - 1)$ in the denominator since it represented the smallest number (i.e., $2 - 1$ as opposed to $4 - 1$). The Cramer's V calculation for the hypothetical test of independence would therefore be

$$\text{Cramer's } V = \sqrt{\frac{26.52}{160(2-1)}}$$

$$= 0.407$$

The judgment for the magnitude of Cramer's V does not always use the guidelines I presented for the other effect size measures (0.10 for small, 0.30 for medium, and 0.50 for large). This is because you must take into account the adjustment to the formula caused by the shape of the table. Once again, Cohen (1988) provides the adjusted set of guidelines. I refer you to Cohen's book for the complete set of figures.

In our example, because I used a 2×4 table, I could use the same 0.1, 0.3, and 0.5 guidelines for judging the effect size for Cramer's V as I did for C. Larger tables will have reduced magnitude effect size criteria that determine small, medium, and large effects. For example, if my table had been a 3 × 4, the effect size criteria for a large effect would be 0.354. In this event, if I had calculated chi-square to be the same 0.407, the effect size would have been determined to be large instead of medium. As is it however, you can conclude that the fictitious study using a 2 × 4 table showed a medium effect size.

REPEATED MEASURES CHI-SQUARE: MCNEMAR TEST

Recall that I made a distinction with other statistical procedures between those that used independent samples and those that used dependent samples. I identified dependent sample designs as those in which one group is somehow linked structurally to the other. Thus, in experimental designs, a group measured twice (e.g., pre-test and post-test) would need to be treated differently than other group measures because the *same group of subjects would be measured twice.*

If the *T* test was used to detect a difference between two dependent samples in an experiment, for example (i.e., pre–post, Time 1 – Time 2, matched samples), you would need to use a special *T* test that "factored out" the relatedness so the *T* test could determine the unique differences that remained between the two samples. The same thing would be true for ANOVA procedures that measured the same group twice in a design.

You may recall that I referred to these kinds of measures in several ways:

- Repeated measures tests
- Dependent sample tests
- Paired sample tests
- Within-subject tests

I will talk about these dependent measures (especially dependent *T* and within-subject ANOVA) in a subsequent chapter because it is so important to research. Chi-square also has a special "within-subject" design that I mention here to give you an idea of what repeated measures are and how chi-square can be used with experimental designs.

Recall that an experiment introduces a treatment (i.e., manipulation of the independent variable) and then takes a measure of the outcome (dependent) variable to observe the effect of the treatment. Chi-square can be used with categorical data in these experimental designs.

Suppose a researcher was interested in the denial by patients who were initially diagnosed with type II diabetes. Since their eventual management of the condition would appear to require their resolve to face the diagnosis and change their eating and exercise patterns, it might be important to find ways to change their attitudes.

The researcher in question might have proposed a new "orientation procedure" consisting of a combination of counseling group therapy. With one group of patients initially diagnosed with type II diabetes, the researcher decided to assess the patients'

TABLE 14.10   The Dependent Sample Chi-Square for the Resolve Study

		Post	
		Not Resolved	Resolved
Pre			
	Resolved	a = 1	b = 9
	Not Resolved	c = 0	d = 17

level of resolve using a standardized instrument.[3] After the orientation procedure, the researcher again administered the resolve instrument to see what changes in resolve might have occurred since the beginning of the procedure.

Table 14.10 shows the table of data the researcher used for the repeated measures chi-square analysis. With this type of design, the researcher measured the same patients at different times (beginning and end of procedure). Therefore, the researcher had to use a special dependent measures chi-square test called the McNemar test. As you can see from Table 14.10, I labeled the cells "a"–"d." There was 1 patient (the upper left cell labeled "a") resolved at the beginning of the procedure but not at the end. By contrast, there were 17 patients not resolved at the beginning but resolved at the end of the procedure (shown in cell "d"). The formula and example solution for this special test is

$$\chi^2_{\text{McNemar}} = \frac{(a-d)^2}{a+d}$$
$$= \frac{(1-17)^2}{1+17}$$
$$= 14.22$$

In this study, the researcher rejected the null hypothesis since 14.22 exceeded the exclusion value ($\chi^2_{0.05,1} = 3.84$). The treatment (orientation procedure) had an effect on the patients such that significantly more of the patients were resolved at the end of the procedure. The φ of 0.73 for this study indicated a large effect size. Phi squared indicated that over 53% of the results of the resolve outcome were explained by categorizing the values of the intervention in this way ($\varphi^2 = 0.73^2 = 0.533$).

The Repeated Measures Chi-Square Table

As you can see, the focus in the cells is the change from cell a to cell d. That is, you need to determine the difference between *how many patients "had" the condition before but not after and the number of patients who did not have the condition at*

---

[3] Assume the (as far as I know) fictitious resolve instrument resulted in identifying a level of resolve high enough to render the judgment by experts as representing appropriate realism for approaching life difficulties.

TABLE 14.11   Changing the Dependent Sample Chi-Square Categories

		Post	
Pre		Resolved	Not Resolved
	Resolved	a = 9	b = 1
	Not Resolved	c = 17	d = 0

the beginning but did afterward. If the null hypothesis is accurate, these two cells should be relatively equal. If the treatment had an effect, these two cells would show differences. (If the procedure results in resolve, then cell *d* would be much larger than cell *a*.) The formula essentially compares the differences between the two cells as a proportion of the total frequency of the two cells.

The McNemar formula changes depending on how you create the table. Just remember that the two critical cells are the ones I identified earlier. Here is an example of changing the table and how the formula would change. If you changed the position of the "post" conditions as shown in Table 14.11, the formula would change to recognize the important two cells.

If you set the table up this way, the two critical cells are now "*b*" and "*c*" since you need to detect the difference between patients who "had" the condition before but not after (cell b) compared to the number of patients who did not have the condition at the beginning but did afterward (cell c). As you can see, you get the same calculated value (14.22), but you must be careful to set the table up to reflect these differences:

$$\chi^2_{\text{McNemar}} = \frac{(b-c)^2}{b+c}$$

$$= \frac{(1-17)^2}{1+17}$$

$$= 14.22$$

USING SPSS® AND EXCEL WITH CHI-SQUARE

Both SPSS and Excel will assist with chi-square analyses although SPSS provides a more thorough summary of findings and is easier to use. I will demonstrate both programs using another example. Table 14.12 shows the frequency data from a hypothetical sample ($N = 200$) placed in the appropriate cells. The data report the frequency of hospitals from a region of the country that indicate whether funding was allocated and/or spent for professional development (training in) of a new technique for sterilization of a certain surgical procedure. To what extent do the hospitals expend funding for which it is intended?

You can calculate this problem manually according to the method I described earlier (chi-square test of independence). Since this is a 2×2 table, you can use the "special" formula to calculate χ^2 if you do not want to calculate expected frequencies. The manually calculated answer is $\chi^2 = 16.87$, $p < 0.05$ (since $\chi^2_{0.05,1} = 3.841$).

USING SPSS® FOR THE CHI-SQUARE TEST OF INDEPENDENCE

You can use the "Crosstabs" command in SPSS to create a chi-square analysis. I will demonstrate this procedure, and then I will show an alternate procedure which is best when you input the data table directly into SPSS.

Coding the Data File

SPSS uses a coding method to locate and use frequency data for chi-square. For an example of this method, see Figure 10.5 showing the 2XANOVA data file structure for the sex–sleep–health problem. Referring to Table 14.12 for the current example, you can create a table whereby both of the study variables are assigned numbers (1 and 2, in this example) according to the location of the table cells. The data for each of the cells is listed in a separate column of the data file according to the cell locations. For example, if a hospital indicated that they did not allocate funding for professional development for the sterilization procedure, both of the cells in the "Allocated – No" column are given the number "1." Both of the cells in the column for "Allocated – Yes" are given a "2." Next, both of the row cells for "Spent – No" are assigned a "1," and both of the row cells for "Spent – Yes" are allocated a "2."[4]

Using this method, you can list the data values for the chi-square example as shown in Table 14.13. For example, cell "d" of Table 14.12 shows 70 hospitals. This number is represented in Table 14.13 as the bottom row. Thus, 70 hospitals are in the second column (Allocated – Yes, 2) and the second row (Spent – Yes, 2), representing the second column and the second row.

Weighting Cases

SPSS prepares a contingency table with the data you specify and provides a range of analyses.

TABLE 14.12 The Chi-Square Values for the Hypothetical Problem

	Allocated - No	Allocated - Yes	Totals (M_r)
Spent - No	53	61	114
Spent - Yes	16	70	86
Totals (M_c)	69	131	(Grand Total) GT = 200

[4] You should provide "Value" labels on the Variable View of the SPSS® screen that correspond to these cell number designations. If you do, the output tables will be listed with the variable labels, making it easier to interpret.

**TABLE 14.13   The Database
for the Chi-Square Example**

Allocated	Spent	Number
1	1	53
1	2	16
2	1	61
2	2	70

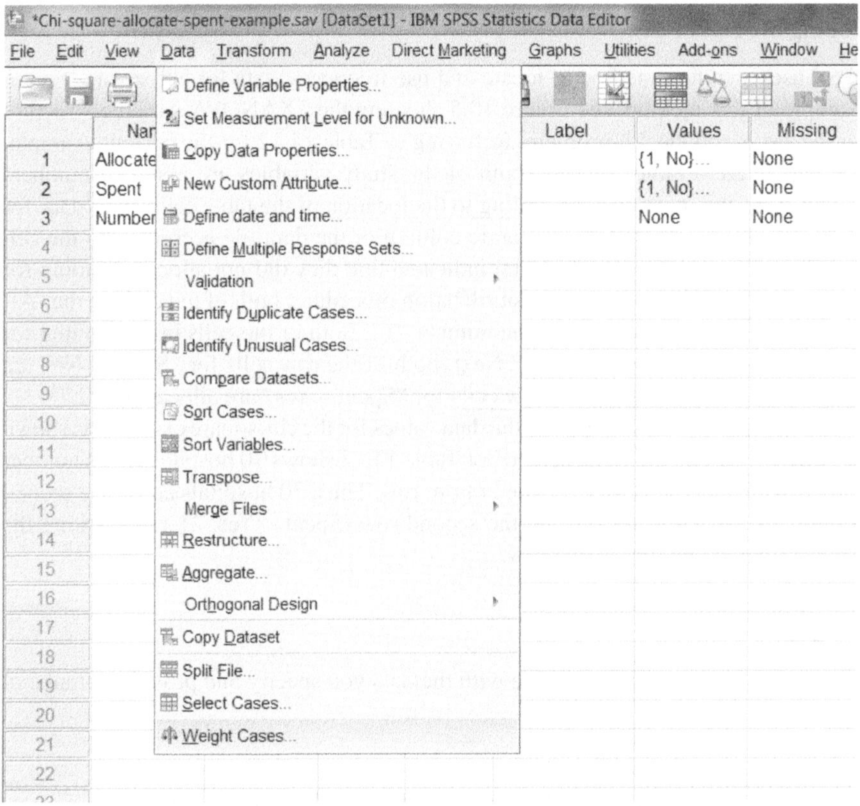

Figure 14.2   The SPSS® "Weight Cases" specification window.

Once the data are listed according to this method, and before you specify the Crosstabs procedure, you must "weight" the cases. Figure 14.2 shows the menu choice for this process. This allows the program to connect the frequency data ("Number") to the variables coded as (in this case) "1" and "2."

Once you select the "Weight Cases" option, SPSS returns the window shown in Figure 14.3, which calls for the procedure to weight cases by the variable I indicated as listing the actual data for the study. As you can see, I called for the program to

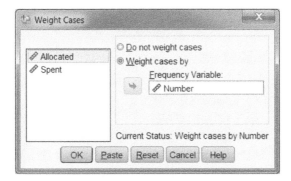

Figure 14.3 The SPSS® "Weight Cases" specification window.

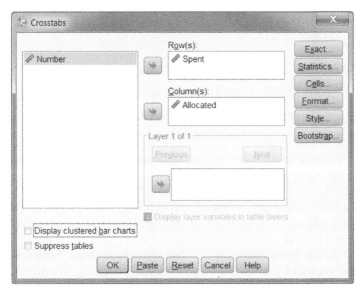

Figure 14.4 The SPSS® Crosstabs specification window.

use the "Number" variable to specify the data according to the coded variables. Once you make this choice, you can use the Crosstabs menus to run the chi-square test procedure.

The Crosstabs Procedure

Starting with the database in which you code the data file, you can choose the Crosstabs procedure through the main menu choices: "Analyze – Descriptive – Crosstabs." Figure 14.4 shows the Crosstabs menu that results from this choice.

As you can see in Figure 14.4, I listed the column variable (Allocated) and the row variable (Spent) according to how I set the data up in Table 14.12. In this example, I

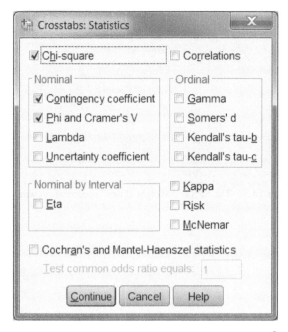

Figure 14.5   The "Crosstabs: Statistics" menu in SPSS®.

am using "Allocated" as the "independent" variable and the row variable "Spent" to be the "dependent" variable for this analysis according to the protocol I discussed earlier.

The "Statistics … " button shown in Figure 14.4 allows the researcher to choose which statistical analyses are desired. Figure 14.5 shows this window in which I call for the overall chi-square statistics and a series of effect size measures for nominal data: C, φ, and Cramer's V.

You also need to choose the "Cells … " button just beneath the "Statistics … " button shown in Figure 14.4. In the resulting menu, you can specify how the percentages are created, among other things. Figure 14.6 shows this menu choice in which I called for column percentages given the protocol I discussed earlier. You can call for "expected counts" or frequencies as well (e.g., to check your manual calculations), but I do not do so for this example.

This series of choices results in SPSS output showing the chi-square analyses needed for significance tests and effect sizes. Figure 14.7 presents the resulting contingency table showing observed frequencies and column percentages for the example data.

As you can see, the Figure 14.7 output looks like the original table of values shown in Table 14.12. The percentages in Figure 14.7 are calculated according to columns, since I am using Allocation as the "independent" variable in this example. The researcher thus interprets the findings of the study across the values of the independent variable (Allocated) within rows of the dependent variable (Spent). These are the percentages used to interpret the study results once the statistical significance and effect sizes are discussed. Figure 14.8 shows the chi-square test results from SPSS.

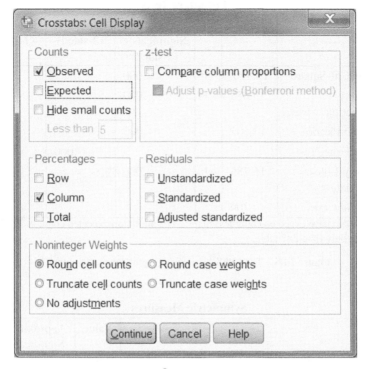

Figure 14.6   The SPSS® "Crosstabs: Cell Display" menu.

Spent * Allocated Crosstabulation

			Allocated		Total
			No	Yes	
Spent	No	Count	53	61	114
		% within Allocated	76.8%	46.6%	57.0%
	Yes	Count	16	70	86
		% within Allocated	23.2%	53.4%	43.0%
Total		Count	69	131	200
		% within Allocated	100.0%	100.0%	100.0%

Figure 14.7   The SPSS® crosstabs contingency table.

Chi-Square Tests

	Value	df	Asymptotic Significance (2-sided)	Exact Sig. (2-sided)	Exact Sig. (1-sided)
Pearson Chi-Square	16.870[a]	1	.000		
Continuity Correction[b]	15.658	1	.000		
Likelihood Ratio	17.607	1	.000		
Fisher's Exact Test				.000	.000
Linear-by-Linear Association	16.785	1	.000		
N of Valid Cases	200				

[a]0 cells (0.0%) have expected count less than 5. The minimum expected count is 29.67.
[b]Computed only for a 2x2 table.

Figure 14.8   The SPSS® chi-square significance test output.

Symmetric Measures

		Value	Approximate Significance
Nominal by Nominal	Phi	.290	.000
	Cramer's V	.290	.000
	Contingency Coefficient	.279	.000
N of Valid Cases		200	

Figure 14.9   The SPSS® effect size measures.

As you can see in Figure 14.8, the "Pearson chi-square" analysis shows a statistically significant chi-square result ($\chi^2 = 16.87$, $p < 0.0001$). This is the same result I reported for the manually calculated value. There are several other tests appropriate for chi-square analyses that I will not cover in this book. I will only point out that the Yates continuity correction factor is shown as "continuity correction" = 15.66, ($p < 0.000$). While I do not advocate the use of this result, you can note that the value, which is only created for the 2×2 table, is less than the chi-square value because it is a more conservative estimate. In any case, this value is also statistically significant.

Figure 14.9 reports the effect sizes for the study. As you recall, I specified these in the Crosstabs procedure. Since this is a 2×2 table, you can use φ which indicates a value of 0.29. According to the guidelines I presented, this is (nearly) a "medium" effect size. If you square φ, you can interpret the value as the percent of variance in Spent accounted for by Allocated. Thus, about 8.4% of the variance in Spent is accounted for by Allocated ($\varphi^2 = 0.29^2 = 0.084$).

Interpreting the Contingency Table

As I mentioned earlier, you need to interpret the analyses from the percentages in the contingency table once you have established a statistically significant finding. If you look at Figure 14.7, you will see that I followed the protocol of using the columns to create percentages that equal 100% so that you can "interpret within columns of the independent variable across rows of the dependent variable."[5]

In this example, the researcher might conclude the following:

- Just over half the percentage of hospitals that allocate funding for the surgical procedure actually spend the funds for training (53.4% vs. 23.2%, respectively).
- Slightly less than half (46.6%) the hospitals allocated funding for training (vs. 76.8% that do not) that is not spent for that purpose. Alternatively, one might conclude that when hospitals do not allocate funds, they are much less likely to designate training (Spend) funds (76.8–46.6%).

USING EXCEL FOR CHI-SQUARE ANALYSES

You can obtain the results from the chi-square test of significance in Excel *once you have created the contingency table from the database*.[6] For example, Table 14.12 shows the contingency table of data resulting from the researcher counting and coding each of the 200 observations according to the category values of Allocated (1 or 2) and Spent (1 or 2).

The Excel CHISQ.TEST Function

When the contingency table cells are recorded, you can use the Chi Test function to obtain results for the test of independence. Since this does not use the "special" (2×2) formula, you must calculate the expected frequencies so Excel can compare observed and expected frequencies.

Figure 14.10 shows the "CHISQ.TEST" function that you can obtain through the "Formulas – Statistical – CHISQ.TEST" menus. As you can see, I identified the cells for actual and expected frequencies from my spreadsheet. The CHITEST function immediately returns the results for the chi-square test immediately below the cell range windows. In this case, Excel returned the value "3.85457E−05," indicating that the chi-square test of independence was statistically significant at the $p = 0.00004$ level. Thus, the calculated chi-square value fell far into the exclusion values of the chi-square distribution indicating a likely nonchance finding.

---

[5]Remember this method depends on where you specify the independent variable. As I mentioned earlier, you can also place the independent variable in rows, in which case you would specify row percentages to equal 100%, resulting in the injunction, "interpret within rows of the independent variable across columns of the dependent variable."

[6]If you have a large database, this is cumbersome, but you can use the "Count" function to help create the table of values.

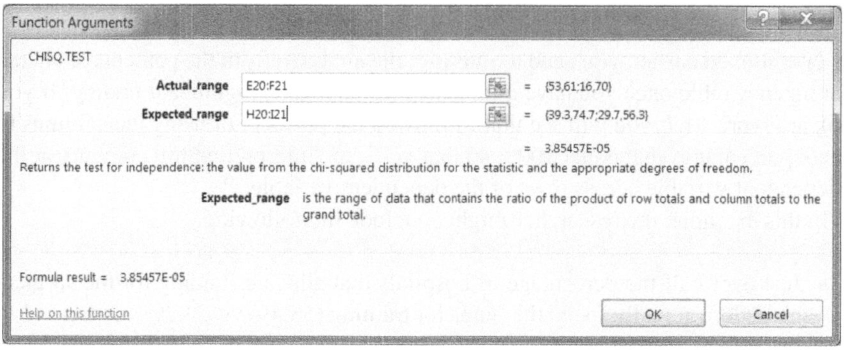

Figure 14.10   The CHISQ.TEST function in Excel for chi-square analysis.

Notice that Excel does not return the actual calculated χ^2 (16.87), nor any indication of effect size. This makes it difficult to report effect size! You can use other Excel functions to return the probability of the finding according to the chi-square distribution if you have already calculated χ^2. Use the "Formulas – Statistical – CHISQ.DIST.RT" menus to create the window shown in Figure 14.11.

As you can see, I simply placed the value of calculated chi-square value of "16.87" in the "X" window and specified "1" for "Deg. Freedom" since the table is a 2×2. The function immediately returns the same probability value (or virtually equal since I used a rounded result from manual calculations) as I obtained with CHISQ.TEST.

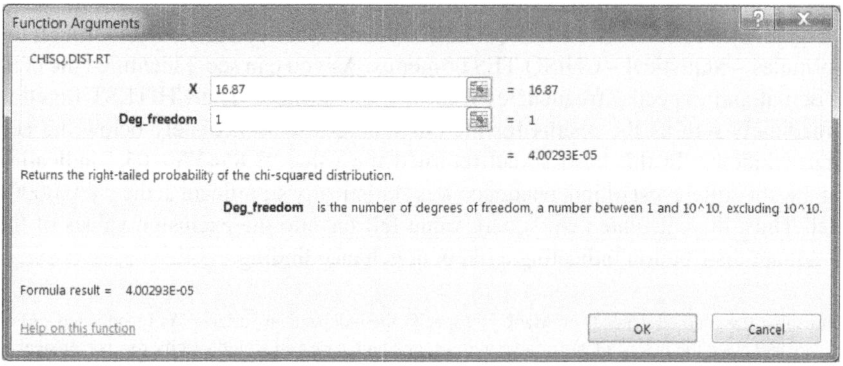

Figure 14.11   The Excel CHIDIST function to identify the chi-square probability.

TERMS AND CONCEPTS

Chi-square test of independence:	Chi-square analyses involving frequencies from more than one study variable.
Contingency coefficient:	An effect size measure for chi-square analyses. This measure is essentially a correlation with nominal data and is used to show the strength of association among study variables.
Contingency table:	Presentation of data in rows and columns to show how data in rows are contingent upon or connected to the data in column cells. Also called "Crosstabs" or "Cross-tabulation analysis."
Cramer's *V*:	An effect size measure for the chi-square test of independence with tables that exceed the 2×2 arrangement (i.e., that have more than two rows and/or categories).
Goodness of fit:	Chi-square analyses that compare *actual* frequency data to *expected* data distributions.
McNemar test:	A special chi-square test used with repeated measures designs.
Phi coefficient:	An effect size measure based upon chi-square and typically used in studies with 2×2 tables. When phi is squared in 2×2 tables, it expresses the proportion of variance in one variable explained by the other.
Yates' correction for continuity:	A method for adjusting 2×2 chi-square table data that have small sample sizes or small expected cell frequencies.

DATA LAB AND EXAMPLES (WITH SOLUTIONS)

The lab for chi-square is from a small study I conducted a number of years ago in a subsidized housing development. The residents of this housing district were all low income, and there was a significant amount of crime prior to an intervention in which services were increased to residents and a new community policing model was established. This sample of residents ($N = 140$) answered a questionnaire that assessed, among other things, their fear of crime and whether they had been the victim of a crime. The survey was conducted after the intervention had taken place, so crime levels were decreasing.

The two variables in the analysis are:

- "Victim" – Whether respondents indicated they had been the victim of a crime
- "Fear" – Assessment of whether their fear of crime was high or low

Problem

Conduct a chi-square analysis on the data in Table 14.14 and summarize your findings.

TABLE 14.14 The Example Data

	Victim?	
Fear	No	Yes
Low	48	33
High	20	39

DATA LAB: SOLUTIONS

Since this data table represents the "special" 2×2 chi-square table, you can use the alternate formula for manual calculations. Once I do this, I will use SPSS and Excel to perform the test of independence.

Manual Calculations

The following are the manual calculations for the data in Table 14.14 using the alternate formula:

$$\chi^2 = \frac{N(ad - bc)^2}{(a+b)(c+d)(a+c)(b+d)}$$
$$= \frac{140(1872 - 660)^2}{(81)(59)(68)(72)}$$
$$= 8.79$$

You can now compare the actual χ^2 (8.79) to the tabled value $\chi^2_{0.05,1} = 3.841$. With these results, you can reject the null hypothesis ($p < 0.05$) and conclude that there is a statistically significant difference between the categories of victim and fear.

The effect size is φ for this table, calculated as follows:

$$\varphi = \sqrt{\frac{\chi^2}{N}}$$
$$= \sqrt{\frac{8.79}{140}}$$
$$= 0.25$$

The effect size is small to medium and indicates that I can explain about 6% (0.25^2) of the variance in one variable as a result of the other.

Using SPSS® for Chi-Square Solutions

Figure 14.12 shows the SPSS spreadsheet with the variable specification for the chi-square analysis. Once you create the data in this fashion, you can weight the cases by the Data variable which will allow you to use the Crosstabs menu to complete the analysis.

Figure 14.13 shows the results of the chi-square analysis. As you can see, $\chi^2 = 8.789$, and $p = 0.003$. Both of these findings confirm the manual calculations.

Figure 14.14 shows the effect size calculations. Recall that you can use phi for this 2×2 table. The calculated $\varphi = 0.25$, which is the same value I calculated manually earlier.

You can use the next part of the output for interpretation. Figure 14.15 shows the Crosstabs output for the contingency table according to the layout of the data. I called

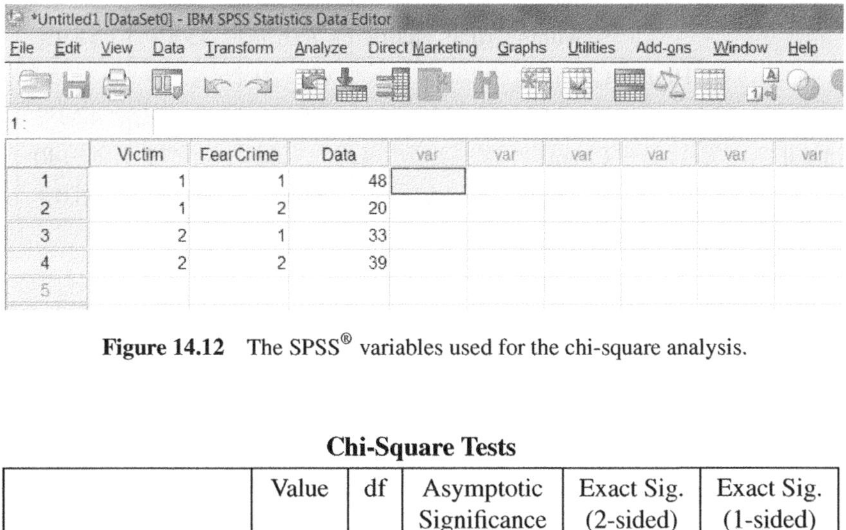

	Victim	FearCrime	Data	var	var	var	var	var	var
1	1	1	48						
2	1	2	20						
3	2	1	33						
4	2	2	39						
5									

Figure 14.12   The SPSS® variables used for the chi-square analysis.

Chi-Square Tests

	Value	df	Asymptotic Significance (2-sided)	Exact Sig. (2-sided)	Exact Sig. (1-sided)
Pearson Chi-Square	8.789[a]	1	.003		
Continuity Correction[b]	7.803	1	.005		
Likelihood Ratio	8.909	1	.003		
Fisher's Exact Test				.004	.002
Linear-by-Linear Association	8.727	1	.003		
N of Valid Cases	140				

[a]0 cells (0.0%) have expected count less than 5. The minimum expected count is 28.66.
[b]Computed only for a 2x2 table.

Figure 14.13   The SPSS® chi-square findings.

Symmetric Measures

		Value	Approximate Significance
Nominal by Nominal	Phi	.251	.003
	Cramer's V	.251	.003
	Contingency Coefficient	.243	.003
N of Valid Cases		140	

Figure 14.14 The SPSS® effect size findings.

FearCrime * Crime Victim Crosstabulation

			Crime Victim		Total
			No	Yes	
FearCrime	Low	Count	48	33	81
		% within Crime Victim	70.6%	45.8%	57.9%
	High	Count	20	39	59
		% within Crime Victim	29.4%	54.2%	42.1%
Total		Count	68	72	140
		% within Crime Victim	100.0%	100.0%	100.0%

Figure 14.15 The SPSS® contingency table output for the crosstabs analysis.

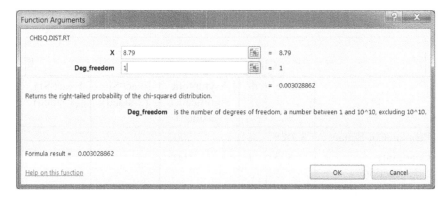

Figure 14.16 The Excel CHISQ.DIST.RT results for the test of independence.

for column percentages in order to use the protocol of placing the predictor variable in columns and the outcome variable in rows.

As you can see from Figure 14.15, when respondents have been victims of a crime, they are much more likely to have a high fear of crime. Over 54% of victims have a high fear of crime compared to 29.4% of those not victimized. This difference in fear persists even when crime is on the decline as it was in our study.

TABLE 14.15 The Contingency Table with Expected Frequencies

Fear	Victim? (Observed)	
	No	Yes
Low	48	33
High	20	39
Fear	**Victim? (Expected)**	
Low	39.3	41.7
High	28.7	30.3

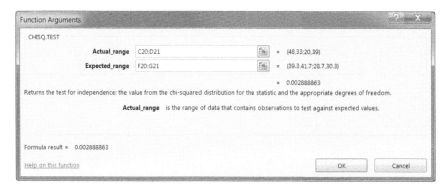

Figure 14.17   The Excel CHISQ.TEST function using observed and expected frequencies.

Using Excel for the Analyses

As I demonstrated earlier in this chapter, you can use Excel to perform the test of independence by using the CHISQ.DIST.RT function as shown in Figure 14.16. As you can see, this function returns the value of $p = 0.003$, indicating a very small probability of concluding a chance finding with these data.

Alternatively, you can use the CHISQ.TEST function by calculating the expected frequencies so you can enter them from the spreadsheet into the CHISQ.TEST function menu. Table 14.15 shows the contingency table with the expected frequencies in separate cells. You need to create the table in this fashion so that you can easily use the CHISQ.TEST function. Figure 14.17 shows the CHISQ.TEST function with the observed and expected frequencies placed in the appropriate windows ("Actual_range" and "Expected_range," respectively).

Figure 14.17 shows the results of the test of independence just below the observed and expected windows. As you can see, $p = 0.003$.

15

REPEATED MEASURES PROCEDURES: T_{DEP} AND ANOVA$_{\text{WS}}$

I have mentioned several times in this book that the researcher needs to consider a statistical procedure carefully before using it. The greatest power and confidence relies on using the correct statistical procedure with the available data according for the research design.

In this chapter, I am returning to two statistical procedures that statisticians have adapted for use with "repeated measures" data. I discussed the independent T test and the general analysis of variance (ANOVA) procedure in earlier chapters, both of which were designed for independent samples. While there are other such procedures, the "dependent T test" and the "within-subject ANOVA" represent important procedures that researchers can use in experimental and post facto designs in which the data are "linked" in some way.

Recall that I made a distinction between statistical procedures that used independent samples and those that used dependent samples. In Chapter 8, I identified dependent sample designs as those in which one group is somehow linked structurally to the other. Thus, in experimental designs, a group measured twice (e.g., pretest and posttest) would need to be treated differently than other group measures because the *same group of subjects would be measured twice.*

If a researcher used a T test to detect a difference between two dependent samples in an experiment (i.e., pre–post, Time1–Time2, matched samples), they would need to use a special T test that factored out the <u>relatedness,</u> so the T test would reveal the unique differences that remained between the two samples. The same thing would be true for ANOVA procedures that measured the same group twice.

Using Statistics in the Social and Health Sciences with SPSS® and Excel®, First Edition.
Martin Lee Abbott.
© 2017 John Wiley & Sons, Inc. Published 2017 by John Wiley & Sons, Inc.

As I noted in Chapter 14 in which I discussed the dependent sample chi-square (McNemar's test), these kinds of measures have several names:

- Repeated measures tests
- Dependent sample tests
- Paired sample tests
- Within-subject tests

INDEPENDENT AND DEPENDENT SAMPLES IN RESEARCH DESIGNS

Independent and dependent sample data can be used in both experimental and post facto designs. Dependent samples are most commonly encountered in experimental or quasi-experimental designs in which a sample group is given a pretest and then administered a posttest after some intervention. It is used in some post facto research to measure a group on some attitude measure at different times.

Table 15.1 shows several possibilities for independent and dependent samples in research and post facto designs. This table highlights the dependent T test since there are only two groups. A similar table could be created for three or more groups that would emphasize the within-subjects ANOVA.

As I noted in Chapter 8, independent samples mean that choosing subjects for one group has nothing to do with choosing subjects for the other group. Thus, if I randomly select Bob and assign him randomly to group 1 (the experimental group

TABLE 15.1 Independent and Dependent Sample in Experimental and Post Facto Designs

	Experimental Designs	Post Facto Designs
Two Independent Samples (Between Subjects)	T_{ind} comparing Post test differences of two groups of *different subjects* after an intervention	T_{ind} comparing existing data on two groups of *different members*
	Example: Do the 'sensitivity to violence' (STV) measures differ between two randomly chosen groups after one group watches a violent movie?	*Example: Do STV measures differ between Trauma workers and GP's?*
Two Dependent Samples (Within Subjects)	T_{dep} comparing Pre—Post differences or Time 1—Time2 differences of the *same group of subjects* after an intervention	T_{dep} test comparing *matched group* differences on an existing measure or outcome
	Example: Is the post test STV score higher than the pre test PFV scores of one group that watches a violent movie?	*Example: Do the STV scores differ between two groups of doctors (one in the urban core and one in the suburbs) matched on time as a physician?*

that watches a violent movie), it has nothing to do with the fact that I choose Sally and assign her randomly to group 2 (the group that does not see the violent movie). The random selection of these group members is a very important assumption because it assures the researcher that there are no built-in linkages between the groups' posttest scores. The power of randomization will result in the comparability of two groups chosen in this way.

Dependent samples consist of groups of subjects that have some structured linkage, like using the same people twice in a study. For example, I might use pretest STV scores from both Bob and Sally and *compare these scores with their own posttest STV scores*. Using dependent samples affects the ability of the randomness process to create comparable samples; in such cases, the researcher is assessing *individual* change (before-to-after measures) in the context of the experiment that is assessing *group* change.

Dependent samples also include *matched samples*, a situation in which the researcher purposely assigns people to be in two groups on the basis of some characteristic(s) rather than choosing and assigning subjects randomly to two groups. For example, you might be concerned about gender for a given study and purposely assign equal numbers of men and women to two groups. In this case, the randomness criterion is violated despite the attempt of the researcher to ensure that study groups have matching characteristics on a crucial study influence. This is typically the case where the researcher cannot control the conditions for random selection and assignment.

USING DIFFERENT *T* TESTS

When researchers use dependent samples, they need to use an independent *T* test that has been "adjusted" for the influence of the relatedness of the samples. This adjusted test is called a *dependent sample T test*. Other names for this test are repeated measures *T* test, within-subject *T* test, and paired sample *T* test. Both Excel and SPSS® refer to these as paired sample *T* tests.

There are two ways to calculate the dependent *T* test (T_{dep}). I will introduce both approaches in this chapter, but I will focus primarily on interpreting the SPSS and Excel procedures rather than the manual calculations.

THE DEPENDENT *T* TEST CALCULATION: THE "LONG" FORMULA

The long formula for T_{dep} looks intimidating, but it makes conceptual sense. It is essentially the same as the formula for T_{ind} except that you must adjust the estimated standard error of difference s_D to account for the relatedness in the samples.

As you will recall from Chapter 8, these are the T_{ind} formulas:

$$t = \frac{(M_1 - M_2) - \mu_{M_1 - M_2}}{s_D}$$

$$s_D = \sqrt{s_{m_1}^2 + s_{m_2}^2}$$

The formulas for T_{dep} are the same except for the estimated standard error of difference using the adjusted formula in the following (s_{D_r}):

$$t_{\text{dep}} = \frac{(M_1 - M_2) - \mu_{M_1 - M_2}}{s_{D_r}}$$

The T_{dep} formula thus becomes

$$t_{\text{dep}} = \frac{(M_1 - M_2)}{s_{D_r}}$$

Here is the formula for the adjusted standard error of difference:

$$s_{D_r} = \sqrt{s_{M_1}^2 + s_{M_2}^2 - [\,2r(s_{M_1})(s_{M_2})\,]}$$

As you can see, the only difference is that there is a "second component" included that is subtracted out of the s_D in the T_{ind} formula. I shaded this portion in the formula. Recall that I said that dependent samples are related (correlated) to one another and that the dependent T test must subtract out this relatedness.

If you look at the T_{dep} formula, the shaded portion that measures this relatedness is subtracted out of the formula. The shaded portion includes "r," the Pearson's correlation coefficient. If the two sample groups are related (correlated), this r value will "modify" the measures that are used to calculate the T_{dep} ratio. However, if you have two independent samples, they will not be related, r will equal 0, and the shaded portion will therefore also equal 0. When this is the case, the s_{D_r} will be equivalent to s_D.

EXAMPLE: THE LONG FORMULA

I will use an example to show these calculations briefly. Recall the formulas I used to create the T_{ind} which I will use to assist in creating the T_{dep} values:

$$s_x = \sqrt{\frac{\Sigma X^2 - \frac{(\Sigma X)^2}{N}}{N - 1}} \text{ or } S_x = \sqrt{\frac{SS}{df}}$$

$$s_D = \sqrt{s_{m_1}^2 + s_{m_2}^2} \quad s_{m_1} = \frac{s_1}{\sqrt{n_1}} \quad s_{m_2} = \frac{s_2}{\sqrt{n_2}}$$

The data for this exercise are fictitious. The values represent the amount of time it takes (number of minutes) for lab technicians to complete a routine tissue test, from receipt of the order to logging the results. Time1 (in the two shaded columns) represents the initial information gathered from the 45 lab technicians (from different sections of a large hospital). Next, the lab technicians are given instruction in new procedures for performing the lab test. Time2 (in the nonshaded columns) represents the testing time from the same technicians as in Time1. Since the same lab technicians were assessed at two different times, you would use the T_{dep} to see if the intervention (instruction in the new procedure) was effective.

Table 15.2 shows the data in columns. Because of space limitations, I created two columns each for Time1 and Time2. Use the formulas I included earlier to calculate the paired T ratio.

Table 15.3 shows the relevant calculations for this problem. Confirm the summary calculations and then use them to conduct a T_{dep} test.

Results

$$t_{dep} = \frac{(M_1 - M_2)}{s_{D_r}}$$

$$= \frac{(40.51 - 36.76)}{0.888}$$

$$= 4.223$$

TABLE 15.2   The Study Data

Time1	Time2	Time1	Time2
11	6.0	41	35.0
4	2.0	62	47.0
11	11.0	29	29.0
18	9.0	55	50.0
30	23.0	46	49.0
7	12.0	39	38.0
12	10.0	41	40.0
42	42.0	45	46.0
32	20.0	49	58.0
17	5.0	41	35.0
24	24.0	54	56.0
46	37.0	50	53.0
26	28.0	52	58.0
28	31.0	50	49.0
44	39.0	56	57.0
44	30.0	62	60.0
38	38.0	57	39.0
45	39.0	54	48.0
35	34.0	79	70.0
45	36.0	64	62.0
39	31.0	47	41.0
40	37.0	64	50.0
48	40.0		

TABLE 15.3   The Calculated Elements of the Study Data

	Time1	Time2
Means	40.51	36.76
SS	12291.244	12102.311
s_x	16.714	16.585
s_m	2.492	2.472
s_D	3.51	
R	0.936	
s_{D_r}	0.888	

The paired T ratio for this study is 4.223. When you compare this to the tabled value of T to determine whether it is a significant ratio, use $df = N - 1$, where N is the *number of pairs of data*. Therefore, $T_{dep0.05,44} = 2.021$. Therefore, since the calculated $T_{dep} = 4.223$, you can reject the null hypothesis ($p < 0.05$). The difference between Time1 and Time2 is statistically different. The lab technicians took less time conducting the tissue test. Time2 data suggest lower times for each lab technician.

Effect Size

You can use the same effect size formula for the T_{dep} as you did for the single sample T test (in Chapter 7). The difference is that N is the number of pairs of data. Using 0.2, 0.5, and 0.8 as the criteria for small, medium, and large, as you did in Chapter 7, you can judge the calculated effect size for this finding ($d = 0.63$) as a medium effect:

$$d = \frac{T_{dep}}{\sqrt{N}}$$
$$= \frac{4.223}{\sqrt{45}}$$
$$= 0.63$$

THE DEPENDENT T TEST CALCULATION: THE "DIFFERENCE" FORMULA

There is another way of manually calculating paired data that is shorter and follows a procedure you have already learned. As you recall from Chapter 7, I discussed the process for calculating the single sample T ratio. The formulas I used were

$$t = \frac{M - \mu}{s_m} \qquad s_m = \frac{s_x}{\sqrt{N}}$$

You can use this method to calculate a T ratio for paired data by subtracting values in one set of scores from paired values in the other set of scores to yield a single set of "difference" scores. Once you have the difference scores, you can use the formulas earlier to calculate the result. You can see how I included the "difference" scores into the single sample T formula in the following to use it with our difference change scores:

$$t = \frac{M - \mu}{s_m} \quad \text{becomes} \quad T_{dep} = \frac{M_{diff} - 0}{s_{m-diff}}$$

One matter of note in the altered formula that uses the difference scores is the "0" in the place occupied by the population mean in the single sample T formula. This simply refers to the fact that the population of all "differences between related group scores" will be 0 since some differences will be negative and some will be positive. This would create a 0 sum. Therefore, the formula compares the *sample* mean difference score to the *population of difference scores*, the latter of which is 0:

$$T_{dep} = \frac{M_{diff} - 0}{S_{m-diff}}$$

$$SS_{diff} = \sum D^2 - \frac{\left(\sum D\right)^2}{N}$$

$$S_{diff} = \sqrt{\frac{SS_{diff}}{N-1}}$$

$$S_{m-diff} = \frac{S_{diff}}{\sqrt{N}}$$

The bottom line is that you can use the same formula you used with the single sample *T* test with only slight variations. In this way, you do not have to calculate the Pearson's *r* value as you did in the "long" formula. By creating difference scores, you "subtract out the relatedness."

The two approaches (long formula and difference formula) yield the same T_{dep} value. With larger data sets, you will likely use SPSS and Excel to make the calculations, so you do not need to be concerned at this point with the different formulas.

Here is how the difference formulas and procedure would work using the data in Table 15.2. Table 15.4 shows the summary calculations which you can use to conduct the T_{dep} test. Remember that the df for this calculation is $N - 1$ (pairs).

The T_{dep} Ratio from the Difference Method

When you use this method, use the modified formula in the following to calculate the T_{dep}:

$$\begin{aligned} T_{dep} &= \frac{M_{diff} - 0}{S_{m-diff}} \\ &= \frac{3.756 - 0}{0.887} \\ &= 4.234 \end{aligned}$$

TABLE 15.4 The Difference Procedure for Calculating T_{dep}

Time1	Time2
Mean	3.756
$\sum D$	169
$\sum D^2$	2193
SS_{diff}	1558.31
S_{diff}	5.95
S_{m-diff}	0.887

TABLE 15.5   The T_{ind} Comparison with T_{dep}

$T_{ind} = 1.07$	$T_{dep} = 4.234$
$T_{.05,88} = 2.00$	$T_{.05,44} = 2.021$
Decision: Do not reject H_0	Reject H_0, $p < .05$

If you compare the T_{dep} value from the difference method, you will find that it is equivalent to the T_{dep} calculated from the long method, with some rounding discrepancy.

T_{DEP} AND POWER

As I have stated several times, *the maximum efficiency of statistical procedures is reached when the researcher uses the appropriate statistical measure with the study data*. To see how this works in the example study earlier, conduct T_{ind} with the data and compare the results to the T_{dep} result. Table 15.5 shows the comparison. As you can see, if you had not used the appropriate formula (T_{dep}), you would not have been able to reject the null hypothesis. However, since you did use T_{dep}, you rejected the null hypothesis and concluded that the training for the tissue test procedure was effective.

CONDUCTING THE T_{DEP} ANALYSIS USING SPSS®

The T_{dep} analysis with SPSS is straightforward. The T_{dep} analysis is accessed by using the "Analyze – Compare Means – Paired-Sample T Test" menu. This will create the window shown in Figure 15.1.

As you can see in Figure 15.1, I simply used the arrow button to indicate Time1 as Variable1 and Time2 as Variable2 for the analysis. This is all that is necessary. The

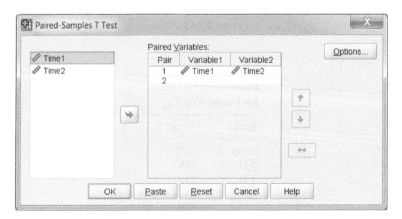

Figure 15.1   The SPSS® T_{dep} specification window.

Paired Samples Statistics

		Mean	N	Std. Deviation	Std. Error Mean
Pair 1	Time1	40.51	45	16.714	2.492
	Time2	36.76	45	16.585	2.472

Figure 15.2 The SPSS® descriptive output for T_{dep}.

default formulas and specifications will produce the analyses needed. When I choose "OK," SPSS produces a series of output tables that I will use to complete the T_{dep} analysis. I show these output tables in Figures 15.2–15.4.

Figure 15.2 shows the descriptive findings from the data. As you can see the s_m values (2.492 and 2.472) are produced and can be used with the long formula to check manual calculations.

Figure 15.3 shows the correlation analysis between Time1 and Time2 which is necessary for the long formula calculation. In any case, it is important to note even if you choose to calculate the T_{dep} manually with the difference method.

Figure 15.4 shows the T_{dep} test findings. You can compare these to the manual calculations earlier. Note that the s_{D_r} value (0.888 in the manual calculations) is shown as "Std. Error Mean." The T_{dep} value (4.233) is shown with the calculated significance ($p = 0.000$). The mean shown in the first column of data is the "difference in means" ($40.51 - 36.76 = 3.75$) from Time1 and Time2 that is used in the numerator of the T_{dep} formula. The "95% confidence interval of the difference" values (1.968–5.543) indicates the confidence brackets that will contain the true population difference (i.e., Time1–Time2 difference) 95% of the time. Note that df = 44, indicating "pairs – 1."

Paired Samples Correlations

		N	Correlation	Sig.
Pair 1	Time1 & Time2	45	.936	.000

Figure 15.3 The SPSS® correlation output for T_{dep}.

Paired Samples Test

		Paired Differences							
					95% Confidence Interval of the Difference				
				Std. Error					
		Mean	Std. Deviation	Mean	Lower	Upper	t	df	Sig. (2-tailed)
Pair 1	Time1 - Time2	3.756	5.951	.887	1.968	5.543	4.233	44	.000

Figure 15.4 The SPSS® T_{dep} test summary.

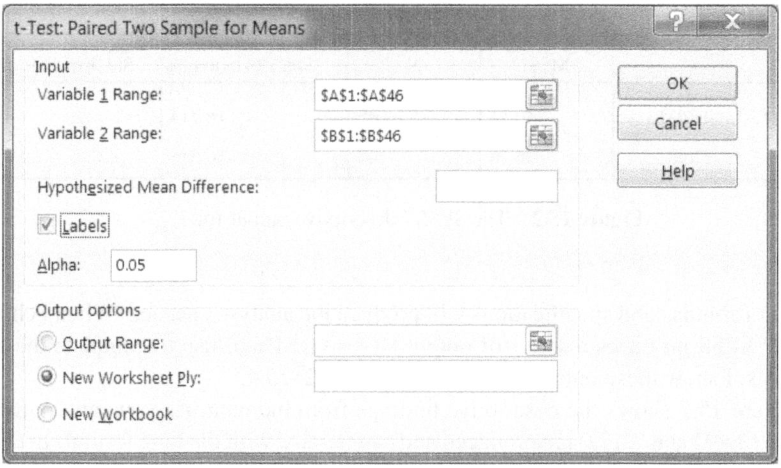

Figure 15.5   The Excel T_{dep} specification window.

CONDUCTING THE T_{DEP} ANALYSIS USING EXCEL

The Excel procedure is created through the Data – Data Analysis – "t-Test: Paired Two Sample for Means" menu. When you make this choice, the screen in Figure 15.5 appears. As you can see, I specified the location of the data in the two "Variable Range" windows, and I indicated that the data included the variable label by checking the "Labels" box.

When you make this selection, Excel returns the findings shown in Figure 15.6. As you can see, the T_{dep} value of 4.23 is shown (shaded cell), and the correlation (0.94) is shown. The values below the T_{dep} figure show the results of the hypothesis test(s) with their respective exclusion values. For example, the cell that includes "$P(T <= t)$ one tail" indicates that T_{dep} is significant at "0.00" (i.e., beyond $p < 0.05$) for the one-tailed T test which sets the exclusion value at 1.68. The last two cells confirm the significance level ("0.00" or beyond $p < 0.05$) with a two-tailed test in which exclusion value $= 2.02$.

WITHIN-SUBJECT ANOVA (ANOVA$_{WS}$)

I now consider another extension of ANOVA. This time, I will discuss within-subject ANOVA that focuses on repeated measures applied to the subjects of one group. The one-way ANOVA (Chapter 9) and the factorial ANOVA (Chapter 10) treatments of ANOVA focused on "between-subject" applications. That is, do sample groups differ on some outcome measure? As you recall, I explored the differences in health resulting from different sleep conditions (one-way ANOVA) and then extended this to include the differences between males and females (factorial ANOVA) by including the second factor (sex).

t-Test: Paired Two Sample for Means

	Time1	Time2
Mean	40.51	36.76
Variance	279.35	275.05
Observations	45.00	45.00
Pearson Correlation	0.94	
Hypothesized Mean Difference	0.00	
df	44.00	
t Stat	4.23	
P(T<=t) one-tail	0.00	
t Critical one-tail	1.68	
P(T<=t) two-tail	0.00	
t Critical two-tail	2.02	

Figure 15.6 The T_{dep} findings from Excel paired two sample test.

TABLE 15.6   The Experimental Design

Pre Test Scores	Experimental Group Treatment	Post Test Scores
Pre Test Scores	Comparison Group(s)	Post Test Scores

EXPERIMENTAL DESIGNS

Table 15.6 shows the "classic" experimental design in which two groups (randomly selected in the "true" experiment and not in the "quasi-experiment") are compared on posttest scores after some intervention. The experimental group receives an intervention, and the control or comparison group does not receive the intervention. *If the posttest scores differ between the groups, the implication is that the treatment is responsible.*

An example might be the factorial ANOVA (Chapter 10) in which I analyzed sleep conditions (factor 1) and sex (factor 2) as influences on health. To do this, I assumed that the experiment included randomization of subjects so that I did not have to include the pretests. The assumption is that if subjects are randomly chosen, the groups' pretest measures will be equal and therefore will not need to be included in the analyses. I simply compared the posttest (learning) scores for men and women in the different noise conditions.

There is also value in knowing how the individual subjects of each group change across the time of the experiment. If the experimental treatment is effective, it should "cause" changes in individuals' posttest scores compared to their pretest scores.

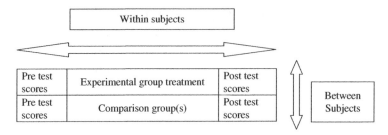

Figure 15.7   The mixed design that includes within-subject and between-group elements.

TABLE 15.7   Data for Within-Subject Study with Three Categories

	Time1	Time2	Time3
Subject 1	11	6	3
Subject 2	4	2	3
Subject 3	11	11	4
.			
	Mean Time1	Mean Time2	Mean Time3

It is often difficult to achieve full randomization, so you cannot assume the pretest measures of different treatment groups (experimental and comparison groups) will be equal. Therefore, you need to take into account the differences that happen from pretest to posttest <u>within</u> both (all) treatment groups. *The experimental design that does not include full randomization therefore may include both within-subject and between-subject measures.* This is known as a "mixed design." Figure 15.7 shows how this works.

In this chapter, I discuss the within-subject element of this design because it is often the case that research simply focuses on how one group of subjects change over time. To extend the example from the T_{dep} section earlier, this might mean conducting tissue test times *assessments three times for each subject* in the experiment. Table 15.7 shows how this design looks.

Since I now have three measures for each lab technician, I extend the T_{dep} test to a <u>within-subject ANOVA</u>. This procedure will detect differences for each lab technician among the three tissue test assessments. Since the three assessments are based on the same technicians, you must use a statistical procedure that factors out the <u>sameness</u> so that you can see what the resulting differences are among the three assessments. Will the training session result in declining times for the tissue test procedures across the three assessments?

POST FACTO DESIGNS

Within-subject procedures can be used with post facto designs as well since you are not necessarily assuming experimental manipulation. You might simply be interested

TABLE 15.8   The Within-Subject Example Data

Time1	Time2	Time3	Time1	Time2	Time3
11	6	3	41	35	40
4	2	3	62	47	40
11	11	4	29	29	40
18	9	6	55	50	40
30	23	7	46	49	41
7	12	8	39	38	41
12	10	9	41	40	41
42	42	9	45	46	44
32	20	12	49	58	47
17	5	18	41	35	48
24	24	20	54	56	49
46	37	21	50	53	49
26	28	22	52	58	51
28	31	27	50	49	52
44	39	30	56	57	52
44	30	32	62	60	56
38	38	33	57	39	57
45	39	34	54	48	62
35	34	36	79	70	62
45	36	36	64	62	62
39	31	37	47	41	63
40	37	38	64	50	75
48	40	40			

in whether a group of students' AP course assessments are consistent across a certain time period (e.g., semester) or if they are erratic for some reason. The key issue is how the same students (or matched group of students) compare to themselves across different data collection periods or conditions.

WITHIN-SUBJECT EXAMPLE

Table 15.8 shows the data I will use for this example. As you can see, it is the same data I used for the T_{dep} example with an additional assessment period for each lab technician (Time3). For the purposes of this example, I will consider the time periods as 1-month intervals with the training session taking place immediately after the Time1 assessment. Will the training approach produce consistent results (lower tissue test times) over the time periods?

USING SPSS® FOR WITHIN-SUBJECT DATA

For this example, I will not present the manual calculations but focus on the use of the statistical program to produce the findings. Excel does not have a straightforward method for calculating the one-way $ANOVA_{ws}$. I will therefore focus on the SPSS program which has detailed procedures for this design. I will discuss the procedure using the data in Table 15.8.

The output for $ANOVA_{ws}$ is quite complex. Therefore, I present only the basic output to show how to interpret the primary findings.

Sphericity

One of the assumptions of ANOVA$_{ws}$ is that the variances among the subjects' (in this case) three time periods be approximately equal. That is, the variance between Time1 and Time2 should be equal, the variance between Time2 and Time3 should be equal, and the variance between Time1 and Time3 should be equal. This is like the assumption I discussed for one-way ANOVA that was assessed by the Levene's test. With the ANOVA$_{ws}$ you assess the variances to make sure they are equivalent by the "Mauchly's test of sphericity" and then proceed with the analyses depending on whether you have met or violated the assumptions.

THE SPSS® PROCEDURE

You create the specification for the ANOVA$_{ws}$ through the "Analyze – General Linear Model – Repeated Measures" menu. This creates the window shown in Figure 15.8. As you can see, I specified at the top that the within-subject factor I will use is Time and that it has three measurements (specified in the "Number of Levels" window).

When I select "Define" the window shown in Figure 15.9 will appear. This summarizes my specification in the "Within-Subjects Variables" window. As you can see, there are several choices I can make to further specify the model on the right side of this window.

Choosing the "Contrasts" button allows the user to specify that the comparison of conditions is based on repeated measures. Figure 15.10 shows this "Repeated Measures: Contrasts" window. As you can see, I clicked on "Time" and then chose the

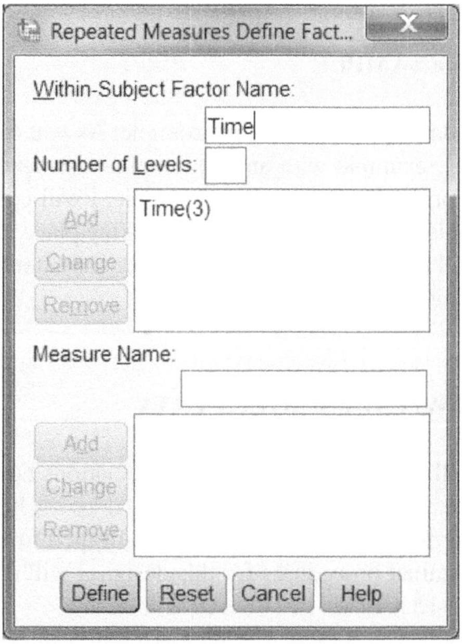

Figure 15.8 The SPSS® specification window for the ANOVA$_{ws}$ procedure.

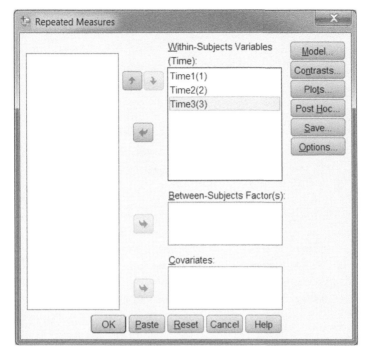

Figure 15.9 The SPSS® "Repeated Measures" window.

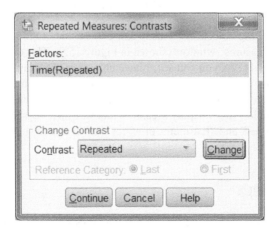

Figure 15.10 The "Contrasts" window for specifying repeated contrasts.

"Change Contrast" button which allowed me to choose "Repeated" and then click-ing "Change" to make sure the change registered in the window. This is shown in Figure 15.10 where the "Factors" window shows "Time(Repeated)."

Returning to the main "Repeated Measures" window shown in Figure 15.9, you can choose the "Plots" button to specify Time on the "Horizontal Axis." I will show this result in the following.

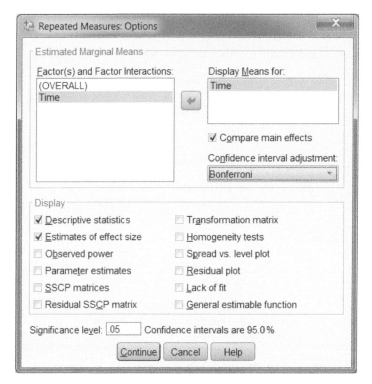

Figure 15.11   The "Options" menu for the ANOVA$_{ws}$ procedure.

When I make these selections, I next can choose the "Options" button in the main "Repeated Measures" window (shown in Figure 15.9). This creates the window shown in Figure 15.11. As you can see, I have chosen to "Display Means for" Time by moving it to the right side window. I also checked the "Compare main effects" box and specified the "Bonferroni" adjustment from the "Confidence interval adjust-ment" button just below the "Display Means" window. Under "Display" I checked the "Descriptive statistics" and "Estimates of effect size" boxes to show the appropriate results in the output.

THE SPSS® OUTPUT

In this book, I will provide only a basic look at the SPSS ANOVA$_{ws}$ analyses and how to create general interpretations. As the research design increases in complexity, how-ever, so does the design specification and output. You will need to consult additional sources if you choose to elaborate on the one-way ANOVA$_{ws}$ design shown here.

Figure 15.12 shows the descriptive table that includes the means of the three time conditions for the 45 subjects. You can see that the SD measures are generally equal, but the SD measure for Time3 is slightly larger. When you test the equivalence in variances (through the Mauchly's test of sphericity), you will assess whether this difference will be problematic.

Descriptive Statistics

	Mean	Std. Deviation	N
Time1	40.51	16.714	45
Time2	36.76	16.585	45
Time3	35.49	18.817	45

Figure 15.12   The "Descriptive Statistics" output.

Mauchly's Test of Sphericity[a]

Measure: MEASURE_1

Within Subjects Effect	Mauchly's W	Approx. Chi-Square	df	Sig.	Epsilon[b]		
					Greenhouse-Geisser	Huynh-Feldt	Lower-bound
Time	.694	15.697	2	.000	.766	.788	.500

Tests the null hypothesis that the error covariance matrix of the orthonormalized transformed dependent variables is proportional to an identity matrix.

a. Design: Intercept
Within Subjects Design: Time

b. May be used to adjust the degrees of freedom for the averaged tests of significance. Corrected tests are displayed in the Tests of Within-Subjects Effects table.

Figure 15.13   The Mauchly's test of sphericity results.

The output for Mauchly's test of sphericity is shown in Figure 15.13. The critical value to look for is the "Sig." value shown in the middle of the table. In this case, the results show that there are significant differences among the variance measures of the three time conditions. Thus, there is a violation of the sphericity condition. These can be very sensitive tests, so I will take note of the violation in the analysis of the remaining output.

The Omnibus Test

Figure 15.14 shows the output for the within-subject effects of time. The first "group" of findings under time shows four different rows of output. The first "Sphericity Assumed" is like the one-way ANOVA F test in which there are equal variances. As you can see, this test is significant ($F = 7.830$, $p < 0.01$). If there are no sphericity violations, you would use this value to make the conclusions.

However, since there is a violation of sphericity, you would need to use an "adjusted" F test value. As you can see from Figure 15.14, SPSS provides three such adjusted tests. The "Greenhouse–Geisser" test is shown in the second row and is a commonly used conservative test. As you can see, this F value is the same, but the significance level is slightly different due to the adjustment for sphericity. The result is the same however. Time is a significant repeated measure condition ($F = 7.830$, $p = 0.002$).

Tests of Within-Subjects Effects

Measure: MEASURE_1

Source		Type III Sum of Squares	df	Mean Square	F	Sig.	Partial Eta Squared
Time	Sphericity Assumed	613.970	2	306.985	7.830	.001	.151
	Greenhouse-Geisser	613.970	1.532	400.870	7.830	.002	.151
	Huynh-Feldt	613.970	1.576	389.624	7.830	.002	.151
	Lower-bound	613.970	1.000	613.970	7.830	.008	.151
Error(Time)	Sphericity Assumed	3450.030	88	39.205			
	Greenhouse-Geisser	3450.030	67.390	51.195			
	Huynh-Feldt	3450.030	69.335	49.759			
	Lower-bound	3450.030	44.000	78.410			

Figure 15.14   The within-subject effects output for Time.

Multivariate Tests

	Value	F	Hypothesis df	Error df	Sig.	Partial Eta Squared
Pillai's trace	.359	12.020[a]	2.000	43.000	.000	.359
Wilks' lambda	.641	12.020[a]	2.000	43.000	.000	.359
Hotelling's trace	.559	12.020[a]	2.000	43.000	.000	.359
Roy's largest root	.559	12.020[a]	2.000	43.000	.000	.359

Each F tests the multivariate effect of Time. These tests are based on the linearly independent pairwise comparisons among the estimated marginal means.

a. Exact statistic

Figure 15.15   The effect size output for ANOVA$_{WS}$.

Effect Size

Figure 15.15 shows the multivariate test results. These reveal the *effect size* findings for this study and are not impacted by sphericity. I have not discussed these so far, but many researchers use "Wilks' lambda" as the effect size measure for ANOVA$_{WS}$ in this situation. Wilks' lambda (Λ) is based on measuring unexplained variance, so the smaller the value, the stronger the effect.

As you can see from Figure 15.15, $\Lambda = 0.641$ and is significant ($p < 0.0001$). You will also notice that in this test, Λ is complimentary to partial eta squared which is not based on error but on the size of the regression (i.e., partial $\eta^2 = 1 - \Lambda$). As you can see, partial $\eta^2 = 0.359$ and Wilks' lambda $= 0.641$, suggesting that the impact of the training on tissue test results across time conditions is considered large (using the criteria I suggested in Chapter 10).

Post Hoc Analyses

Just as I showed with the ANOVA tests in Chapter 9, you must perform post hoc analyses when the omnibus test is significant. Figure 15.16 shows the pairwise comparisons output that indicates which time conditions differ. As you can see, all the comparisons are significantly different except the difference between Time2 and Time3.

Pairwise Comparisons

Measure: MEASURE_1

(I) Time	(J) Time	Mean Difference (I-J)	Std. Error	Sig.b	95% Confidence Interval for Differenceb	
					Lower Bound	Upper Bound
1	2	3.756*	.887	.000	1.968	5.543
	3	5.022*	1.453	.001	2.094	7.951
2	1	−3.756*	.887	.000	-5.543	-1.968
	3	1.267	1.526	.411	-1.809	4.342
3	1	−5.022*	1.453	.001	-7.951	-2.094
	2	−1.267	1.526	.411	-4.342	1.809

Based on estimated marginal means

*. The mean difference is significant at the .05 level.

b. Adjustment for multiple comparisons: Least Significant Difference (equivalent to no adjustments).

Figure 15.16 The post hoc output for the study.

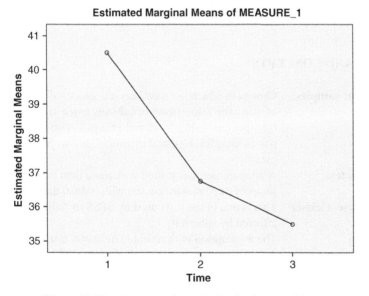

Figure 15.17 The comparison plot for the time conditions.

You can see that the differences among the means of the time conditions are large except for Time2–Time3 (1.267). The plot in Figure 15.17 provides visual comparisons in the plotting of the means. As you can see, there are large differences (less time for tissue tests) between Time1 and Time2, and between Time1 and Time3, but the difference between Time2 and Time3 is smaller and not significant.

The Interpretation

Taking all the output into account, it appears that training lab technicians does lower their time for tissue tests across the time conditions in this hypothetical study. Each time period indicates less time for the tests, especially after the training. The primary differences are between the initial assessment (Time1) and both of the subsequent assessments (Time2 and Time3). The effects are not different between the latter two assessments (Time2–Time3).

NONPARAMETRIC STATISTICS

In past chapters, I presented the nonparametric counterparts of some parametric tests. Thus, for the independent sample T test, I discussed the Mann–Whitney U test, and I presented a section on the Kruskal–Wallis test when I discussed the one-way ANOVA procedure.

Both of the repeated measures tests in the current chapter have nonparametric counterparts as well. With *two* related (dependent) samples of ordinal data, the researcher would use the Wilcoxon test. If there are *more than two* dependent samples of less than interval data, the researcher would use the Friedman test. Both of these are available in SPSS and can be accessed with the same "analyze" menu I demonstrated with the Mann–Whitney U and Kruskal–Wallis tests.

TERMS AND CONCEPTS

Dependent samples:	Groups in which the members are structurally related, such as using the same group of subjects twice in an experiment (pre–post) or using "matched groups." Also known as paired samples, repeated measures, and within-subject measures.
Friedman test:	A nonparametric test used with more than two dependent samples (repeated measures) with ordinal data.
Greenhouse–Geisser test:	This is one of the tests used by SPSS to "adjust" values affected by sphericity.
Sphericity:	The assumption with repeated measures tests (like ANOVA$_{WS}$) that the variance of group differences is equal.
Wilcoxon test:	A nonparametric test used with two dependent samples (repeated measures) with ordinal data.
Wilks' lambda:	An effect size measure based on the amount of unexplained variance. Small results are considered stronger than large results.

APPENDIX A

SPSS® BASICS[1]

This book explores statistical procedures using SPSS®. Appendix A includes descriptions of the important procedures and basic functions of SPSS. I introduce the specific data management and analysis menus of SPSS in each of the chapters of the book that discuss the different statistical procedures for data analysis.

In order to help you make use of SPSS, I will use the data I introduced in Table 2.7, combined with a second variable "Respondent Sex." Table A.1[2] shows these two sets of data, which represent a random sample of the BRFSS database on the GENHLTH question "Would you say that in general your health is … " and the question regarding Respondent Sex. The sample of 50 cases is listed in Table A.1 in two columns for space consideration.

USING SPSS®

In a book such as this, it is important to understand the nature and uses of a statistical program like SPSS. There are several statistical software packages available for management and analysis of data; however, in my experience SPSS is a versatile and responsive program. Because it is designed for a great many statistical procedures, we cannot hope to cover the full range of tools within SPSS in our treatment. I will

---

[1]Some material in this Appendix is adapted from Abbott (2011), *Understanding Educational Statistics Using Microsoft Excel and SPSS®*.
[2]Centers for Disease Control and Prevention (CDC). *Behavioral Risk Factor Surveillance System Survey Data*. Atlanta, Georgia: U.S. Department of Health and Human Services, Centers for Disease Control and Prevention, 2013.

Using Statistics in the Social and Health Sciences with SPSS® and Excel®, First Edition.
Martin Lee Abbott.
© 2017 John Wiley & Sons, Inc. Published 2017 by John Wiley & Sons, Inc.

TABLE A.1   BRFSS Responses to the General Health and Respondent Sex Questions

GENHLTH	SEX	GENHLTH	SEX
4	2	1	2
1	1	3	2
2	1	1	1
3	1	2	2
2	1	3	1
2	1	2	1
2	2	3	1
1	1	1	2
3	1	3	1
2	1	1	2
2	1	4	1
3	2	1	1
2	2	2	2
2	2	4	2
2	1	3	2
1	1	3	2
5	2	5	2
2	1	5	1
4	1	4	2
1	2	3	2
4	2	2	1
2	2	5	1
3	1	3	2
2	2	3	1
1	2	2	2

cover, in as much depth as possible, the general procedures of SPSS, especially those that provide analyses for the statistical procedures we discuss in this book. The wide range of SPSS products is available for purchase online (http://www.SPSS®.com/).

The calculations and examples in this book require a basic familiarity with SPSS. Generations of social science students and evaluators have used this statistical software, making it somewhat a standard in the field of statistical analyses. In the following sections, I will make use of SPSS output with actual data in order to explore the power of statistics for discovery. I will illustrate the SPSS menus so it is easier for you to negotiate the program. The best preparation for the procedures we discuss, and for research in general, is to become acquainted with the SPSS data managing functions and menus. Once you have a familiarity with these processes, you can use the analysis menus to help you with more complex methods.

GENERAL FEATURES

Generally, SPSS is a large spreadsheet that allows the evaluator to enter, manipulate, and analyze data of various types through a series of drop-down menus. The screen

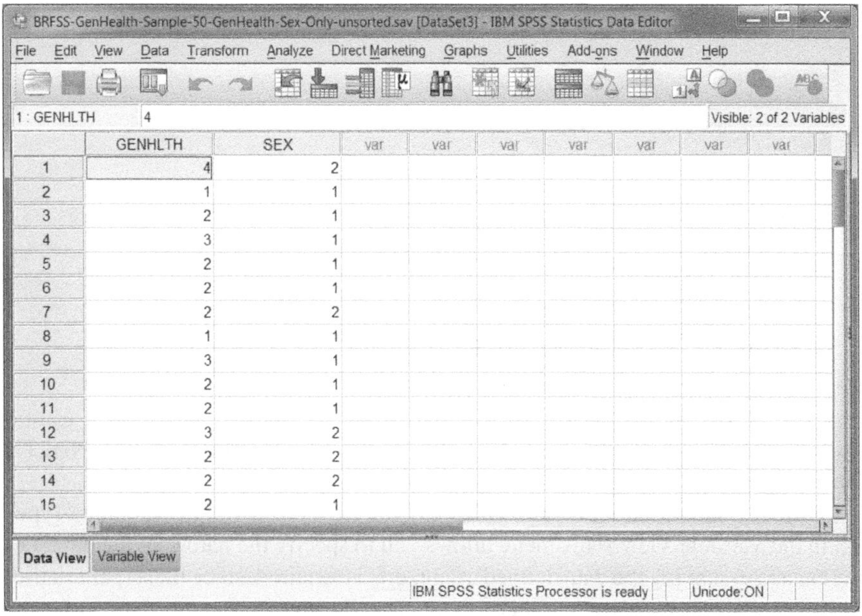

Figure A.1   SPSS® screen showing the data page and drop-down menus.

in Figure A.1 shows the opening page where data can be entered.[3] This screen shows the data from Table A.1 as it appears when entered into the data spreadsheet. (Please note that only the first 15 cases are shown in the interests of space.) The tab on the bottom left of the screen identifies this as the "Data View" so you can see the data as they are entered.

A second view of the data is available when first opening the program as indicated by the "Variable View" tab also located in the bottom left of the screen. As shown in Figure A.2, the Variable View (which you can see by the highlighted tab at the bottom left corner of the initial screen) allows you to see how variables are managed: their name, the width of the column, the number of decimals, any variable labels you wish to add, any values assigned to data (e.g., for the SEX variable, this column may indicate that "Male" is given a value of "1," etc.), missing number identifiers, and so on.

The information in these cells can be edited by the use of the drop-down menus in each cell (click on the right side of the cells). One of the important features on this page is the "Type" column, which allows the user to specify whether the variable is "numeric" (i.e., a number), "String" (e.g., a letter), or some other form (a date, currency, etc.). The "Measure" column near the far right side of the screen indicates with different symbols whether the variable is "scale, ordinal, or nominal." Chapter 2 discusses the different scales of measurement, so you should refer to that discussion to clarify how to select the measurement level with which you plan to treat your data. As shown, both GENHLTH and SEX are numerical but treated initially as "nominal."

[3]SPSS® Version 22.

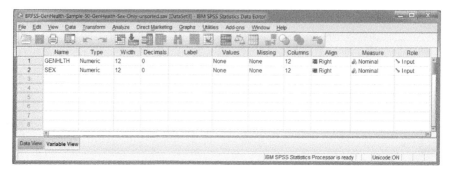

Figure A.2 SPSS® screen showing the variable view and variable attributes.

This designation is appropriate for SEX, but may not be appropriate for GENHLTH depending on how the researcher wishes to treat the data.

Figure A.3 shows the submenu available if you click on the right side of the "Type" cell in the Variable View. This menu allows you to specify the nature of the data. For most analyses, having the data defined as numeric is required, since most (parametric) statistical analyses require a number format. The "String" designation, shown below at the bottom of the choices, allows you to enter data as letters and words, such as quotes from research subjects, names of subject groups, etc. If you use a statistical procedure that requires numbers, make sure the variable is entered as a "numeric" variable or you will receive an error message and your requested procedure will not be executed.

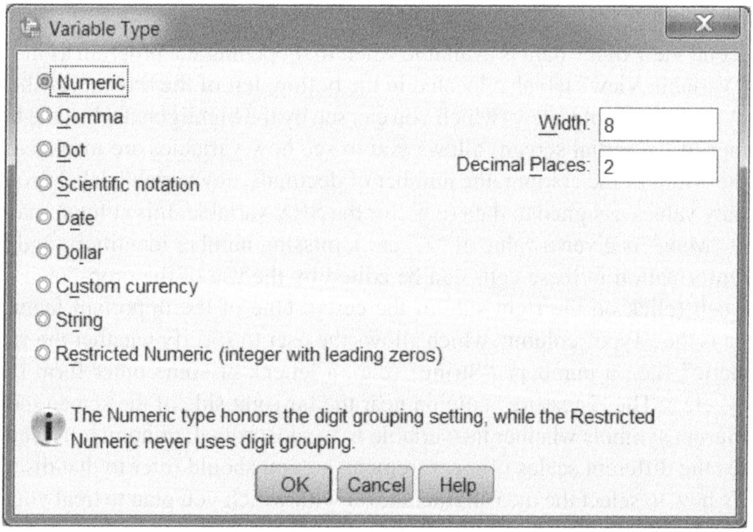

Figure A.3 SPSS® screen showing the submenu for specifying the type of variable used in the data field.

MANAGEMENT FUNCTIONS

In this appendix, I cover the essential functions that will allow you to get started right away with numerical analyses. Before a statistical procedure is created, however, it is important to understand how to manage the data file.

Reading and Importing Data

Data can be entered directly into the "spreadsheet" or it can be read by the SPSS program from different file formats. The most common format for data to be imported to SPSS is through such data programs as Microsoft Excel or simply an ASCII file where data are entered and separated by tabs. Using the drop-down menu commands, "File – Open – Data" will create a screen that enables the user to specify the type of data to be imported (e.g., Excel, Text, etc.). The user will then be guided through an import wizard that will translate the data to the SPSS spreadsheet format.

Figures A.4 and A.5 show the screens that allow you to select among a number of "Files of type:" when you want to import data into SPSS. Figure A.4 shows the initial screen for this process. Choosing "File" at the left of the top menu ribbon will result in the second screen allowing you to "Open" a series of files, one of which is "Data" as shown.

Figure A.5 shows the screen resulting from choosing "Data." As you can see, the small drop-down menu (under "Files of type:" at the bottom of the "Open

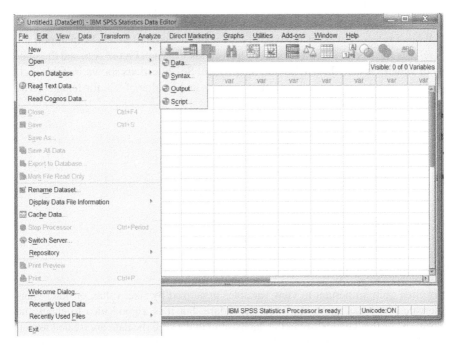

Figure A.4 The SPSS® screens showing the import data choices.

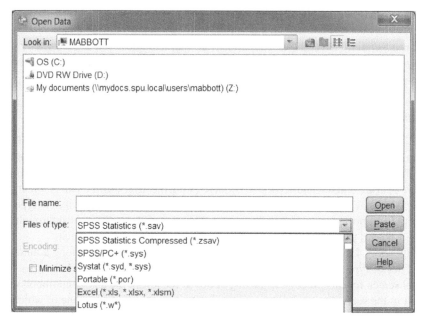

Figure A.5   The SPSS® screens showing the import data choices.

Data" screen) allows you to choose "Excel" among other types of files when you import data.

When I select "Excel" as the type of file I want to read into SPSS, I can import the Excel data file using an import wizard. The result is shown in Figure A.6, and the sample of values on the GENHLTH and Respondent Sex questions shown in Table A.1. The SEX variable uses a value of "1" for males and a value of "2" for females. The response categories for GENHLTH are as follows:

1	Excellent
2	Very good
3	Good
4	Fair
5	Poor

Sort

It is often quite important to view variables organized by size, value, or other characteristics. You can run a statistical procedure, but it is a good idea to check the "position" of the data visibly in the database to make sure the data are treated as you would expect. In order to create this organization, you can "sort" the data entries of a variable in SPSS as you did in Excel.

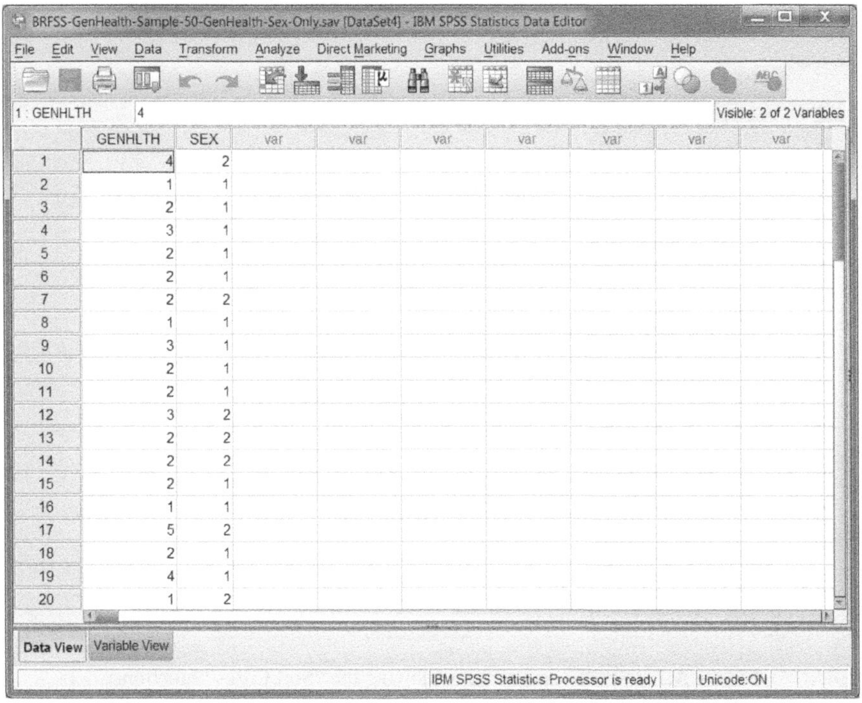

Figure A.6   The SPSS® data file from the imported Excel database.

The data in Figure A.6 are shown "unsorted" or reported directly from the overall database. This "spreadsheet" presents the data in rows (cases) and columns (variables) preparing them for different management and statistical analyses procedures.

In order to sort the data according to some value or characteristic, the researcher can use a series of data management menus to "Sort" the variables shown. In SPSS, the user selects "Data" from the main menu ribbon and then "Sort" from the submenu. This results in the screens shown in Figure A.7.

If we choose to sort the set of data by Respondent Sex, as shown in the submenu on the right side of the panel in Figure A.7, we can specify a sort that is either "Ascending" (alphabetical order beginning with "A" if the variable is a string variable or starting with the lowest value if it is a numerical value) or "Descending." Selecting "Respondent Sex – Ascending" results in the screen shown in Figure A.8. (Using the arrow in the middle of that submenu allows the variable names to shift to the "Sort by:" box.) Compare this screen with the one shown in Figure A.6. As you can see, the values of the GENHLTH variable are now arranged according to the values of Respondent Sex where each respondent has recorded their Sex and their response to the question asking about their general health.

Using this procedure, the researcher can then visually inspect the data to observe any patterns that might exist among the variables. You can also sort the other variables easily in SPSS using the same procedure. Remember that when SPSS performs the

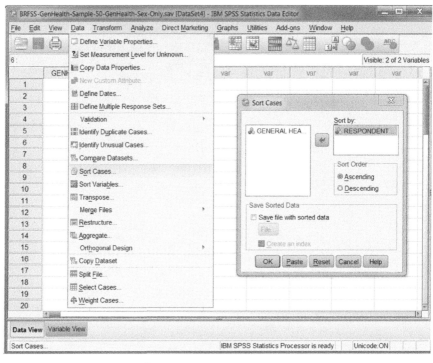

Figure A.7 SPSS® data screens showing the "Sort Cases" function.

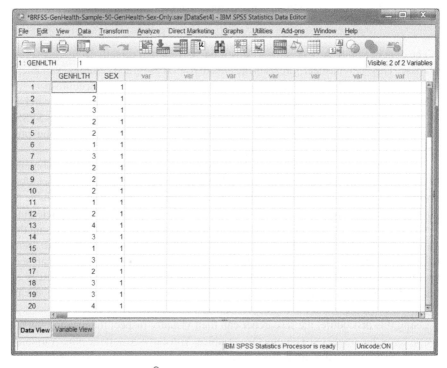

Figure A.8 The SPSS® screen showing variables sorted by Respondent Sex.

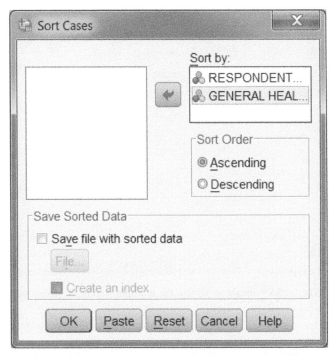

Figure A.9   The SPSS® Sort Cases window showing a sort by multiple variables.

sort procedure, it keeps the variable responses "linked" for each case. That is, in this example, the respondent's sex and their opinion about their health still represent the same respondent. If the sort did not keep the values linked, then the researcher would not know which attitude about health would represent a specific respondent.

SPSS allows multiple sorts in which the values of one variable are sorted according to the sorted value of the first variable. Figure A.9 shows this specification in SPSS in which the database is sorted first by Respondent Sex and then by GENHLTH. (Figure A.9 also indicates the nature of the variable (string or numeric) by the small symbols next to each variable.)

Figure A.10 shows the database now sorted by both variables. The first variable specified in the sort menu is sorted first, and then the additional variables in the sort are arranged by sorted values within the categories of the first variable sorted. The additional variable values are thus "nested" in the variables preceding them.

ADDITIONAL MANAGEMENT FUNCTIONS

SPSS is quite versatile at handling large data sets. There are several useful functions that perform specific operations to make the analyses and subsequent interpretation of data easier. These functions evolved with constant use by researchers since SPSS

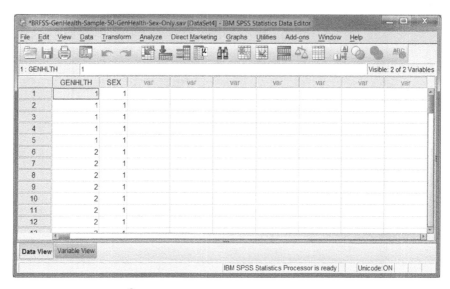

Figure A.10 The SPSS® database sorted by multiple variables (Respondent Sex and GENHLTH).

is designed specifically for many advanced statistical procedures. I will not cover all of these, but the following sections highlight some important operations.

Split File

A useful command for students and researchers that we will use in the subsequent chapters is "Split File," which allows the user to arrange output specifically for the different values of a variable. Using our "sort" example from Figure A.6, we could use the "Split File" command to create two separate files according to the Respondent Sex variable and then call for separate statistical analyses on the other variable, GENHLTH.

By choosing the "Data" drop-down menu, you can select "Split File" from a range of choices that enable you to perform operations on my existing data. Figure A.11 shows the submenu for "Data" with "Split File" near the bottom.

When you choose "Split File," you can then select which variable to use to create the separate data files. This is the "Organize output by groups" button shown in Figure A.11. As you can see, if you choose this button, you can specify "Gender" by clicking on it in the left column and moving it to the "Groups Based on:" box by clicking the arrow button.

Figure A.12 shows that I selected the option "Organize output by groups" and then clicked on the variable "Respondent Sex" in the left panel to move it to the right panel (using the arrow button in the middle). By these choices, I issued the command to create (in this case) two separate analyses for whatever statistical procedure I call for next since there are two values for the Respondent Sex variable ("1" for males and "2" for females). When you perform a split file procedure in SPSS, it does not

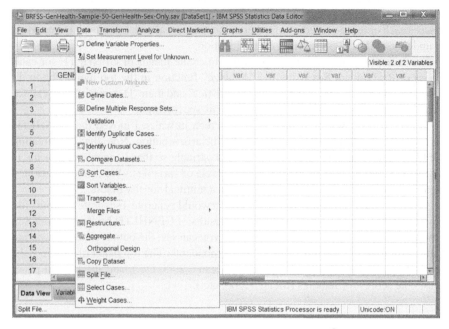

Figure A.11   The "Split File" option in SPSS®.

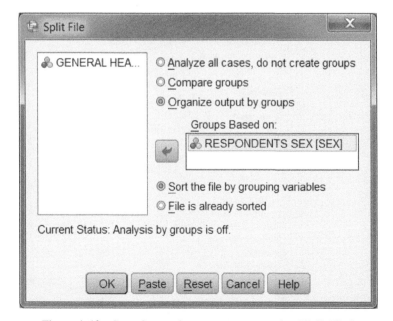

Figure A.12   Steps for creating separate output using "Split File."

change the database; rather, it creates separate output according to whatever statistical procedure you want to examine (e.g., descriptive statistics, correlation, etc.). I will discuss each of these procedures further in the chapters ahead. For now, it is important to understand that SPSS has this useful function.

For example, you could use "Split File" to create <u>means</u> of GENHLTH for categories of Respondent Sex using the "Analyze" function in the top menu ribbon. In this case, you would select "Descriptive Statistics" and then "Descriptives" to call for a calculation of means. Figure A.13 shows this specification.

Figure A.14 shows the resulting menu screen in which I moved the GENHLTH variable into the "Variables" window using the arrow button. Note that I am treating the GENHLTH variable as being an interval variable so that I can create a mean. (I discuss in Chapter 2 the difference among levels of variables.) We cannot generate a mean value for "Respondent Sex" since it is a nominal-level variable.

In this example, choosing the "OK" button would generate a separate "output" file (apart from the data file) showing separate results of GENHLTH by Respondent Sex groups. Figure A.15 shows these results. As you can see, the output contains separate listings for males ("1") and female ("2") respondents. The top panel of Figure A.15 shows the GENHLTH results for males (Mean = 2.48, etc.), and the bottom panel shows the scores for females (Mean = 2.60, etc.).

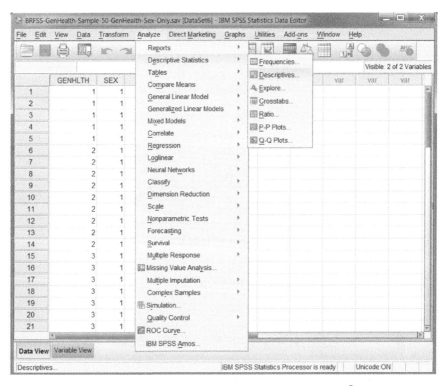

Figure A.13 Menus for creating mean values in SPSS®.

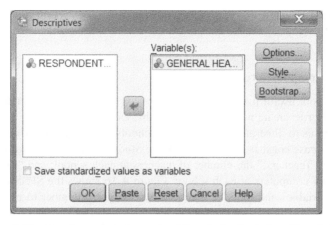

Figure A.14   Creating mean values using "Descriptive Statistics – Descriptives."

RESPONDENTS SEX = 1					
Descriptive Statistics[a]					
	N	Minimum	Maximum	Mean	Std. Deviation
GENERAL HEALTH	25	1	5	2.48	1.159
Valid N (listwise)	25				

RESPONDENTS SEX = 2					
Descriptive Statistics[b]					
	N	Minimum	Maximum	Mean	Std. Deviation
GENERAL HEALTH	25	1	5	2.60	1.225
Valid N (listwise)	25				

[a]RESPONDENTS SEX = 1.
[b]RESPONDENTS SEX = 2.

Figure A.15   Split File output ("Descriptives") for Respondent Sex and GENHLTH in SPSS®.

Please note that when you use this procedure, it is necessary to "reverse" the "Split File" procedure after you have created the desired output. Otherwise, you will continue to get "split results" with every subsequent statistical analysis you call for. SPSS will continue to provide split file analyses until you "turn it off" by selecting the first option, "Analyze all cases, do not create groups" at the top of the option list in the "Split File" submenu. You can see this option near the top of the submenu in Figure A.12.

Transform/Compute (Creating Indexes)

One of the more useful management operations is the "Compute" function, which allows the user to create new variables. For this example, I am using a very small number of cases to illustrate this procedure (schools from across the United States). The example case consists of three variables: "Students," the number of students at each school; "Teachers," the number of teachers at each school; and "Computers," the number of computers at each school. Figure A.16 shows the SPSS data screen with these variables and the "ID" variable that assigns a number to each case for identification.

If you wish to report the number of computers available per students at the schools (the ratio), you can compute a new variable using the menus in SPSS. At the main menu (see Figure A.1), you can access this function by selecting the "Transform" and then "Compute Variable" option (see Figure A.17).

When you select this option, Figure A.18 shows a dialog box in which you can create a formula. As you can see, I created a new variable name, "StudentPerComputer," since I am creating a new variable from using two existing variables. Place the name of the new variable in the top left slot, "Target Variable," and then you can create the formula by using the arrow key to move the existing variables from the "Type & Label" panel to the "Numeric Expression" field. As you can see, I simply indicated, using the symbol key, "/" to divide the number of students by the number of computers. Selecting the "OK" tab at the bottom of the screen initiates the procedure and saves the new variable.

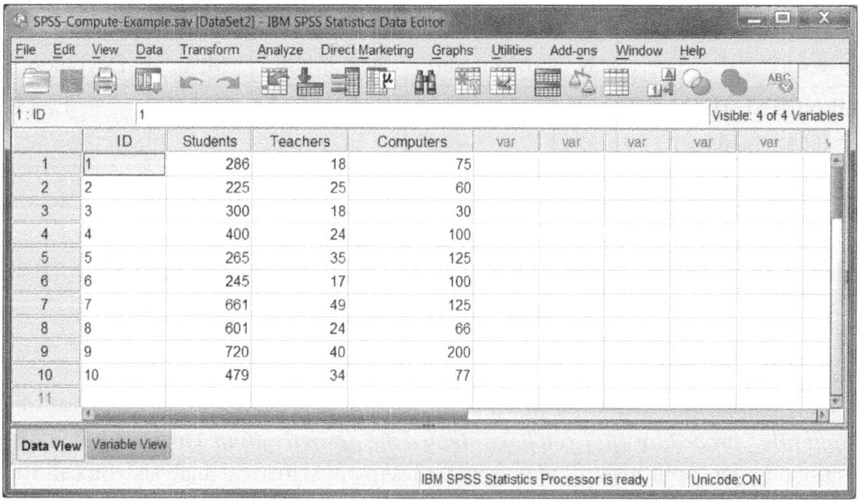

Figure A.16   SPSS® screen showing example data for "Compute" function.

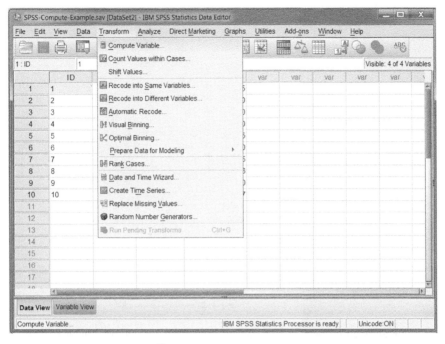

Figure A.17 SPSS® screen showing "Transform/Compute" menus.

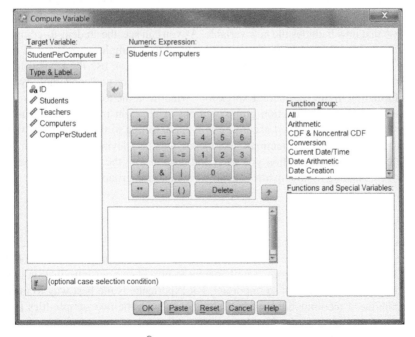

Figure A.18 SPSS® screen showing "Compute Variable" function.

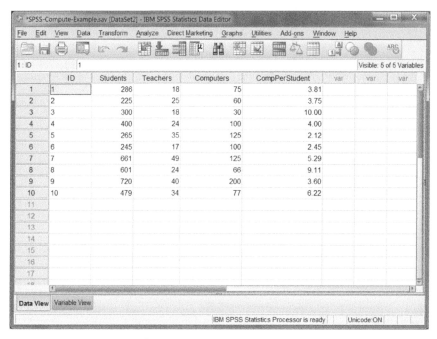

Figure A.19 SPSS® screen showing the database with the new variable.

This procedure will result in a new variable with values that represent the ratio of students to computers at the example schools. Figure A.19 shows the resulting database that now includes the new variable. As you can see, the student-to-computer ratio ranges from 2.12 to 10.00, quite a disparity at the example schools.

As you can see from the screen in Figure A.18, you can use the keypad in the center of the dialog box for entering arithmetic operators, or you can simply type in the information in the "Numeric Expression" window at the top. You will also note that there are several "Function group" options at the right in a separate window. These are operations grouped according to type. Scrolling to the bottom allows the user to specify "statistical functions" like means, standard deviations, and so on. You can select whichever operation you need and enter it into the Numeric Expression window by clicking on the up arrow next to the Function group window.

Merge

The merge function is one of the most useful but the most misunderstood functions from SPSS. I have yet to see any accurate treatment of the appropriate steps for this procedure in any resource book. I will attempt to provide a brief introduction to the procedure here because it is so important, but experience is the best way to master the technique. I recommend that you follow along with the two sample files I will discuss and then try it on the data that you generate (at first, you can make values up and use the procedures I discuss in the following text).

The merge function allows you to add information to one file from another using a common identifier on which the procedure is "keyed." In this example, I will show how to create one file that combines variables located on separate data files using a common "index" variable; in this case the index variable is "ID." Perhaps one file has a school ID number and the number of "Computers" variable we created in the last example, while a second file has a school ID (the same school IDs as the other file) and the number of "Students" and number of "Teachers" variables. The merge function allows you to combine variables by adding the variables from one of the files to the other using the common ID number.

You can approach the merge in several ways, but my preferred method is to choose one file as the "master" to which the separate information is brought. After the transfer, you can save this file separately as the master file since it will contain both sets of information. SPSS allows you to specify which information to bring to the separate file in a dialog box.

In this example, I will merge two separate files with a common school ID number ("ID"). Figures A.20 and A.21 show the separate data files. The first contains the variables "Students" and "Teachers," whereas the second file has the "Computers" variable. The object is to create a master file containing all three variables.

The first step is to make sure both "ID" variables are sorted (Ascending) and saved in the same way. (See the previous section on sorting variables.) This variable is the one on which the sort is keyed, and the merge cannot take place if the variables are sorted differently within the different files, if there are duplicate numbers, missing numbers, and so on.

Second, in the file you identify as the master file (File 1 in this example), choose "Data – Merge Files" and then "Add Variables" as shown in the dialog box in Figure A.22. This will allow you to move entire variables from another file into this one. The other option "Add Cases" allows you to append all the cases in one file to the cases in the other file, a completely different function.

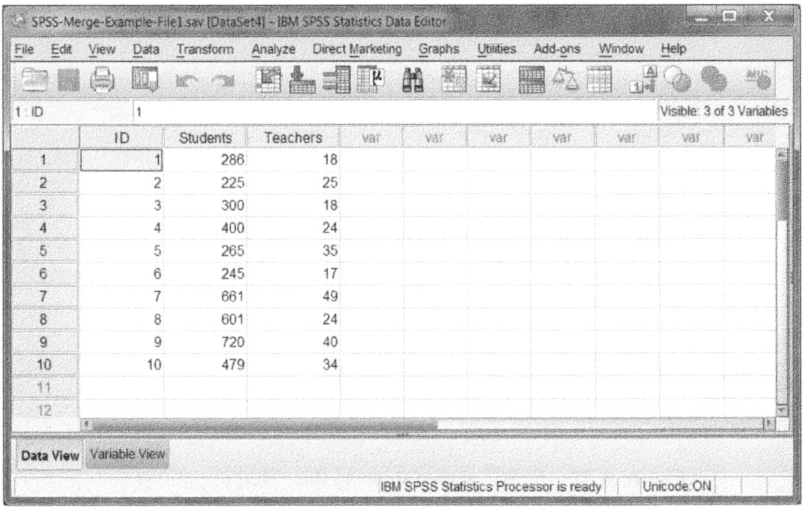

Figure A.20 Data File 1 for merge example.

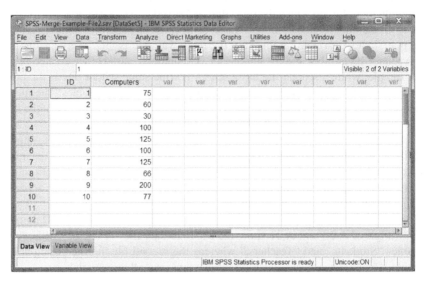

Figure A.21   Data File 2 for merge example.

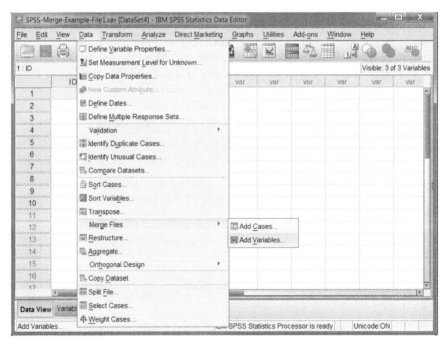

Figure A.22   SPSS® screen showing the "Merge" options.

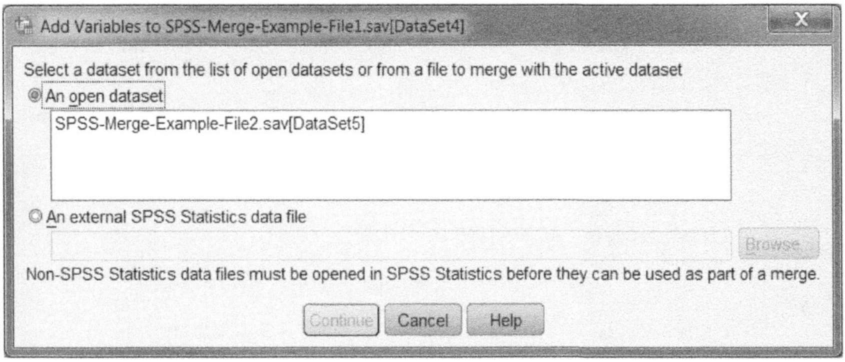

Figure A.23 SPSS® screen listing the available data files to merge.

When you ask to "add variables," the dialog box shown in Figure A.23 appears, which enables you to choose the data file from which you wish to move the desired variable into the master file. As shown in Figure A.23, click on the file shown ("SPSS-Merge-Example-File2") to identify the second database from which we will extract variables to add to the master. In this example, Data File 2 includes the "Computers" variable as shown in Figure A.21.

The next dialog box that appears is shown in Figure A.24, in which you can specify which variable is the "key variable" on which to base the merge. In the current

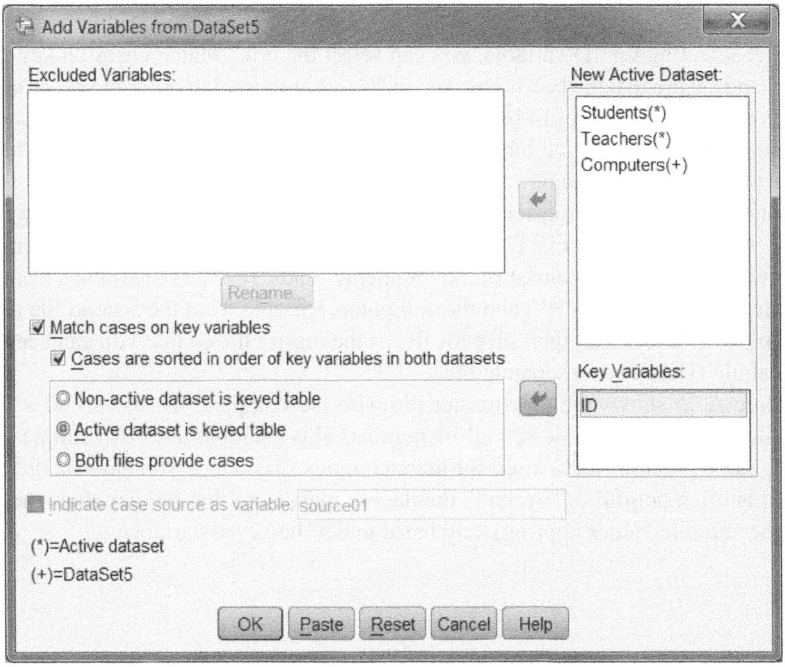

Figure A.24 SPSS® screen used to identify the "key variable" for the merge.

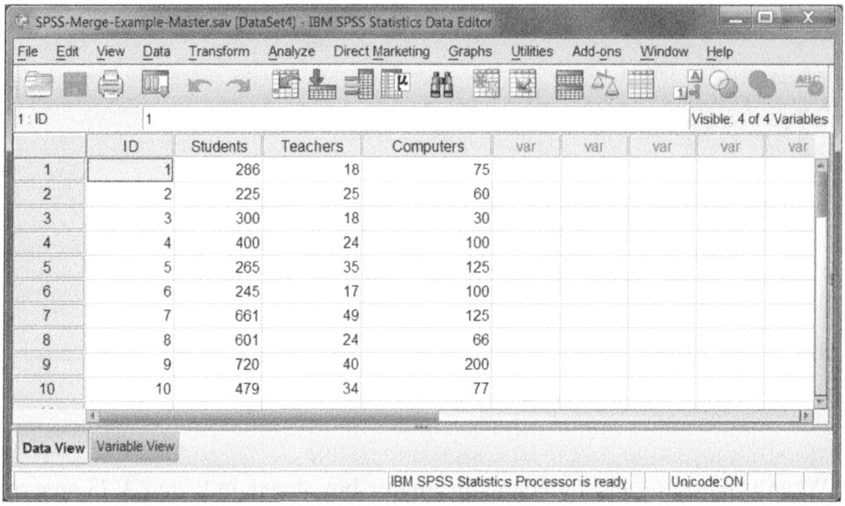

Figure A.25 SPSS® screen showing the merged ("master") file.

example, I have used the first file containing "ID," "Students," and "Teachers" as the master file and called for a merge <u>from</u> the second file containing "ID" and "Computers." The "ID" variable can be chosen from the top dialog box ("Excluded Variables") and moved to the "Key Variables" box on the lower right panel using the arrow key. It is the only variable listed in the "Excluded Variables" box because it is found in both files.

After selecting the ID variable, you can select the box "Match cases on key variables" and ensure that the box is checked in "Cases are sorted in order of key variables in both datasets." The box just below allows you to identify the "master file" by choosing "Active dataset is keyed table." This tells SPSS that you want the second file to be the one from which the new variable is to be chosen and placed in the master file. You can see that the new master file will consist of the variables listed in the top right dialog window ("New Active Dataset") when the merge is complete. In this example, the new master file will consist of the "Students" and "Teachers" variables from the first file (indicated by an "*") and the computers variable from the second file (indicated by a "+"). You can then save the file as the master file so that you can keep the original file (Data 1) as a separate file.

Figure A.25 shows the new master file with the complete list of variables from both files keyed to the same school ID number. This example used two simple files, but the same process can be used for more complex files. Once you have merged the files, it is often helpful to "eyeball" the data to make sure that the variables merged with the variable values appropriately listed under the keyed variable.

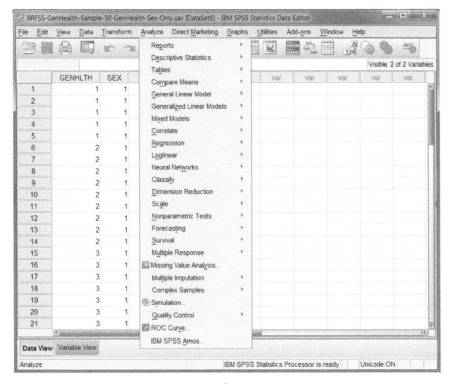

Figure A.26 The SPSS® "Analyze" menu options.

Analysis Functions

Over the course of this book, you will have extensive practice at conducting statistical procedures with SPSS. All of these are accessible through the opening "Analyze" drop-down menu as shown in Figure A.13. The screen in Figure A.26 shows the contents of the "Analyze" menu. We will not be able to cover all of these in this book, but you will have the opportunity to explore several of the submenu choices.

APPENDIX B

EXCEL BASICS[1]

Microsoft Excel® is a powerful application for education researchers and students studying educational statistics. Excel worksheets can hold data for a variety of uses and therefore serve as a database. We will focus primarily on its use as a spreadsheet, however. This book discusses how students of statistics can use Excel menus to create specific data management and statistical analysis functions.

I will use Microsoft Office Excel 2013 for all examples and illustrations in this book.[2] Like other software, Excel changes occasionally to improve performance and adapt to new standards. As I write, other versions are projected; however, most all of my examples use the common features of the application that are not likely to undergo radical changes in the near future.

I cannot hope to acquaint the reader with all the features of Excel in this book. My focus is therefore confined to the statistical analysis and related functions called into play when using the data analysis features. I will introduce some of the general features in this appendix and cover the statistical applications in more depth in the procedure chapters.

DATA MANAGEMENT

The opening spreadsheet presents the reader with a range of menu choices for entering and managing data. Like other spreadsheets, Excel consists of rows and columns for

[1]Some material in this appendix is adapted from Abbott (2011), *Understanding Educational Statistics Using Microsoft Excel and SPSS*®.
[2]Used with permission from Microsoft.

Using Statistics in the Social and Health Sciences with SPSS® and Excel®, First Edition.
Martin Lee Abbott.
© 2017 John Wiley & Sons, Inc. Published 2017 by John Wiley & Sons, Inc.

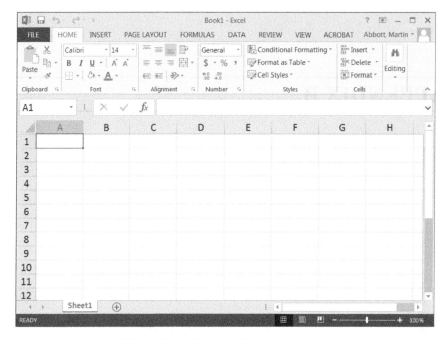

Figure B.1   The initial Excel spreadsheet.

entering and storing data of various kinds. Typically, rows represent cases in statistical analyses, and columns represent variables. According to the Microsoft Office website, the spreadsheet can contain over 1,000,000 rows and over 16,000 columns. We will not approach either of these limits; however, you should be aware of the capacity in the event you are downloading a large database from which you wish to select a portion of data. One practical feature to remember is that researchers typically use the first row of data to record variable names in each of the columns of data. Therefore, the total data set contains (rows − 1) cases, which takes this into account.

Figure B.1 shows the spreadsheet with its menus and navigation bars. I will cover much of the available spreadsheet capacity over the course of discussing our statistical topics throughout the book. Here are some basic features.

Data Sheets

Figure B.1 shows a "Sheet" tab on the bottom of the spreadsheet. This is a tab naming this spreadsheet. You may add sheets to this Excel file by selecting the "plus" button and work on them individually or linked. Many separate worksheets can be contained in the overall workbook file. Although the sheets can be used independently to store data, the statistical user typically places a data set on one sheet and then uses additional sheets for related analyses. For example, as we will discuss in later chapters, each statistical procedure will generate a separate "output" sheet. Thus, the original sheet of data will not be modified or changed (unless it is specifically linked). The user can locate the separate statistical findings in separate sheets. Each Sheet tab can be named by "right-clicking" on the sheet.

THE EXCEL MENUS

The main Excel menus are located in a ribbon at the top of the spreadsheet beginning with "FILE" and extending several choices to the right. I will comment on these briefly before we look more comprehensively at the statistical features.

Home

The "Home" menu includes many options for formatting and structuring the entered data, including a font group, alignment group, cells group (for such features as insert/delete options), and other such features.

One set of submenus is particularly useful for the statistical user. These are listed in the "Number" category located in the ribbon at the bottom of the main set of menus. The default format of "Number" is typically "General" shown in the highlighted box (see Figure B.1). If you select this drop-down menu, you will be presented with a series of possible formats for your data among which is the choice "Number" – the second choice in the submenu. If you click this option, Excel returns the data in the cell as a number with two decimal points.

When you select the "Number" button at the bottom of the category box, you can select from several choices that allow you to refine the nature of the data entered, as shown in Figure B.2. (The additional choices for data formats are located in the "Category:" box located on the left side of this submenu.) We will primarily use this "Number" format since we are analyzing numerical data, but we may have occasion to use additional formats. You can use this submenu to create any number of decimal places by using the "Decimal places:" box. You can also specify different ways of handling negative numbers by selecting among the choices in the "Negative numbers:" box.

Insert Tab

I will return to this menu many times over the course of our discussion. Primarily, we will use this menu to create the visual descriptions of our analyses (graphs and charts).

Page Layout

This menu is helpful for formatting functions and creating the desired "look and feel" of the spreadsheet.

Formulas

The "Formulas" menu is a very important part of the statistical arsenal of Excel. We will discuss specific functions as we get to them in the course of our study; for

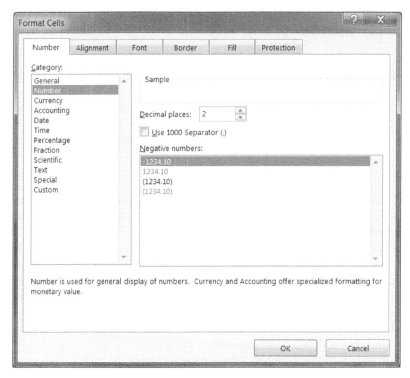

Figure B.2   The variety of cell formats available in the "Number" submenu.

now, I will point out that the first section of this menu is the "Function Library" that contains a great many categories of functions (i.e., "Financial," "Logical," "Text," etc.). Selecting any of these results in a submenu of choices for formulas specific to that category of use. There are at least two ways to create statistical formulas, which we will discuss in this book:

1. *"More Functions" tab*This tab presents the user with additional categories of formulas, one of which is "Statistical." As you can see when you select this tab, there are a great many choices for handling data. Essentially, these are embedded formulas for creating specific statistical output. For example, "AVERAGE" is one of the first formulas listed when you choose "More Functions" and then select "Statistical." This formula returns the mean value of a set of selected data from the spreadsheet.

2. *"Insert Functions" tab*A second way to access statistical (and other) functions from the Function Library is using the "Insert Function" submenu that, when selected, presents the user with the screen shown in Figure B.3. As you can see, I chose "AVERAGE" which appears in the highlighted bar.

Choosing this feature is the way to "import" the function to the spreadsheet. As you can see, there are a variety of ways to choose a desired function. The "Search

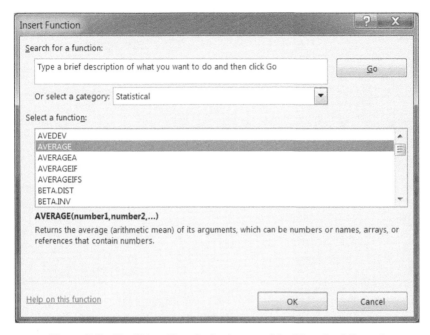

Figure B.3   The "Insert Function" submenu of the "Function Library."

for a function:" box allows the user to describe what they want to do with their data. When selected, the program will present several choices in the "Select a function:" box immediately below it, depending on which function you queried.

The "Or select a category:" box lists the range of function categories available. The statistical category of functions will be shown if double-clicked (as shown in Figure B.3). Accessing the list of statistical functions through this button will result in the same list of functions obtainable through the "More Functions" tab.

When you use the categories repeatedly, as we will use the "Statistical" category repeatedly, Excel will show the functions last used in the "Select a function:" box.

Data

This is the main menu for discussion in this book. Through the submenu choices, the statistical student can access the data analysis procedures, sort and filter data in the spreadsheet, and provide a number of data management functions important for statistical analysis. Figure B.4 shows the submenus of the "Data" menu (highlighted).

The following are some of the more important submenus that I will explain in detail in subsequent chapters.

Sort and Filter   The "Sort" submenu allows the user to rearrange the data in the spreadsheet according to a specific interest or statistical procedure. For example, if you had a spreadsheet with two variables, General Health and Sex, you could use the "Sort" key to arrange the values of the variables according to Sex. (You might

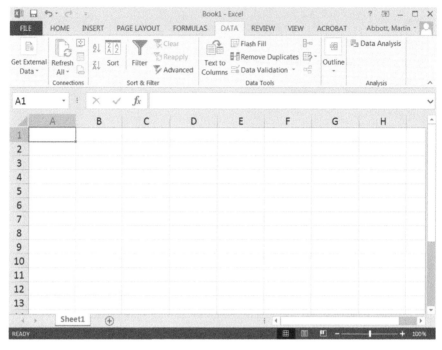

Figure B.4 The submenus of the "Data" menu.

recognize these data from the example in Appendix A, Table A.1.)[3] Doing this would result in Excel arranging the Sex categories, "1" (male) and "2" (female) in ascending or descending order (alphabetically depending on whether you proceed from "smallest to largest" or from "largest to smallest") with the values of the other variable(s) linked to this new arrangement. Thus, a visual scan of the data would allow you to see how the cases of the variables change as you proceed from Sex category 1 to category 2 (male and female) respondents. The following two figures show the results of this example.

Figure B.5 shows the first fourteen cases (the category name occupies the top cell, so the 15th line in the spreadsheet is case #14) on the unsorted variables. As you can see from Figure B.5, you cannot easily discern a pattern to the data depending on whether males or females have higher or lower values on GENHLTH scores in this sample.[4] Sorting the data according to the Sex variable may help to indicate relationships or patterns in the data that are not immediately apparent. Figure B.6 shows the same variables sorted according to SEX (sorted "smallest to largest" resulting in the male scores listed first).

[3]Centers for Disease Control and Prevention (CDC). *Behavioral Risk Factor Surveillance System Survey Data*. Atlanta, Georgia: U.S. Department of Health and Human Services, Centers for Disease Control and Prevention, 2013.

[4]The example data represent a very small number of cases, so there is no attempt to make research conclusions about the variables shown.

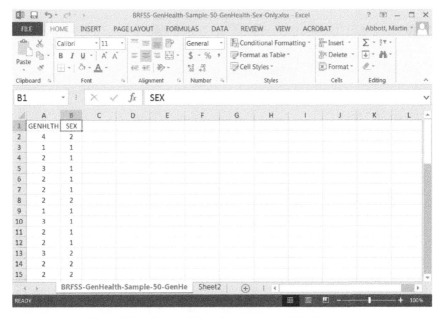

Figure B.5 Unsorted data for the two-variable database.

Figure B.6 shows the data arranged according to the categories of the Sex variable. Viewed in this way, you can detect some general patterns. It appears, generally, that female students indicated generally higher scores on GENHLTH than males. Of course, this small sample is not a good indicator of the overall relationship between Sex and general health.

An important operational note for sorting is to first "select" the entire database before you sort any of the data fields (by clicking on the box above the numbered cases and to the left of the lettered variables). If you do not sort the entire database, you can inadvertently only sort one variable, which may result in the values of this variable disengaging from its associated values on adjacent variables. In these cases, the values for each case may become mixed. Selecting the entire database before any sort ensures that the values of a given variable remain fixed to the values of all the variables for each of the cases. The "Filter" submenu is useful in this regard. Excel adds drop-down menus next to each variable when the user selects this submenu. When you use the menus, you can specify a series of ways to sort the variables in the database without "disengaging" the values on the variables.

You can also perform a "multiple" sort in Excel using the "Sort" menu. Figure B.7 shows the submenu presented when you choose "Sort." As you can see from the screen, choosing the "Add Level" button in the upper left corner of the screen results in a second sort line ("Then by") allowing you to specify a second sort variable. This would result in a sort of the data first by SEX, and then the values of GENHLTH would be presented low to high within both categories of SEX.

Excel also records the nature of the variables. Under the "Order" column on the far right of Figure B.7, the variables chosen for sorting are listed as "Smallest to

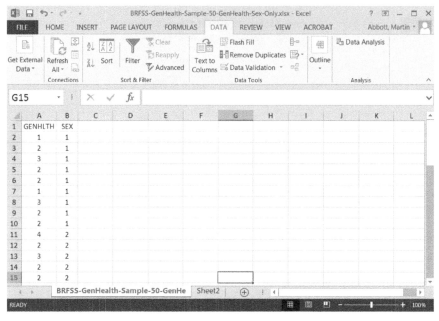

Figure B.6   Using the "Sort" function to arrange values of the variables.

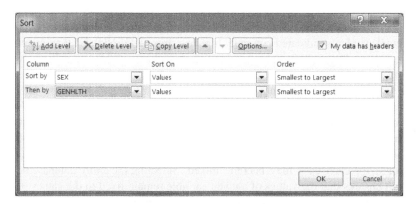

Figure B.7   The Excel submenu showing a sort by multiple variables.

Largest," indicating they are numeric or represent numbers rather than letters. Text variables are composed of values (either letters or numbers) that are treated as letters and not used in calculations. If the SEX values in Figure B.6 had been listed as "Male" and "Female" and not coded as 1 or 2 in the original data set, Excel might treat the values differently in calculations (since letters cannot be added, subtracted, etc.). In this case I would want to ensure that the "1" and the "2" would be treated as a number. Be sure to format the cells properly (from the "Number" group in the "Home" menu) so that you can be sure the values are treated as you intend them to be treated in your analyses.

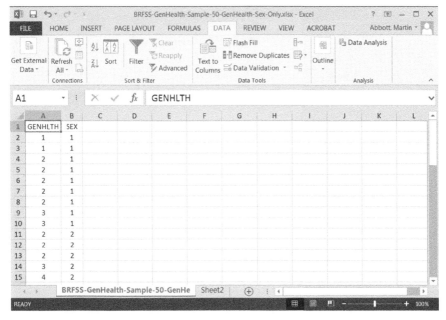

Figure B.8   The Excel screen showing the results of a multiple sort.

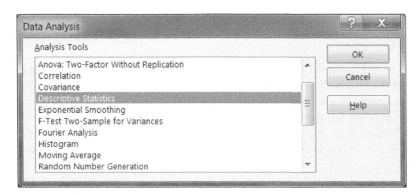

Figure B.9   The "Data Analysis" submenu containing statistical analysis procedures.

Figure B.8 shows the resulting sort. Here you can see that the data were first sorted by SEX, and then the values of GENHLTH were presented low to high in value within both SEX categories.

Data Analysis   This submenu choice (located in the "Data" tab in the "Analysis" group) is the primary statistical analysis device we will use in this book. Figure B.4 shows the "Data Analysis" submenu in the upper right corner of the menu bar. Choosing this option results in the box shown in Figure B.9.

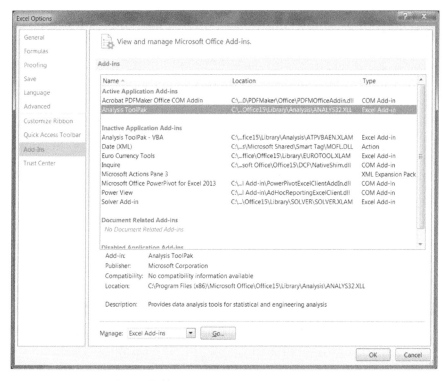

Figure B.10   The "Add-In" options for Excel.

Figure B.9 shows the statistical procedures available in Excel. The scroll bar to the right of the screen allows the user to access several additional procedures. We will explore many of these procedures in later chapters.

You may not see the "Data Analysis" submenu displayed when you choose the "Data" menu on the main Excel screen. That is because it is often an "add-in" program. Not everyone uses these features so Excel makes them available as an "adjunct."[5]

If your Excel screen does not show the "Data Analysis" submenu in the right edge of the menu bar when you select the "Data" menu, you can add it to the menu. Select the "Office Button" in the upper left corner of the screen, and then you will see an "Excel Options" button in the lower center of the screen. Choose this and you will be presented with several options in a column on the left edge of the screen. "Add-Ins" is one of the available choices, which, if you select it, presents you with the screen shown in Figure B.10. I selected "Add-Ins" and the screen in Figure B.10 appeared with "Analysis ToolPak" highlighted in the upper group of choices. When you select this option (you might need to restart Excel to give it a chance to add), you should be

---

[5]MAC users may not have access to the "Data Analysis" features since they were removed in previous versions. There may be programs available that perform similar functions, but refer to the Excel website for assistance.

able to find the "Data Analysis" submenu on the right side of the "Data" menu. This will allow you to use the statistical functions we discuss in the book.

Review and View Menus

These two tabs available from the main screen have useful menus and functions for data management and appearance. I will make reference to them as we encounter them in later chapters.

USING STATISTICAL FUNCTIONS

The heart of the statistical uses of Excel is in the "Data Analysis" submenu shown in Figure B.9. I introduce many of these statistical tools in the book chapters describing different statistical procedures. However, before we delve into those specific topics, I want to point out other ways that we can build statistical formulas directly into the spreadsheet.

I described several ways in the "Formulas" section earlier that users can enter statistical formulas directly from the available submenus. As I mentioned, there are several statistical formulas available that we use extensively in this book. Most are single procedure formulas like calculating "AVERAGE" or "STDEV" (standard deviation). Other procedures are more complex like the "FTEST" that calculates the equivalence in variance in two sets of data.

Entering Formulas Directly

A very important use of Excel is to "embed" formulas directly into the worksheet so that you can devise whatever calculation you need. The functions we discussed earlier are simply common calculations that have been arranged so that if you have repeated need for a certain calculation, you can use them more quickly than entering the formulas manually.

Selecting the "=" key in any cell notifies Excel that what follows is a <u>user-created formula</u>. Thereafter, you can enter the calculation you want as a string of characters. For example, using the sample of GENHLTH and SEX values shown in Figure B.5, the following commands (user-created formulas) would yield the average value for GENHLTH scores: =Sum(A2:A15)/14.

Figure B.11 shows how this looks in Excel. In this example, there are three main components of the formula:

- "=" informs Excel that the user is entering a formula.
- "Sum(A2:A15)" calls for adding the values together from cell A2 to A15.
- "/14" divides the summed GENHLTH scores by 14 (the total number of scores), yielding the average GENHLTH score (2.214).

The results of entering the formula are shown in cell F4 in Figure B.11 (or whatever cell you used to enter the formula). The formula you entered is shown in the

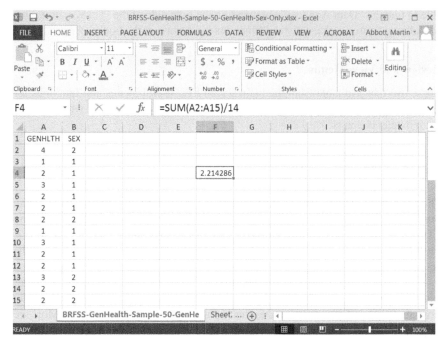

Figure B.11 Entering user-generated formulas in Excel.

formula bar directly above the spreadsheet. As you can see, it appears exactly as I described earlier. The "answer" of the formula appears in the cell selected (F4 in the example in Figure B.11). You can edit this formula line if you wish to include additional cases, and the formula will automatically adjust the calculation to reflect the change in values.

There are several ways to get the same result for most formulas you might wish to enter. For example, you could use the menu system I described earlier to enter a function to create the "AVERAGE," which is what we did using our own formula. Look at Figure B.3 again, and you will see that "AVERAGE" (listed in the column on the left side of the screen) is one of the choices from the "Functions" menu.

Using the "SUM" Button

Another way to help create your own formulas is to use the "$\sum$" button shown on the "Home" tab at the far right of the menu ribbon. Look at Figure B.5 and you will see this symbol at the right side of the figure. The symbol means "sum of," and we will use it extensively in our discussion in later chapters since it is such an important function for statistical analyses. Figure B.12 shows the result of clicking this symbol when the cursor is in cell F6. As you can see, when you select the symbol, it creates a formula calling for summing a series of cells you select in the spreadsheet (shown in a dashed box around the selected values). In the example that follows, I selected the

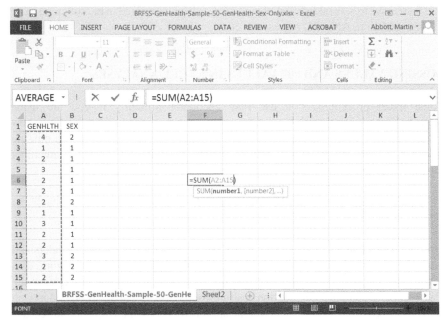

Figure B.12 Using the $\sum$ button to create a formula.

string of GENHLTH values (cells A2–A15) with the cursor, which Excel then added to the formula.

Figure B.12 also shows a "ScreenTip" box that appears when you choose the "$\sum$" button. Directly below the selected cell where the formula is entered, you will see the "help" bar explanation of the function: "SUM(**number1**,[number2, …])." This shows that the sum symbol enters the "SUM" function wherein the numbers from the selected cells are added sequentially.

I used the $\sum$ button in this example to demonstrate that it is helpful if you are building your own formula. Had we wanted to complete the formula for the average value of the GENHLTH values, we would simply place the "/14" figure at the end of the "SUM" function listed in the formula window. This would create the same formula we created directly shown in Figure B.11.

DATA ANALYSIS PROCEDURES

The "Data Analysis" submenu is a more comprehensive and extensive list of statistical procedures available in Excel. Typically, this involves several related and linked functions and specialized formulas that statisticians and researchers use repeatedly. These are more complex than each separate function (e.g., average, standard deviation, etc.) and in fact may use several functions in the computation of the formulas. We start the book showing "Descriptive Statistics" (a "Data Analysis" submenu choice) and then move to several inferential procedures also represented in the submenu (e.g., *t* test, correlation, ANOVA, regression, etc.).

MISSING VALUES AND "0" VALUES IN EXCEL ANALYSES

Some Excel procedures you use may encounter difficulty if you are using large data sets or have missing cases. In particular, you need to be careful about how to handle *missing cases and zeros*. Some procedures do not work well with missing values in the data set. Also, be careful about how "0" values are handled. Remember missing cases are not "0" values, and vice versa.

USING EXCEL WITH "REAL DATA"

Over the book chapters, I introduce you to several databases that we use to understand the different statistical procedures. I find that it is always better to use real-world data when I teach statistics since students and researchers must, at some point, leave the classroom and venture into situations calling for the use of statistical procedures on actual research problems. I take this same approach in my book *Understanding Educational Statistics* (Abbott, 2011) in which I demonstrate the use of several statistical procedures using data from actual databases and/or my own evaluation data.

APPENDIX C

STATISTICAL TABLES

TABLE C.1   Z-Score Table (Values Shown are Percentages – %)

z	0		0.01		0.02		0.03		0.04		0.05	
0.0	0.000	50.000	0.399	49.601	0.798	49.202	1.197	48.803	1.595	48.405	1.994	48.006
0.1	3.983	46.017	4.380	45.620	4.776	45.224	5.172	44.828	5.567	44.433	5.962	44.038
0.2	7.926	42.074	8.317	41.683	8.706	41.294	9.095	40.905	9.483	40.517	9.871	40.129
0.3	11.791	38.209	12.172	37.828	12.552	37.448	12.930	37.070	13.307	36.693	13.683	36.317
0.4	15.542	34.458	15.910	34.090	16.276	33.724	16.640	33.360	17.003	32.997	17.364	32.636
0.5	19.146	30.854	19.497	30.503	19.847	30.153	20.194	29.806	20.540	29.460	20.884	29.116
0.6	22.575	27.425	22.907	27.093	23.237	26.763	23.565	26.435	23.891	26.109	24.215	25.785
0.7	25.804	24.196	26.115	23.885	26.424	23.576	26.730	23.270	27.035	22.965	27.337	22.663
0.8	28.814	21.186	29.103	20.897	29.389	20.611	29.673	20.327	29.955	20.045	30.234	19.766
0.9	31.594	18.406	31.859	18.141	32.121	17.879	32.381	17.619	32.639	17.361	32.894	17.106
1.0	34.134	15.866	34.375	15.625	34.614	15.386	34.850	15.151	35.083	14.917	35.314	14.686
1.1	36.433	13.567	36.650	13.350	36.864	13.136	37.076	12.924	37.286	12.714	37.493	12.507
1.2	38.493	11.507	38.686	11.314	38.877	11.123	39.065	10.935	39.251	10.749	39.435	10.565
1.3	40.320	9.680	40.490	9.510	40.658	9.342	40.824	9.176	40.988	9.012	41.149	8.851
1.4	41.924	8.076	42.073	7.927	42.220	7.780	42.364	7.636	42.507	7.493	42.647	7.353
1.5	43.319	6.681	43.448	6.552	43.574	6.426	43.699	6.301	43.822	6.178	43.943	6.057
1.6	44.520	5.480	44.630	5.370	44.738	5.262	44.845	5.155	44.950	5.050	45.053	4.947
1.7	45.543	4.457	45.637	4.363	45.728	4.272	45.818	4.182	45.907	4.093	45.994	4.006
1.8	46.407	3.593	46.485	3.515	46.562	3.438	46.638	3.363	46.712	3.288	46.784	3.216
1.9	47.128	2.872	47.193	2.807	47.257	2.743	47.320	2.680	47.381	2.619	47.441	2.559
2.0	47.725	2.275	47.778	2.222	47.831	2.169	47.882	2.118	47.932	2.068	47.982	2.018
2.1	48.214	1.786	48.257	1.743	48.300	1.700	48.341	1.659	48.382	1.618	48.422	1.578
2.2	48.610	1.390	48.645	1.355	48.679	1.321	48.713	1.287	48.745	1.255	48.778	1.222
2.3	48.928	1.072	48.956	1.044	48.983	1.017	49.010	0.990	49.036	0.964	49.061	0.939
2.4	49.180	0.820	49.202	0.798	49.224	0.776	49.245	0.755	49.266	0.734	49.286	0.714
2.5	49.379	0.621	49.396	0.604	49.413	0.587	49.430	0.570	49.446	0.554	49.461	0.539
2.6	49.534	0.466	49.547	0.453	49.560	0.440	49.573	0.427	49.585	0.415	49.598	0.402
2.7	49.653	0.347	49.664	0.336	49.674	0.326	49.683	0.317	49.693	0.307	49.702	0.298
2.8	49.744	0.256	49.752	0.248	49.760	0.240	49.767	0.233	49.774	0.226	49.781	0.219
2.9	49.813	0.187	49.819	0.181	49.825	0.175	49.831	0.169	49.836	0.164	49.841	0.159
3.0	49.865	0.135	49.869	0.131	49.874	0.126	49.878	0.122	49.882	0.118	49.886	0.114

Using Statistics in the Social and Health Sciences with SPSS® and Excel®, First Edition.
Martin Lee Abbott.
© 2017 John Wiley & Sons, Inc. Published 2017 by John Wiley & Sons, Inc.

TABLE C.1   Continued

z	0.06		0.07		0.08		0.09	
0.0	2.392	47.608	2.790	47.210	3.188	46.812	3.586	46.414
0.1	6.356	43.644	6.749	43.251	7.142	42.858	7.535	42.465
0.2	10.257	39.743	10.642	39.358	11.026	38.974	11.409	38.591
0.3	14.058	35.942	14.431	35.569	14.803	35.197	15.173	34.827
0.4	17.724	32.276	18.082	31.918	18.439	31.561	18.793	31.207
0.5	21.226	28.774	21.566	28.434	21.904	28.096	22.240	27.760
0.6	24.537	25.463	24.857	25.143	25.175	24.825	25.490	24.510
0.7	27.637	22.363	27.935	22.065	28.230	21.770	28.524	21.476
0.8	30.511	19.489	30.785	19.215	31.057	18.943	31.327	18.673
0.9	33.147	16.853	33.398	16.602	33.646	16.354	33.891	16.109
1.0	35.543	14.457	35.769	14.231	35.993	14.007	36.214	13.786
1.1	37.698	12.302	37.900	12.100	38.100	11.900	38.298	11.702
1.2	39.617	10.383	39.796	10.204	39.973	10.027	40.147	9.853
1.3	41.309	8.692	41.466	8.534	41.621	8.379	41.774	8.226
1.4	42.786	7.215	42.922	7.078	43.056	6.944	43.189	6.811
1.5	44.062	5.938	44.179	5.821	44.295	5.705	44.408	5.592
1.6	45.154	4.846	45.254	4.746	45.352	4.648	45.449	4.551
1.7	46.080	3.920	46.164	3.836	46.246	3.754	46.327	3.673
1.8	46.856	3.144	46.926	3.074	46.995	3.005	47.062	2.938
1.9	47.500	2.500	47.558	2.442	47.615	2.385	47.670	2.330
2.0	48.030	1.970	48.077	1.923	48.124	1.876	48.169	1.831
2.1	48.461	1.539	48.500	1.500	48.537	1.463	48.574	1.426
2.2	48.809	1.191	48.840	1.160	48.870	1.130	48.899	1.101
2.3	49.086	0.914	49.111	0.889	49.134	0.866	49.158	0.842
2.4	49.305	0.695	49.324	0.676	49.343	0.657	49.361	0.639
2.5	49.477	0.523	49.492	0.508	49.506	0.494	49.520	0.480
2.6	49.609	0.391	49.621	0.379	49.632	0.368	49.643	0.357
2.7	49.711	0.289	49.720	0.280	49.728	0.272	49.736	0.264
2.8	49.788	0.212	49.795	0.205	49.801	0.199	49.807	0.193
2.9	49.846	0.154	49.851	0.149	49.856	0.144	49.861	0.139
3.0	49.889	0.111	49.893	0.107	49.897	0.104	49.900	0.100

Source: Pearson (1914).

TABLE C.2   Exclusion Values for the *T*-Distribution

one-tailed	0.4	0.25	0.1	0.05	0.025	0.01	0.005	0.0025
two-tailed	0.8	0.5	0.2	0.1	0.05	0.02	0.01	0.005
Degrees of Freedom								
1	0.325	1.000	3.078	6.314	12.706	31.821	63.657	127.320
2	0.289	0.816	1.886	2.920	4.303	6.965	9.925	14.089
3	0.277	0.765	1.638	2.353	3.182	4.541	5.841	7.453
4	0.271	0.741	1.533	2.132	2.776	3.747	4.604	5.598
5	0.267	0.727	1.476	2.015	2.571	3.365	4.032	4.773
6	0.265	0.718	1.440	1.943	2.447	3.143	3.707	4.317
7	0.263	0.711	1.415	1.895	2.365	2.998	3.499	4.029
8	0.262	0.706	1.397	1.860	2.306	2.896	3.355	3.833
9	0.261	0.703	1.383	1.833	2.262	2.821	3.250	3.690
10	0.260	0.700	1.372	1.812	2.228	2.764	3.169	3.581
11	0.260	0.697	1.363	1.796	2.201	2.718	3.106	3.497
12	0.259	0.695	1.356	1.782	2.179	2.681	3.055	3.428
13	0.259	0.694	1.350	1.771	2.160	2.650	3.012	3.372
14	0.258	0.692	1.345	1.761	2.145	2.624	2.977	3.326
15	0.258	0.691	1.341	1.753	2.131	2.602	2.947	3.286
16	0.258	0.690	1.337	1.746	2.120	2.583	2.921	3.252
17	0.257	0.689	1.333	1.740	2.110	2.567	2.898	3.222
18	0.257	0.688	1.330	1.734	2.101	2.552	2.878	3.197
19	0.257	0.688	1.328	1.729	2.093	2.539	2.861	3.174
20	0.257	0.687	1.325	1.725	2.086	2.528	2.845	3.153
21	0.257	0.686	1.323	1.721	2.080	2.518	2.831	3.135
22	0.256	0.686	1.321	1.717	2.074	2.508	2.819	3.119
23	0.256	0.685	1.319	1.714	2.069	2.500	2.807	3.104
24	0.256	0.685	1.318	1.711	2.064	2.492	2.797	3.091
25	0.256	0.684	1.316	1.708	2.060	2.485	2.787	3.078
26	0.256	0.684	1.315	1.706	2.056	2.479	2.779	3.067
27	0.256	0.684	1.314	1.703	2.052	2.473	2.771	3.057
28	0.256	0.683	1.313	1.701	2.048	2.467	2.763	3.047
29	0.256	0.683	1.311	1.699	2.045	2.462	2.756	3.038
30	0.256	0.683	1.310	1.697	2.042	2.457	2.750	3.030
40	0.255	0.681	1.303	1.684	2.021	2.423	2.704	2.971
60	0.254	0.679	1.296	1.671	2.000	2.390	2.660	2.915
120	0.254	0.677	1.289	1.658	1.980	2.358	2.617	2.860
∞	0.253	0.674	1.282	1.645	1.960	2.326	2.576	2.807

Source: Pearson and Hartley (1962).

TABLE C.3   Critical (Exclusion) Values for the Distribution of F

		\multicolumn{12}{c}{df in the Numerator (Between)}										
	Exclusion Level	1	2	3	4	5	6	7	8	9	10	11	12
1	0.05	161	200	216	225	230	234	237	239	241	242	243	244
	0.01	4052	4999	5403	5625	5764	5859	5928	5981	6022	6056	6082	6106
2	0.05	18.51	19.00	19.16	19.25	19.30	19.33	19.36	19.37	19.38	19.39	19.40	19.41
	0.01	98.49	99.00	99.17	99.25	99.30	99.33	99.36	99.37	99.39	99.40	99.41	99.42
3	0.05	10.13	9.55	9.28	9.12	9.01	8.94	8.88	8.84	8.81	8.78	8.76	8.74
	0.01	34.12	30.82	29.46	28.71	28.24	27.91	27.67	27.49	27.34	27.23	27.13	27.05
4	0.05	7.71	6.94	6.59	6.39	6.26	6.16	6.09	6.04	6.00	5.96	5.93	5.91
	0.01	21.20	18.00	16.69	15.98	15.52	15.21	14.98	14.80	14.66	14.54	14.45	14.37
5	0.05	6.61	5.79	5.41	5.19	5.05	4.95	4.88	4.82	4.78	4.74	4.70	4.68
	0.01	16.26	13.27	12.06	11.39	10.97	10.67	10.45	10.29	10.15	10.05	9.96	9.89
6	0.05	5.99	5.14	4.76	4.53	4.39	4.28	4.21	4.15	4.10	4.06	4.03	4.00
	0.01	13.74	10.92	9.78	9.15	8.75	8.47	8.26	8.10	7.98	7.87	7.79	7.72
7	0.05	5.59	4.74	4.35	4.12	3.97	3.87	3.79	3.73	3.68	3.63	3.60	3.57
	0.01	12.25	9.55	8.45	7.85	7.46	7.19	7.00	6.84	6.71	6.62	6.54	6.47
8	0.05	5.32	4.46	4.07	3.84	3.69	3.58	3.50	3.44	3.39	3.34	3.31	3.28
	0.01	11.26	8.65	7.59	7.01	6.63	6.37	6.19	6.03	5.91	5.82	5.74	5.67
9	0.05	5.12	4.26	3.86	3.63	3.48	3.37	3.29	3.23	3.18	3.13	3.10	3.07
	0.01	10.56	8.02	6.99	6.42	6.06	5.80	5.62	5.47	5.35	5.26	5.18	5.11
10	0.05	4.96	4.10	3.71	3.48	3.33	3.22	3.14	3.07	3.02	2.97	2.94	2.91
	0.01	10.04	7.56	6.55	5.99	5.64	5.39	5.21	5.06	4.95	4.85	4.78	4.71
11	0.05	4.84	3.98	3.59	3.36	3.20	3.09	3.01	2.95	2.90	2.86	2.82	2.79
	0.01	9.65	7.20	6.22	5.67	5.32	5.07	4.88	4.74	4.63	4.54	4.46	4.40
12	0.05	4.75	3.88	3.49	3.26	3.11	3.00	2.92	2.85	2.80	2.76	2.72	2.69
	0.01	9.33	6.93	5.95	5.41	5.06	4.82	4.65	4.50	4.39	4.30	4.22	4.16
13	0.05	4.67	3.80	3.41	3.18	3.02	2.92	2.84	2.77	2.72	2.67	2.63	2.60
	0.01	9.07	6.70	5.74	5.20	4.86	4.62	4.44	4.30	4.19	4.10	4.02	3.96
14	0.05	4.60	3.74	3.34	3.11	2.96	2.85	2.77	2.70	2.65	2.60	2.56	2.53
	0.01	8.86	6.51	5.56	5.03	4.69	4.46	4.28	4.14	4.03	3.94	3.86	3.80
15	0.05	4.54	3.68	3.29	3.06	2.90	2.79	2.70	2.64	2.59	2.55	2.51	2.48
	0.01	8.68	6.36	5.42	4.89	4.56	4.32	4.14	4.00	3.89	3.80	3.73	3.67
16	0.05	4.49	3.63	3.24	3.01	2.85	2.74	2.66	2.59	2.54	2.49	2.45	2.42
	0.01	8.53	6.23	5.29	4.77	4.44	4.20	4.03	3.89	3.78	3.69	3.61	3.55

df in the Denominator

Source: Snedecor and Cochran (1980).

TABLE C.3   Continued

		df in the Numerator (Between)											
	Exclusion Level	1	2	3	4	5	6	7	8	9	10	11	12
17	0.05	4.45	3.59	3.20	2.96	2.81	2.70	2.62	2.55	2.50	2.45	2.41	2.38
	0.01	8.40	6.11	5.18	4.67	4.34	4.10	3.93	3.79	3.68	3.59	3.52	3.45
18	0.05	4.41	3.55	3.16	2.93	2.77	3.66	2.58	2.51	2.46	2.41	2.37	2.34
	0.01	8.28	6.01	5.09	4.58	4.25	4.01	3.85	3.71	3.60	3.51	3.44	3.37
19	0.05	4.38	3.52	3.13	2.90	2.74	2.63	2.55	2.48	2.43	2.38	2.34	2.31
	0.01	8.18	5.93	5.01	4.50	4.17	3.94	3.77	3.63	3.52	3.43	3.36	3.30
20	0.05	4.35	3.49	3.10	2.87	2.71	2.60	2.52	2.45	2.40	2.35	2.31	2.28
	0.01	8.10	5.85	4.94	4.43	4.10	3.87	3.71	3.56	3.45	3.37	3.30	3.23
21	0.05	4.32	3.47	3.07	2.84	2.68	2.57	2.49	2.42	2.37	2.32	2.28	2.25
	0.01	8.02	5.78	4.87	4.37	4.04	3.81	3.65	3.51	3.40	3.31	3.24	3.17
22	0.05	4.30	3.44	3.05	2.82	2.66	2.55	2.47	2.40	2.35	2.30	2.26	2.23
	0.01	7.94	5.72	4.82	4.31	3.99	3.76	3.59	3.45	3.35	3.26	3.18	3.12
23	0.05	4.28	3.42	3.03	2.80	2.64	2.53	2.45	2.38	2.32	2.28	2.24	2.20
	0.01	7.88	5.66	4.76	4.26	3.94	3.71	3.54	3.41	3.30	3.21	3.14	3.07
24	0.05	4.26	3.40	3.01	2.78	2.62	2.51	2.43	2.36	2.30	2.26	2.22	2.18
	0.01	7.82	5.61	4.72	4.22	3.90	3.67	3.50	3.36	3.25	3.17	3.09	3.03
25	0.05	4.24	3.38	2.99	2.76	2.60	2.49	2.41	2.34	2.28	2.24	2.20	2.16
	0.01	7.77	5.57	4.68	4.18	3.86	3.63	3.46	3.32	3.21	3.13	3.05	2.99
26	0.05	4.22	3.37	2.98	2.74	2.59	2.47	2.39	2.32	2.27	2.22	2.18	2.15
	0.01	7.72	5.53	4.64	4.14	3.82	3.59	3.42	3.29	3.17	3.09	3.02	2.96
27	0.05	4.21	3.35	2.96	2.73	2.57	2.46	2.37	2.30	2.25	2.20	2.16	2.13
	0.01	7.68	5.49	4.60	4.11	3.79	3.56	3.39	3.26	3.14	3.06	2.98	2.93
28	0.05	4.20	3.34	2.95	2.71	2.56	2.44	2.36	2.29	2.24	2.19	2.15	2.12
	0.01	7.64	5.45	4.57	4.07	3.76	3.53	3.36	3.23	3.11	3.03	2.95	2.90
29	0.05	4.18	3.33	2.93	2.70	2.54	2.43	2.35	2.28	2.22	2.18	2.14	2.10
	0.01	7.60	5.42	4.54	4.04	3.73	3.50	3.33	3.20	3.08	3.00	2.92	2.87
30	0.05	4.17	3.32	2.92	2.69	2.53	2.42	2.34	2.27	2.21	2.16	2.12	2.09
	0.01	7.56	5.39	4.51	4.02	3.70	3.47	3.30	3.17	3.06	2.98	2.90	2.84
32	0.05	4.15	3.30	2.90	2.67	2.51	2.40	2.32	2.25	2.19	2.14	2.10	2.07
	0.01	7.50	5.34	4.46	3.97	3.66	3.42	3.25	3.12	3.01	2.94	2.86	2.80
34	0.05	4.13	3.28	2.88	2.65	2.49	2.38	2.30	2.23	2.17	2.12	2.08	2.05
	0.01	7.44	5.29	4.42	3.93	3.61	3.38	3.21	3.08	2.97	2.89	2.82	2.76
36	0.05	4.11	3.26	2.86	2.63	2.48	2.36	2.28	2.21	2.15	2.10	2.06	2.03
	0.01	7.39	5.25	4.38	3.89	3.58	3.35	3.18	3.04	2.94	2.86	2.78	2.72
38	0.05	4.10	3.25	2.85	2.62	2.46	2.35	2.26	2.19	2.14	2.09	2.05	2.02
	0.01	7.35	5.21	4.34	3.86	3.54	3.32	3.15	3.02	2.91	2.82	2.75	2.69

df in the Denominator (left side vertical label)

Source: Snedecor and Cochran (1980).

TABLE C.3 Continued

		df in the Numerator (Between)											
	Exclusion Level	1	2	3	4	5	6	7	8	9	10	11	12
40	0.05	4.08	3.23	2.84	2.61	2.45	2.34	2.25	2.18	2.12	2.07	2.04	2.00
	0.01	7.31	5.18	4.31	3.83	3.51	3.29	3.12	2.99	2.88	2.80	2.73	2.66
42	0.05	4.07	3.22	2.83	2.59	2.44	2.32	2.24	2.17	2.11	2.06	2.02	1.99
	0.01	7.27	5.15	4.29	3.80	3.49	3.26	3.10	2.96	2.86	2.77	2.70	2.64
44	0.05	4.06	3.21	2.82	2.58	2.43	2.31	2.23	2.16	2.10	2.05	2.01	1.98
	0.01	7.24	5.12	4.26	3.78	3.46	3.24	3.07	2.94	2.84	2.75	2.68	2.62
46	0.05	4.05	3.20	2.81	2.57	2.42	2.30	2.22	2.14	2.09	2.04	2.00	1.97
	0.01	7.21	5.10	4.24	3.76	3.44	3.22	3.05	2.92	2.82	2.73	2.66	2.60
48	0.05	4.04	3.19	2.80	2.56	2.41	2.30	2.21	2.40	2.08	2.03	1.99	1.96
	0.01	7.19	5.08	4.22	3.74	3.42	3.20	3.04	2.90	2.80	2.71	2.64	2.58
50	0.05	4.03	3.18	2.79	2.56	2.40	2.29	2.20	2.13	2.07	2.02	1.98	1.95
	0.01	7.17	5.06	4.20	3.72	3.41	3.18	3.02	2.88	2.78	2.70	2.62	2.56
55	0.05	4.02	3.17	2.78	2.54	2.38	2.27	2.18	2.11	2.05	2.00	1.97	1.93
	0.01	7.12	5.01	4.16	3.68	3.37	3.15	2.98	2.85	2.75	2.66	2.59	2.53
60	0.05	4.00	3.15	2.76	2.52	2.37	2.25	2.17	2.10	2.04	1.99	1.95	1.92
	0.01	7.08	4.98	4.13	3.65	3.34	3.12	2.95	2.82	2.72	2.63	2.56	2.50
65	0.05	3.99	3.14	2.75	2.51	2.36	2.24	2.15	2.08	2.02	1.98	1.94	1.90
	0.01	7.04	4.95	4.10	3.62	3.31	3.09	2.93	2.79	2.70	2.61	2.54	2.47
70	0.05	3.98	3.13	2.74	2.50	2.35	2.23	2.14	2.07	2.01	1.97	1.93	1.89
	0.01	7.01	4.92	4.08	3.60	3.29	3.07	2.91	2.77	2.67	2.59	2.51	2.45
80	0.05	3.96	3.11	2.72	2.48	2.33	2.21	2.12	2.05	1.99	1.95	1.91	1.88
	0.01	6.96	4.88	4.04	3.56	3.25	3.04	2.87	2.74	2.64	2.55	2.48	2.41
100	0.05	3.94	3.09	2.70	2.46	2.30	2.19	2.10	2.03	1.97	1.92	1.88	1.85
	0.01	6.90	4.82	3.98	3.51	3.20	2.99	2.82	2.69	2.59	2.51	2.43	2.36
125	0.05	3.92	3.07	2.68	2.44	2.29	2.17	2.08	2.01	1.95	1.90	1.86	1.83
	0.01	6.84	4.78	3.94	3.47	3.17	2.95	2.79	2.65	2.56	2.47	2.40	2.33
150	0.05	3.91	3.06	2.67	2.43	2.27	2.16	2.07	2.00	1.94	1.89	1.85	1.82
	0.01	6.81	4.75	3.91	3.44	3.14	2.92	2.76	2.62	2.53	2.44	2.37	2.30
200	0.05	3.89	3.04	2.65	2.41	2.26	2.14	2.05	1.98	1.92	1.87	1.83	1.80
	0.01	6.76	4.71	3.88	3.41	3.11	2.90	2.73	2.60	2.50	2.41	2.34	2.28
400	0.05	3.86	3.02	2.62	2.39	2.23	2.12	2.03	1.96	1.90	1.85	1.81	1.78
	0.01	6.7	4.66	3.83	3.36	3.06	2.85	2.69	2.55	2.46	2.37	2.29	2.23
1000	0.05	3.85	3.00	2.61	2.38	2.22	2.10	2.02	1.95	1.89	1.84	1.80	1.76
	0.01	6.66	4.62	3.80	3.34	3.04	2.82	2.66	2.53	2.43	2.34	2.26	2.20
∞	0.05	3.84	2.99	2.60	2.37	2.21	2.09	2.01	1.94	1.88	1.83	1.79	1.75
	0.01	6.63	4.60	3.78	3.32	3.02	2.80	2.64	2.51	2.41	2.32	2.24	2.18

df in the Denominator

Source: Snedecor and Cochran (1980).

TABLE C.4   Tukey's Range Test (Upper 5% Points)

k = Num. of Groups	2	3	4	5	6	7	8	9	10
MS_w df									
1	18.00	27.00	32.80	37.10	40.40	43.10	45.40	47.40	49.10
2	6.09	8.30	9.80	10.90	11.70	12.40	13.00	13.50	14.00
3	4.50	5.91	6.82	7.50	8.04	8.48	8.85	9.18	9.46
4	3.93	5.04	5.76	6.29	6.71	7.05	7.35	7.60	7.83
5	3.64	4.60	5.22	5.67	6.03	6.33	6.58	6.80	6.99
6	3.46	4.34	4.90	5.31	5.63	5.89	6.12	6.32	6.49
7	3.34	4.16	4.68	5.06	5.36	5.61	5.82	6.00	6.16
8	3.26	4.04	4.53	4.89	5.17	5.40	5.60	5.77	5.92
9	3.20	3.95	4.42	4.76	5.02	5.24	5.43	5.60	5.74
10	3.15	3.88	4.33	4.65	4.91	5.12	5.30	5.46	5.60
11	3.11	3.82	4.26	4.57	4.82	5.03	5.20	5.35	5.49
12	3.08	3.77	4.20	4.51	4.75	4.95	5.12	5.27	5.40
13	3.06	3.73	4.15	4.45	4.69	4.88	5.05	5.19	5.32
14	3.03	3.70	4.11	4.41	4.64	4.83	4.99	5.13	5.25
15	3.01	3.67	4.08	4.37	4.60	4.78	4.94	5.08	5.20
16	3.00	3.65	4.05	4.33	4.56	4.74	4.90	5.03	5.15
17	2.98	3.63	4.02	4.30	4.52	4.71	4.86	4.99	5.11
18	2.97	3.61	4.00	4.28	4.49	4.67	4.82	4.96	5.07
19	2.96	3.59	3.98	4.25	4.47	4.65	4.79	4.92	5.04
20	2.95	3.58	3.96	4.23	4.45	4.62	4.77	4.90	5.01
24	2.92	3.53	3.90	4.17	4.37	4.54	4.68	4.81	4.92
30	2.89	3.49	3.84	4.10	4.30	4.46	4.60	4.72	4.83
40	2.86	3.44	3.79	4.04	4.23	4.39	4.52	4.63	4.74
60	2.83	3.40	3.74	3.98	4.16	4.31	4.44	4.55	4.65
120	2.80	3.36	3.69	3.92	4.10	4.24	4.36	4.48	4.56
∞	2.77	3.31	3.63	3.86	4.03	4.17	4.29	4.39	4.47

Source: Pearson and Hartley (1962).

TABLE C.5 Critical (Exclusion) Values for Pearson's Correlation Coefficient, *r*

one-tailed	0.05	0.025	0.01	0.005	0.0025	0.0005
two-tailed	0.1	0.05	0.02	0.01	0.005	0.001
Degrees of Freedom						
1	0.988	0.9969	0.9995	0.999877	0.9999692	0.99999877
2	0.9000	0.950	0.9800	0.99000	0.99500	0.99900
3	0.805	0.878	0.9343	0.9587	0.9740	0.99114
4	0.729	0.811	0.882	0.9172	0.9417	0.9741
5	0.669	0.754	0.833	0.875	0.9056	0.9509
6	0.621	0.707	0.789	0.834	0.870	0.9249
7	0.582	0.666	0.750	0.798	0.836	0.898
8	0.549	0.632	0.715	0.765	0.805	0.872
9	0.521	0.602	0.685	0.735	0.776	0.847
10	0.497	0.576	0.658	0.708	0.750	0.823
11	0.476	0.553	0.634	0.684	0.726	0.801
12	0.457	0.532	0.612	0.661	0.703	0.780
13	0.441	0.514	0.592	0.641	0.683	0.760
14	0.426	0.497	0.574	0.623	0.664	0.742
15	0.412	0.482	0.558	0.606	0.647	0.725
16	0.400	0.468	0.543	0.590	0.631	0.708
17	0.389	0.456	0.529	0.575	0.616	0.693
18	0.378	0.444	0.516	0.561	0.602	0.679
19	0.369	0.433	0.503	0.549	0.589	0.665
20	0.360	0.423	0.492	0.537	0.576	0.652
25	0.323	0.381	0.445	0.487	0.524	0.597
30	0.296	0.349	0.409	0.449	0.484	0.554
35	0.275	0.325	0.381	0.418	0.452	0.519
40	0.257	0.304	0.358	0.393	0.425	0.490
45	0.243	0.288	0.338	0.372	0.403	0.465
50	0.231	0.273	0.322	0.354	0.384	0.443
60	0.211	0.250	0.295	0.325	0.352	0.408
70	0.195	0.232	0.274	0.302	0.327	0.380
80	0.183	0.217	0.257	0.283	0.307	0.357
90	0.173	0.205	0.242	0.267	0.290	0.338
100	0.164	0.195	0.230	0.254	0.276	0.321

Source: Pearson and Hartley (1962).

TABLE C.6   Critical Values of the χ^2 (Chi-Square) Distribution

			p Value		
Degrees of freedom (k)	0.1	0.05	0.02	0.01	0.001
1	2.706	3.841	5.412	6.635	10.827
2	4.605	5.991	7.824	9.210	13.815
3	6.251	7.815	9.837	11.345	16.266
4	7.779	9.488	11.668	13.277	18.467
5	9.236	11.070	13.388	15.086	20.515
6	10.645	12.592	15.033	16.812	22.457
7	12.017	14.067	16.622	18.475	24.322
8	13.362	15.507	18.168	20.090	26.125
9	14.684	16.919	19.679	21.666	27.877
10	15.987	18.307	21.161	23.209	29.588
11	17.275	19.675	22.618	24.725	31.264
12	18.549	21.026	24.054	26.217	32.909
13	19.812	22.362	25.472	27.688	34.528
14	21.064	23.685	26.873	29.141	36.123
15	22.307	24.996	28.259	30.578	37.697
16	23.542	26.296	29.633	32.000	39.252
17	24.769	27.587	30.995	33.409	40.790
18	25.989	28.869	32.346	34.805	42.312
19	27.204	30.144	33.687	36.191	43.820
20	28.412	31.410	35.020	37.566	45.315

Source: Pearson and Hartley (1962).

REFERENCES

Abbott, M.L. *The Evaluation Prism: Using Statistical Methods to Discover Patterns*. Hoboken, NJ: John Wiley & Sons, Inc., 2010.

Abbott, M.L.. *Understanding Educational Statistics Using Microsoft Excel and SPSS®*. Hoboken, NJ: John Wiley & Sons, Inc., 2011.

Abbott, M.L., Baker, D., Smith, K., and Trzyna, T. *Winning the Math Wars*. Seattle, WA: University of Washington Press, 2010.

Abbott, M.L. and McKinney, J. *Understanding and Applying Research Design*, Hoboken, NJ: John Wiley & Sons, Inc., 2013.

Campbell, D.T. and Stanley, J.C. *Experimental and Quasi-Experimental Designs for Research*. Chicago: Rand McNally,1963.

Centers for Disease Control and Prevention (CDC). "Behavioral Risk Factor Surveillance System" Centers for Disease Control and Prevention, 2013.

Cohen, J. *Statistical Power Analysis for the Behavioral Sciences*. (2nd ed.) Hillsdale, NJ: Lawrence Erlbaum Associates, 1988.

Cohen, J., Cohen, P., West, S.G., and Aiken, L.S. *Applied Multiple Regression/Correlation Analysis for the Behavioral Sciences*. (3rd ed.) Mahwah, NJ: Lawrence Erlbaum Associates, 2003

Hackman, R.J. and Oldham, G.R. *Work Redesign*. Reading, MA: Addison-Wesley, 1980.

Johnson, Steven, *The Ghost Map*. New York, NY: Riverhead Books, 2006.

Marmot, M. *The Status Syndrome*. New York, NY: Holt, 2004.

Nightingale, F. *Notes on Matters Affecting the Health, Efficiency, and Hospital Administration of the British Army*, 1858 (Public domain).

Pedhazur, E.J., *Multiple Regression in Behavioral Research*. New York, NY: Harcourt, 1997.

Playfair, W. *Statistical Breviary*, 1801 (Public domain).

Siegel, S. and Castellan, N.J. *Nonparametric Statistics for the Behavioral Sciences* (2nd ed.) New York, NY: McGraw-Hill, 1988.

Snedecor, G.W. and Cochran, W.G. *Statistical Methods*. Iowa State University Press, 1980.

Snow, J., On the Mode of Communication of Cholera, 1855 (Public domain).

Pearson, K.F.R.S. *Tables for Statisticians and Biometricians Part I*. (3rd ed.). (Public domain), 1914.

Pearson, E.S. and Hartley, H.O. *Biometrika Tables for Statisticians: Volume I*. (2nd ed.) Cambridge, UK: University Press, 1962.

Trzyna, T. and Abbott, M. "Grieving in the Ethnic Literature Classroom," *College Literature, Issue* **18**.(3), 1991, 1–14.

INDEX

additive rule of probability *see* probability, addition rule
aggregate data, 23, 363
alpha error *see* type I error
analysis of variance (ANOVA), 255–296
ANCOVA, 298
  defined, 319
ARDA, 9
average deviation, 61, 63–64
  defined, 70

Bayes' theorem *see* probability, Bayes' theorem
beta, 188, 382, 394–396
  defined, 409
beta coefficient, 418
beta error *see* type II error
biased estimator, 172, 201
bimodal, 27
  defined, 47
bimodal distribution *see* distribution, bimodal
bivariate regression, 371–408 *see also* regression
  assumptions of, 399–404
  and z score, 380–382
Bonferroni method, 292, 293
BRFSS, 8, 18, 28, 509

categorical data, 17, 45, 455, 462, 472
  defined, 47
  with MLR, 420
CDC, 8, 161
centered leverage values, 428
  defined, 448
central limit theorem, 144–148, 167
  defined, 158
central tendency *see* descriptive statistics, central tendency
Chi square, 455–488
  contingency tables, 455–456, 483
  defined, 455, 483
  distribution (*see* distribution, Chi square)
  effect size (*see* effect size)
  expected frequencies, 457–458
  frequencies versus proportions, 461–462
  goodness of fit, 457, 483
  repeated measures (*see* repeated measures, Chi square)
  special 2X2 table, 468–470
  test of independence, 463–70, 483
coefficient of determination *see* effect size, coefficient of determination
Cohen's *d see* effect size, Cohen's *d*

Using Statistics in the Social and Health Sciences with SPSS® and Excel®, First Edition.
Martin Lee Abbott.
© 2017 John Wiley & Sons, Inc. Published 2017 by John Wiley & Sons, Inc.

collinearity statistics, 440, 448
conditional probability *see* probability, conditional.
confidence interval, 195, 227–228, 383, 385–386, 391, 409, 440
defined, 193, 201, 409
contingency coefficient *see* effect size, contingency coefficient
contingency tables *see* Chi square, contingency tables
continuous data, 45, 112, 455
defined, 47
continuous variable, 241, 276, 331
control group, 137, 139, 208–210
defined, 158
convenience sample, 142
defined, 158
Cook's distance values, 428–429, 448
correlation, 329–370 *see also* Pearson's *r*
versus causation, 14, 349
defined, 329
Spearman's rho (*see* nonparametric statistics)
z score method, 342–344, 394
Cramer's *V see* effect size, Cramer's *V*
critical value *see exclusion values*
crosstabs *see* Chi square, contingency tables
cumulative proportions, 81 *see also* percentiles
curvilinear relationship, 334–335, 352, 400–403, 421
defined, 364

data distribution *see* distribution, data
deciles, 57
defined, 70
degrees of freedom
in ANOVA, 264
in Chi square, 460, 466
in correlation, 346
defined, 174, 201
in independent *T* test, 219
in single sample *T* test, 174
dependent events, 111
defined, 127
dependent variables, 139, 209, 211
defined, 158
descriptive statistics, 13–76
central tendency, 23–37, 47, 49–54, 71
contrasted to inferential statistics, 16
defined, 47
graphical methods, 41–47
research applications, 13–16
scales of measurement, 16–22
standard deviation, 60–71
variance (*see* variance)

diagnostics for MLR, 349–352, 423–430
Cook's distance values (*see* Cook's distance values)
distance statistics (*see* distance statistics)
influence statistics (*see* influence statistics)
leverage values (*see* centered leverage values)
dichotomized variable, 17, 48
defined, 364
distance statistics, 428–429, 449
distribution
bimodal, 27, 47
Chi square, 460–461
data, 48
distribution-free tests (*see* nonparametric statistics)
f-, 235–236
frequency, 48
normal, 36–37, 77–79
raw score, 87–90
sampling, of differences, 215–221
sampling, of means, 144–149, 160, 172
t-, 181–182, 201
z (standard normal), 78–83, 99, 112–117
Dunnett test, 271

effect size, 156
Cohen's *d*, 187–189, 228, 239, 245, 268
coefficient of determination, 10, 347–349, 364, 407
contingency coefficient, 462, 483
Cramer's V, 471–472, 483
defined, 158, 201
eta squared, 228–229, 249, 268, 288
partial eta squared, 308, 319, 506
Phi coefficient, 470, 483
practical significance, 156
squared part correlation, 441, 449
Wilks' lambda, 506
empirical probability *see* probability, empirical
eta squared, η^2 *see* effect size, eta squared
EXCEL, 531–544
with ANOVA, 287–289
with bivariate regression, 396–398
with central tendency, 32–35
with chi square, 481–482
with correlation, 357–358
with dependent *t*-test, 498
for equal variance, 232–235
with independent *t* test, 243–245
and percentiles, 59–60
with scattergrams, 339–341
with single sample T test, 199–200
with standard deviation, 66–67
with z scores, 94–99
with Z test, 157–158

exclusion values, 181–182, 184
expected frequency *see* Chi square, expected
    frequencies
experiment *see* research design, experiment
extreme score, 425–428
    defined (outlier), 364
    univariate, 425

f distribution *see* distribution, *f*-
f ratio, 260, 265–266
f test, 260–266
    defined, 293
factor analysis, 79
factorial ANOVA, 297–328
familywise error, 257
    defined, 293
fixed effects modeling, 449
fixed vs. random effects (MLR), 419
frequency distribution *see* distribution, frequency
frequency polygon, 77
    defined, 99
Friedman test *see* nonparametric statistics,
    Friedman test

goodness of fit *see* Chi square, goodness of fit
Greenhouse–Geisser test, 505
group designs, 210
    between, 249
    mixed, 210, 249
    within, 249

heteroscedasticity, 351
    defined, 364
hierarchical regression *see* multiple linear
    regression, hierarchical
histograms, 44–48 *see also* scattergram
    defined, 48
homogeneity of variance, 239
homoscedasticity, 351
    defined, 364
HSD *see post hoc* analyses
hypothesis, 135
    alternative, 155, 158
    defined, 158
    null, 154, 159
hypothesis test, 154–156

independent events, 108, 127
independent variables, 138, 255
    defined, 159
inferential SD, 66–68
    defined, 71
inferential statistics, 16, 143–154
    defined, 48

influence statistics, 429–430
    defined, 449
interaction effects, 299–301, 319
    charting, 300
    defined, 319
    disordinal, 319
    ordinal, 319
interquartile range, 57
    defined, 70
interval data, 20–22, 48
interval estimate *see* confidence interval

joint rule of probability *see* probability,
    multiplication rule.

Kruskal–Wallis test *see* nonparametric statistics,
    Kruskal–Wallis test
kurtosis, 40–41
    defined, 48

levels of measurement *see* scales of measurement
Levene's test, 238–239
    defined, 293
line of best fit *see* regression, line
linear relationship, 334
    defined, 364

main effects *see* factorial ANOVA
mancova, 299, 319
Mann–Whitney U test *see* nonparametric statistics
manova, 299, 319
matched groups, 210
    defined, 249
Mauchley's test of sphericity *see* sphericity
McNemar test. 483 *see also* repeated measures,
    Chi squared
mean, 24–25, 48
mean squares 263–264
measurement *see* scales of measurement
median, 25–26, 48
mixed designs, 210, 249
mode, 26, 48
multicollinearity, 422, 449
multilevel analysis, 421
multiple correlation, 406–407, 409
multiple linear regression, 417–454
    analyzing residuals, 422–423
    assumptions of, 421–423
    with categorical data, 420
    coefficients, 418
    elements of, 417–418
    entry schemes, 420, 437, 442, 447
    hierarchical, 436, 442–443, 449

multiple linear regression (*Continued*)
  squared part correlation (*see* effect size,
    squared part correlation)
  stepwise, 420, 447, 449
multiple regression, 409
multiplication rule of probability (*see* probability,
    multiplication rule)
multivariate, 319
multivariate ANOVA procedures, 298–299
mutually exclusive, 108, 128

nominal data, 17
  defined, 48
nonparametric statistics, 508
  defined, 246, 508
  dependent-samples, 508
  distribution-free tests, 246
  Friedman test, 508
  Kruskal–Wallis test, 289–293
  Mann–Whitney U test, 246–249
  Spearman's rho, 358–363
  Wilcoxon test, 508
  within-subjects ANOVA (*see* within-subjects
    ANOVA)
normal curve, 77–79
  standard (*see* distribution, z)
  and z score, 77–80
normal curve equivalent (NCE) scores, 57
  defined, 70
normal distribution *see* distribution, normal
null hypothesis *see* hypothesis, null

observed frequencies, 459
omnibus test results, 382, 392
  ANOVA, 257, 271
  factorial ANOVA, 306
  regression, 382, 392–393, 404
  within-subjects ANOVA, 505–506
one-tailed test *see* two-tailed and one-tailed tests
ordinal data, 17–22
  defined, 48
outlier *see* extreme score

parameter, 149
  defined, 159
  estimation, 169–171
parametric statistics, 246, 508, 512
part correlation 420, 437, 441 *see also*
    semi-partial correlation
  defined, 441, 449
  squared part correlation, 441–442
partial correlation, 408, 409
partial eta squared *see* effect size, partial eta
    squared

partial regression plots, 449
Pearson's *r*, 332–334, 341–346 *see also*
    correlation
percentiles, 56–57
  calculating, 83–84
  defined, 56, 70
Phi *see* effect size, Phi coefficient
point estimate, 192–193
  defined, 201
pooled variance *see* variance, pooled
population SD, 66–67
  defined 70
post facto research *see* research design, *post facto*
post hoc analyses, 506–508
  defined, 293
  Tukey's HSD test, 271–274
  varieties of, 270–271
power, 188–189, 192
  defined, 201
practical significance *see* effect size
predictor variable *see* regression, predictor
    variables
pretest sensitivity, 211
probability
  addition rule, 108, 127
  Bayes' theorem, 111–112, 127
  combinations, 109–110
  combining probabilities, 107
  conditional, 111, 127
  defined, 128
  elements of, 106–107
  empirical, 107, 127
  exact, 123–126
  multiplication rule, 108, 128
  normal curve (*see* normal curve)
  permutation, 110
  posterior, 128
  prior, 128
  relationship to z score, 112–113
procrustean exercise, 14, 48
proportional reduction in error (PRE), 331
  defined, 364

quartiles, 57
  defined, 70
quasi-experimental design (*see* research design)

r^2 *see* effect size, coefficient of determination
random effects modeling, 449
random sample, 142
  defined, 160
  stratified random sampling, 142
randomization, 136–137
  defined, 160

range, 55–56
  defined, 71
ranks, tied, 360–361
ratio data, 22–23
  defined, 48
real-world data, 7–8, 544
regression
  bivariate (*see* bivariate regression)
  coefficients, 382, 394, 418
  explaining variance, 386–387
  hierarchical (*see* multiple linear regression, hierarchical)
  line, 374–376, 409
  nature of, 372–374
  predictor variables, 159
  slope, 394–395
  standard error of estimate, 383–384, 409
  y intercept, 374–376, 394, 409
  z score formula (*see* bivariate regression, *z* score)
rejecting null hypothesis, 155
repeated measures
  Chi square, 468, 472–474
  dependent t-test, 491–498
  within-subjects ANOVA (*see* within-subjects ANOVA)
research design, 9, 133–135, 167–168, 208–211
  defined, 160
  experiment, 136–140
  post facto, 140–141
  quasi-experimental, 139–140, 160
  sampling, 142 (*see also* sample(s))
  variables (*see* variable)
residuals, 449
residuals analysis, 433–435
  checking assumptions, 433–435
  residuals vs. predicted values, 435
  standardized residuals, 433–434
restricted range, 350
  defined, 364

sample(s)
  convenience, 142
  defined, 142
  dependent, 209–210, 249
  independent, 209–211, 223, 249
  matched, 210, 249, 491
  mixed, 249
  random, 142
  snowball, 142
  stratified random, 142
sampling distribution of means *see* distribution, sampling, of means
sampling distribution of differences *see* distribution, sampling, of differences

semi-partial correlation, 420, 441 *see also* part correlation
scales of measurement, 16–23
  defined, 49
  in descriptive statistics (*see under* descriptive statistics)
  interval data, 20–22
  nominal data, 17
  ordinal data, 17–20
  ratio data, 22–23
scattergram
  in correlation, 334–335
  defined, 364
  in multiple linear regression, 422, 426, 435
  in regression, 375–376
Scheffe test, 271
significance *see* statistical significance
simple effects, 301, 319
skewness, 37–41
  defined, 49
slope *see* regression, slope
sphericity, 502, 504–505, 508
Spearman's rho *see* nonparametric statistics, Spearman's rho
SPSS, 509–530
  with ANOVA, 282–288
  with bivariate regression, 390–395
  with central tendency, 28–34
  with chi square, 474–480
  confidence intervals, 198–199
  with correlation, 352–357
  with curvilinear relationships, 400–404
  with dependent *t*-test, 496–497
  with factorial ANOVA, 311–316
  with independent-samples *t* test, 239–242
  with multiple linear regression, 431–448
  percentiles, 90–93
  with single sample *t* test, 196–200
  with standard deviation, 67–70
  syntax, 310, 315, 319
  within-subjects ANOVA, 501–508
  z score, 90–93
spuriousness, 13–14, 49
squared part correlation *see* effect size, squared part correlation
standard deviation, 60–73
  calculation of, 61–63
  defined, 71
  in descriptive statistics (*see* descriptive statistics)
  estimated, of the population, 201
  estimated, of the sampling distribution of means, 201
  inferential (*see* inferential SD)
  population (*see* population SD)

standard error of estimate *see* regression, standard error of estimate
standard error of the mean, 177–178, 201
standard normal distribution
  see distribution, *z*
standard normal score *see z* score
standardized test, 20
  defined, 49
statistical significance, 156
  defined, 160
stepwise entry method *see* multiple linear regression, stepwise
sum of squares, 64, 260–261

t distribution *see* distribution, t-
t test
  dependent-samples, 491–498
  independent-samples, 207–254
  single sample, 165–206
  versus Z test, 166–167
theory, 134–135
  defined, 160
treatment group, 137
  defined, 160
Tukey's HSD test *see post hoc* analyses
two-tailed and one-tailed tests, 189–194
  defined, 201
type I error (alpha), 183–185, 257, 293
  defined, 201
type II error (beta), 185–188
  defined, 201

univariate, 298, 311–314
  defined, 319
  extreme scores (*see* extreme scores, univariate)

variable
  dependent, 139
  independent, 138–139
  manipulated independent, 138
  nonmanipulated independent, 138
variance
  between, 293
  defined, 71
  in descriptive statistics, 60–61
  pooled, 218–221
  total, 293
  within, 293

Wilcoxon test *see* nonparametric statistics, Wilcoxon test
Wilks' lambda *see* effect size, Wilks' lambda
Winning the Math Wars, 7
within-group designs, 249
within-subjects ANOVA, 319, 498–508

Yates correction for continuity, 469, 483
y-intercept *see* regression, y-intercept

z score, 79–80, 99
  and bivariate regression (*see* bivariate regression, *z* score)
  and correlation (*see* correlation, *z* score)
  defined, 99
  distribution (*see* distribution, *z*)
  and probability (*see* probability, relationship to *z* score)
  table of values, 80–81, 545
z test, 154–157
  elements, 156–157
  hypothesis test (*see* hypothesis test)
  versus *T* test, 166–167

Printed and bound by CPI Group (UK) Ltd, Croydon, CR0 4YY

16/04/2025

14658535-0003